Lung Function in Children and Adolescents
Methods, Reference Values

Progress in Respiration Research

Vol. 22

Series Editor
H. Herzog, Basel

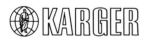

Basel · München · Paris · London · New York · New Delhi · Singapore · Tokyo · Sydney

Lung Function in Children and Adolescents

Methods, Reference Values

A. Zapletal, Prague

Co-authors
M. Šamánek, T. Paul, Prague

59 figures and 283 tables, 1987

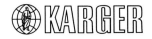

Basel · München · Paris · London · New York · New Delhi · Singapore · Tokyo · Sydney

Progress in Respiration Research

Contents

Preface VII

Studied Healthy Subjects 1

I. Static Lung Volumes and Lung Ventilation 4

Methods 5
Results 7
Discussion 11
Conclusions 12

II. Lung Elasticity 13

Methods 15
Results 20
Discussion 26
Conclusions 31

III. Airway Patency 32

Maximum Expiratory Flow Rates 32
    Methods 38
    Results and Discussion 40
Dynamic Lung Volumes 47
    Methods 49
    Results and Discussion 49
    Conclusions 50
Airflow Resistance 51
Airway Resistance 52
    Method 58
    Results and Discussion 61
Lung (Pulmonary) Resistance 63
    Results and Discussion 64
    Conclusions 65

Contents

Multiple-Breath Nitrogen Lung Washout Curve 66
    Results and Discussion 67
    Conclusions 67

IV. Work of Breathing 68

    Method 73
    Results 75
    Discussion 77
    Conclusions 81

V. Gas Exchange in the Lungs 83

    Alveolar Ventilation, Respiratory Functional Dead Space and Its Ventilation,
        Oxygen Consumption and Elimination of Carbon Dioxide 83
        Methods 84
        Results and Discussion 84
    Lung-Diffusing Capacity (Transfer Factor) 85
        Method and Subjects 90
        Results 91
        Discussion 93
        Conclusions 94

    Summary 95
    References 100
    Addendum 113
        Explanations to Tables 113

Subject Index 219

Preface

During recent years, lung function testing in children has shown considerable progress and nowadays it contributes significantly when establishing diagnoses in children with respiratory diseases. Lung function testing has also become an indispensable diagnostic tool in pediatric cardiology, surgery, sports medicine as well as in other branches of pediatric and adolescent medicine. Numerous new methods have been introduced into the investigation of lung function in children thus making it possible to detect the minor abnormalities of lung function caused by disturbances of the respiratory system. In order to assess whether certain results of lung function tests are normal or pathological, one has to compare them with the reference ('normal') values of the tests also taking their physiological variability into account.

A specific feature of pulmonary function tests in children is the fact that the test values change during growth and development. In the literature, reference values of some basic pulmonary function tests in various groups of children and adolescents have been published repeatedly [2, 4, 10–12, 28, 29, 36, 40, 41, 50–52, 57, 63, 89, 90, 91, 97, 124, 147, 149, 152].

In the present work we report on cross-sectional data of lung function tests obtained in the same group of healthy subjects, i.e. lung volumes and ventilation, results of lung elasticity indices, values of indices used for an assessment of abnormalities in the airway patency, lung mechanical work (work of breathing), and some indices of gas exchange in the lungs.

Methodological procedures and the values for pulmonary function tests from healthy subjects are limited in this publication for the age group between 5 and 18 years. The latter are presented as regression equations in tables, complemented in some cases by their graphic expression. The data are given in traditional as well as SI units in the text (table 82). Main emphasis is put on the detailed description of methodical procedures of lung function testing used in the studied subjects.

With respect to the fact that the methods described are somewhat identical with those used in adults, they are useful not only to pediatricians but also to those performing lung function tests in adolescents and adults.

The book is not written as a textbook but to emphasis our own results as presented in tables and graphs, with the hope of making the evaluation of lung function in patients easier for the investigator. Therefore, not all methods have been described but only those used for the data reported.

The authors are indebted to all colleagues and co-workers of the Cardiopulmonary Laboratory and other departments of the University Hospital Motol in Prague dealing with respiratory problems in children and adolescents, Pediatric Clinic of the Hospital 'Pod Petřínem', as well as to co-workers of the Lung Sanatoriums for Children at Šumperk and Dolný Smokovec, whose cooperation helped in the 'birth' of this publication. The authors acknowledge the help of Dr. B. Zapletalová for her final preparations of the tables. Finally, we would like to thank the publishers, S. Karger, for their continued help and advice during the creation of this publication.

Alois Zapletal

Studied Healthy Subjects

All values of lung function indices presented in this study, except those for gas exchange, were obtained at cross-sectional study from a group of 173 healthy children and adolescents aged 6–18 years and 16 adults aged 21–23 years, and in whom the work of breathing and the volume of isoflow were determined. In the studied basic group of children and adolescents there were 86 boys and 87 girls. Some indices on gas exchange (lung diffusing capacity, alveolar ventilation, etc.) were obtained in another 56 healthy children and adolescents. In some subjects not all the measurements could be performed due to technical reasons, so that the number of tested subjects in the tables and figures is not always the same. Body heights varying between 107 and 182 cm and weights of from 19 to 90 kg were, in all subjects, within the range of normal values for a healthy population [167]. The studied healthy subjects did not suffer from respiratory, heart or other chronic diseases, and were free of any acute illness at the time of examination. They reported themselves for the examination voluntarily. The whole examination was performed between 8 a.m. and 1 p.m. During the testing the children were dressed in light clothing, the temperature of the room varied between 25 and 26°C.

The results obtained were related to body height, age and body surface, and some of them to the static lung volumes of the subjects; simple regression equations were calculated. For each relationship the linear, quadratic and power functions as simple regression equations were computed. The regression equation, expressing the best fitting curve, was obtained by the method of least-squares from the mean [164]. The curve with the smallest sum of least squares was selected as the representative one. This was the regression equation with the highest correlation coefficient and the smallest variation coefficient. The given lung function parameter as a dependent variable (y) is presented as a function of one independent variable (x). The multiple regression equations for lung function parameter with an independent variable including body height, age and body surface or weight for the given relationship were not calculated.

The majority of lung function parameters in our healthy subjects correlated most significantly with their body height (see below).

The majority of the relationships between lung function parameters and the studied somatometric parameters were nonlinear and a power function ($y = a \cdot x^b$) expressed the relationship best. The regression equations with a power function were transformed into the logarithmic type of equations, i.e. $\log y = \log a + b \cdot \log x$, where the logarithm is decadic. Also, the computed 95% confidence limits (± 2 SD from the mean) by means of a power function bounded the distribution of the data for various lung function parameters best (see further). However, the standard deviation of the mean with a positive sign (+SD) is larger than that with a negative sign (−SD). The calculation of the mean value (y) and 95% confience limits, e.g. of vital capacity (in ml), in a girl of body height 150 cm (x) by using a power function is as follows:

Mean value:

Formula: $\log y$ = $-2.2970 + 2.6361 \cdot \log x$
          $\log 150$ =   2.17609
          $\log y$ = $-2.2970 + 5.7363$
          $\log y$ =   3.4393, antilogarithm:
           y =   2,750 ml.

Lower limits (i.e. −2 SD from mean):

SD $\log yx$ = -0.0415
        $\log y$ = $-2.2970 + 5.7363 - 0.083$
        $\log y$ =   3.3564, antilogarithm:
         y =   2,272 ml.

Upper limits (i.e. +2 SD from mean):

SD $\log yx$ = $+0.0415$
        $\log y$ = $-2.2970 + 5.7363 + 0.083$
        $\log y$ =   3.5223, antilogarithm:
         y =   3,328 ml.

In the tables and figures, the mean values of lung function indices are given in relation to body height, age, body surface, lung volumes as well as 95% confidence limits, i.e. ± 2 SD from the mean value, of the studied healthy population. The data of lung function indices from our healthy subjects are given for the range of body height, age, body surface or volumes within those they were measured.

The values of some lung function parameters (indices) are given for both sexes together as well as separately for boys and girls, if a statistically significant difference between sexes was found for a parameter.

The comparison of a certain value of the lung function parameter of a patient with the value of our healthy subjects was carried out on the basis of that relationship from our healthy subjects, expressed by a regression equation, which had the largest correlation and the smallest variation coefficient. Values outside the 95% confidence limits for healthy subjects were considered as pathological. Difference in sex was also taken into account.

The data on lung function parameters (indices, tests) obtained in our studied healthy subjects may also be considered as reference (standard, 'normal') values.

I. Static Lung Volumes and Lung Ventilation

For assessing lung function, it is necessary to know the amount of gas in the different spaces of the lungs, i.e. lung volumes. The measurement of static lung volumes represents the basic indispensable procedure in lung function testing. Knowledge of the various static lung volumes and their interrelationships is required for an estimation of gas mixing in the lungs and all other lung function alterations. Absolute values of the static lung volumes can be normal, reduced or increased; also their relationships can be increased, reduced or normal. Some lung diseases are accompanied by a reduction or increase of only some static lung volumes. The values of the static lung volumes measured are affected by various mechanical properties of the lungs and thorax, control of breathing, etc.

Static lung volumes can be divided into 4 not overlapping primary volumes and 4 capacities comprising two or more primary volumes (fig. 1).

Primary Lung Volumes

Tidal volume (V_T) is the amount of gas inspired or expired during normal breathing cycle.

Inspiratory reserve volume (IRV) is the maximal amount of gas which can be inspired from the end-inspiratory resting level.

Expiratory reserve volume (ERV) is the maximal amount of gas which can be expired from the end-expiratory resting level.

Residual volume (RV) is the amount of gas which remains in the lung after maximal expiration.

Lung Capacities

Total lung capacity (TLC) is the amount of gas in the lungs at the end of maximal inspiration.

Vital capacity (VC) is the maximal amount of gas which can be expired after maximal inspiration, or inspired after maximal expiration, during an unlimited period of time.

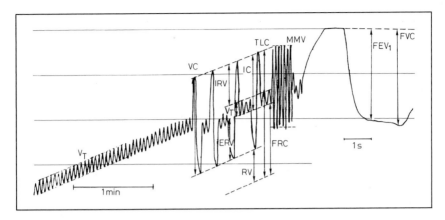

Fig. 1. Spirographic record in a 14-year-old patient, height 164 cm, with idiopathic pulmonary fibrosis (VC = 2,600 ml) and subdivision of static lung volumes. For symbols see text.

Inspiratory capacity (IC) is the maximal amount of gas that can be inspired from the end-expiratory resting level.

Functional residual capacity (FRC) is the amount of gas remaining in the lungs at the end-expiratory resting level.

The values of static lung volumes are given in liters or milliliters.

Lung ventilation represents a process during which the physiological composition of gases in the lungs in a healthy subject is restored by air transport between the lungs and the external environment (atmosphere). Lung ventilation can be assessed from *minute ventilation* (MV) and *maximal voluntary ventilation* (MVV) (or maximum breathing capacity, MBC) values.

Minute ventilation is the amount of gas inspired or expired in a minute. It is obtained by multiplying the tidal volume by the number of breaths in a minute (f). Maximal voluntary ventilation is the amount of gas which a subject can inspire or expire by maximal voluntary effort per minute. The latter values are expressed in liters or milliliters per minute.

Methods

Static lung volumes were determined from the spirographic records and from the functional residual capacity measurements. Ventilation values were measured from the spirographic records.

Spirographic Investigation

The spirographic record was obtained with a 9-liter water spirometer (Resparameter MK 4, Morgan Ltd.; Volutest, Medicor; Universal-Spirograph, Medicor) with subjects in a sitting position in a chair allowing their position at the spirometer to be adjusted.

Smaller children had their legs on a supporting pad, and older children had their feet on the floor. The connection of a subject with the spirometer was provided by a soft plastic mouthpiece fitted into a three-way stopcock. From the spirographic record (fig. 1), vital capacity, inspiratory reserve volume, inspiratory capacity, tidal volume, minute ventilation and maximal voluntary ventilation were measured and corrected for body, temperature, and pressure saturation (BTPS) conditions. At least five VCs were obtained in each subject and the highest one was taken as the representative VC. From such a recording IC, IRV and ERV values were also determined. Breathing frequency and V_T were measured from the technically good part of the spirogram, i.e. when a subject was breathing quietly and regularly. Minute volume was calculated by multiplying the tidal volume value obtained from the record by the number of breaths per minute, MVV was calculated by multiplying the maximum V_T by the number of breaths per 12 to 20-seconds period and then converted for a period of 1 minute.

Functional Residual Capacity Measurement

Helium Dilution Method. The measurement was performed under the same conditions as the spirographic investigation (Resparameter MK 4, Morgan Ltd.). After a dead space measurement of the spirometer with its tubings, the spirometer was flushed with air, and a zero helium concentration was set on a helium analyzer (Cambridge Instrument Company Ltd.). Then 300 ml of helium and 1,000 ml of oxygen were let into the spirometer. A small ventilator in the circuit of the apparatus stirred the gas mixture in the spirometer. After addition of helium into the spirometer, the helium concentration in the spirometer circuit was measured and named as the initial one (%He in). At the end-expiratory level, the subject was connected to the spirometer by turning on the three-way stopcock. The child was connected to the spirometer circuit for 7 min, breathing the mixture of helium and oxygen. CO_2 was absorbed with soda lime and the humidity with silica gel. Oxygen was let into the spirometer continuously so as to avoid changing the position of the spirometer bell. Equilibration of helium concentration in the spirometer and the lungs was reached after the position of the indicator on the helium analyzer was stable (in healthy children usually after 2–3 min). The final helium concentration (%He fin) was read on the analyzer scale at the end of the 7th min of breathing the helium-oxygen mixture. FRC value was calculated according to the following formula:

$$FRC_{He} = Vs \cdot \left(\frac{\%He \ in - \%He \ fin}{\%He \ fin} \right),$$

where Vs is the dead space volume of the spirometer with its tubings, and %He in and %He fin are the initial and final helium concentrations. The volumes of the mouthpiece and stopcock were subtracted from the calculated FRC value. The FRC value obtained was corrected for BTPS conditions.

The dead space of the spirometer with the inlet tubings was measured every day before the start of study, it varied between 2.45 and 2.57 liters according to the amount of water in the spirometer. Determination of the spirometer dead space was performed by letting in 300 ml of helium and 100 ml of oxygen into an empty spirometer. The spirometric bell was reset at the zero position and the helium concentration was measured. The dead space volume of the spirometer with its tubings up to the three-way stopcock (Vs) was calculated according to the following formula:

$$Vs = \frac{Vad \cdot \%He \; fin}{\%He \; in - \%He \; fin},$$

where Vad is the amount of air added into the spirometer, %He in is the initial helium concentration after the spirometer was at zero position, and %He fin is the helium concentration after the addition of 1 liter of air into the spirometric cylinder. The mouthpiece and stopcock volumes amounted to 50 ml. The FRC value determined by the helium-dilution method (FRC_{He}) gives the amount of gas in the lungs, which communicates via the airways with the atmosphere.

Body Plethysmography. For this examination the constant volume body plethysmograph (Siregnost FD-91, Siemens or Body test, Jaeger), was used. Lung volumes measurement by means of body plethysmography, including FRC determination, is described in a special chapter (pp. 56–58). FRC determined in a body plethysmograph (FRC_{box}) includes the amount of gas in the lungs communicating as well as not communicating with the atmosphere through the airways. From the difference of the FRC value determined in a body plethysmograph (thoracic gas volume; TGV) and that determined by the helium-dilution method one can calculate the amount of gas in the lung not communicating with atmospheric air and thus not participating in the gas exchange. This amount of gas is named 'trapped gas' or 'trapped air'.

However, in the patients with a high airway resistance, FRC measured in a body plethysmograph can be overestimated [153, 154, 165] by 3–5%, depending on breathing frequency at FRC_{box} (TGV) measurement, i.e. with increasing frequency more than 1 Hz [154]. The TLC value was determined as the sum of FRC and IC values; the RV value was obtained as TLC minus VC.

Results

The data on static lung volumes, their mutual ratios, percentage of the difference between the functional residual capacity determined by body plethysmography and the helium-dilution method, and on ventilation in healthy studied subjects are given in tables 1–88 and figures 2–5.

All static lung volumes and capacities increased nonlinearly with increasing body height, surface and age. The best correlation of these parameters was found with body height. A more rapid increase of these values starts at 150 cm of body height (fig. 2, 3). VC, IC, IRV, ERV, TLC_{box}, TLC_{He}, FRC_{box} and FRC_{He} values differed significantly between the boys and girls even prior to puberty. The RV/TLC_{box} ratio (i.e. that determined in a body plethysmograph) decreased with increasing body height, surface and age (fig. 4), whereas the RV/TLC_{He} ratio (i.e. that determined by the helium-dilution method) was independent of the body height

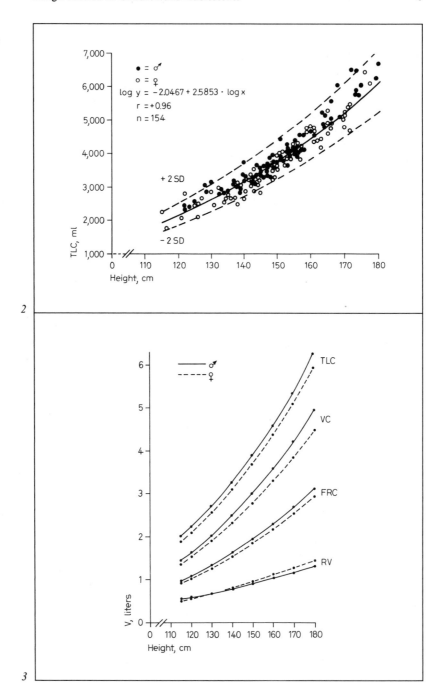

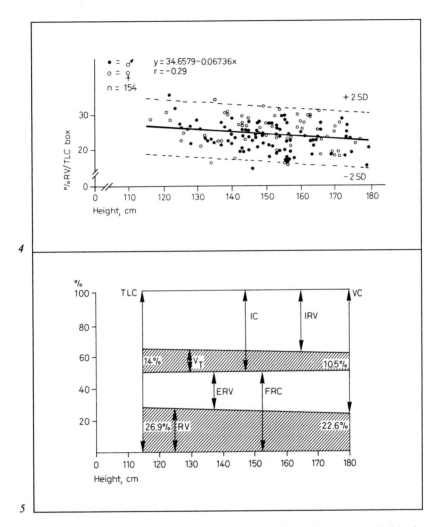

Fig. 2. TLC measured in a body plethysmograph in relation to body height in healthy boys (♂) and girls (♀). Full line represents mean value of the group. Interrupted lines represent upper and lower limits for 95% of values (± 2 SD from the mean) in a given group. r = Correlation coefficient; n = number of subjects.

Fig. 3. Mean values of TLC, VC, FRC, and RV in relation to body height in healthy boys (♂) and girls (♀).

Fig. 4. Ratio RV/TLC (in %) measured in a body plethysmograph in relation to body height in healthy boys and girls. For further explanations, see figure 2.

Fig. 5. Interrelationship of static lung volumes related to body height in healthy boys and girls. For symbols, see text. V_T and RV values (hatched areas) decrease with increasing body height with regard to the other static lung volumes.

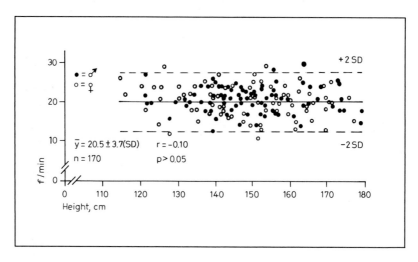

Fig. 6. Breathing frequency per minute (f/min) in relation to body height in healthy boys and girls. ȳ = Mean value.

(mean value: 22.5 ± 4.8%). The FRC/TLC$_{box}$ ratio (i.e. that determined in a body plethysmograph) did not change with body height in the mean value: 49.1 ± 3.5%. The ratio FRC/TLC$_{He}$ increased with body height as did the VC/RV$_{box}$ ratio. The IC/ERV ratio decreased with body height. The average IRV/ERV value amounted to 1.5 ± 0.34. The mutual ratios of static lung volumes changed with growth of the studied subjects (fig. 5). Also the values of tidal volume, minute ventilation and maximum voluntary ventilation increased nonlinearly with increasing body height, surface and age (table 79–88). The proportion of V$_T$ and MV to TLC and VC decreased with increasing body height (fig. 5). The difference between the FRC$_{box}$ and FRC$_{He}$ values expressed as a percentage FRC$_{box}$ increased significantly with decreasing body height in children (table 76–78). The difference between FRC$_{box}$ and FRC$_{He}$ expressed in absolute values (i.e. in ml) was independent of body height (r = 0.06). The FRC$_{box}$ value was, on average, higher than the FRC$_{He}$ value by 84 ± 141 ml. The average percentual difference between FRC$_{box}$ and FRC$_{He}$ amounted to 4.9 ± 7.95% for the whole group. Respiratory frequency per minute (f) in the studied group was independent of body height (fig. 6). Similar dependences of the latter parameters as on the body height were also for body surface and age, though the latter relationships were less significant.

Discussion

The values of the static lung volumes and ventilation in our group of healthy children and adolescents are similar to the majority of those reported in the literature [7, 10–12, 21, 29, 31, 33, 40, 46, 52, 59, 64, 65, 68, 77, 78, 90, 104, 137, 152, 162, 177, 178, 221, 226]. They are nearest to the values published by Polgar and Promadhat [146], who compiled the lung volume values reported in the literature until 1970, and later until 1978 and calculated summary regression equations [149] similar to those in our group. The relation between lung volumes on the one hand and body height, body surface and age on the other, was best expressed by an exponential (logarithmic) function. Sexual differences for the absolute lung volume values were larger in the individuals with the larger body height. The difference in RV values was not significant between sexes due to a greater dispersion. Sexual differences of the lung volumes were smaller with respect to body surface; with respect to age the latter differences were found only for VC.

Greater percentual differences between the FRC_{box} and FRC_{He} values in smaller and younger children may be caused by the relatively larger proportion of gas in the abdominal cavity, which at the plethysmographic measurement is also included into the obtained TGV value and can contribute to higher TGV and thus also FRC_{box} values. The difference between FRC_{box} and FRC_{He} is close to that reported in the literature, i.e. around 100 ml [43]. A certain role in the latter greater differences in smaller children can nevertheless also be due to the greater unevenness of distribution of ventilation in smaller children, causing lower FRC_{He} values. Also, the relatively larger RV/TLC ratio in smaller children can be explained by their uneven distribution of ventilation. Diminishing differences of the FRC/TLC_{box} and FRC/TLC_{He} ratios show a similar trend as the difference of FRC_{box} and FRC_{He} values. The static lung volumes obtained by body plethysmography and the helium-dilution method in healthy children and adolescents show physiological pecularities in the development of static lung volumes. The significance of static lung volume measurements, first of all FRC, TLC and RV, is especially important in patients with obstructive lung diseases, in whom a body plethysmography can measure lung volumes more acurately, i.e. also in lung regions which do not allow proper gas mixing due to airways obstruction. An inert gas (e.g. helium) does not reach the alveoli in a respective region or gas is not eliminated from a lung region (e.g. nitrogen at oxygen breathing). FRC measured by an inert gas technique can therefore be normal or even lower than the predicted value in the patients with obstructive lung diseases. Nevertheless, TGV can also be overestimated if airway resistance and breathing frequency at the TGV measurement are very high since the mouth pressure does not reflect the alveolar pressure properly [153, 154, 165]. The values of the RV/TLC and FRC/TLC ratios, and trapped air can be included into the indirect methods for the assessment of airways patency.

Conclusions

In a group of 173 children and adolescents (86 boys and 87 girls), 6–17 years old, with body heights of 115–180 cm, static lung volumes were determined by spirographic investigation, plethysmographically, and by the helium-dilution method. The values obtained were correlated with body height, age and body surface of the studied subjects. Statistically, the most significant correlation was found between static lung volumes and body height. The relationship of the studied volumes to body height was nonlinear (exponential). Statistically significant differences in VC, IC, IRV, ERV, TLC and FRC values were observed between boys and girls. The FRC/TLC$_{box}$ ratio was 49.2 $\pm$ 4.8% on average. The RV/TLC$_{box}$ ratio decreased with body height, age and body surface, while the FRC/TLC$_{He}$ ratio increased with body height, age and body surface. The V$_T$/TLC and V$_T$/VC ratios decreased with body height, age and body surface.

II. Lung Elasticity

Lung elasticity (LE) represents the mechanical properties of the lungs to be expanded (distended) by pressures surrounding or inflating the lungs and to collapse as soon as the latter pressures disappeared. LE is determined by a number of factors (the number of elastic and collagen fibers of lung tissue, surface tension in the alveoli, pulmonary blood volume, smooth muscles of the bronchi and vessels, etc.).

LE assessment plays an important role in pulmonary and cardiac diseases (affecting the pulmonary circulation), because *by this investigation one can differentiate whether the lung pathological processes lead to compliant (emphysematic) or rigid (fibrotic) lung.* It also provides a possibility to further *separate the restrictive lung diseases* from those *due to intra- and extraparenchymal causes.* LE assessment in children and adolescents is even more significant, because in this way it is possible to reveal already the initial stages of lung fibrosis or emphysema. However, LE evaluation in children and adolescents requires proper and suitable methods for this age range.

Various lung and cardiac diseases have been accompanied by changes of the elastic properties of the lungs already in childhood and adolescence. The assessment of LE in young subjects with such diseases is of greater significance as it provides important information on the basic mechanical characteristics of the diseased organ and helps in the better management of the patients. In spite of the general assumption of the irreversibility of LE due to lung disease [7, 32, 82], one cannot exclude the possibility of favorable effects of various therapeutic regimes concerning LE in still somatically growing children and adolescents with lung disease. The proper assessment of LE abnormalities in pediatric and adolescent lung patients requires, however, the standards (reference values) expressing the developmental aspects of LE.

LE has been assessed in vivo most often functionally from a simultaneous recording of transpulmonary pressure (see below) and lung volume

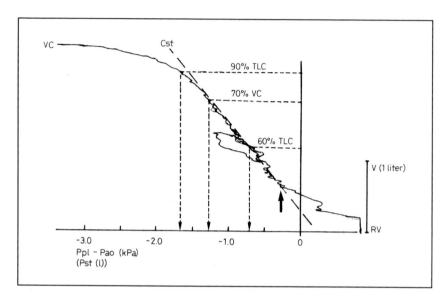

Fig. 7. PV curve of the lungs expressing the dependence of transpulmonary pressure (P_{pl}–P_{ao}) on lung volume during the whole vital capacity (VC) maneuver in a healthy 10-year-old boy, height 145 cm. The curve was obtained during slow expiration at airflow rate of 0.1–0.05 liters/s. The curve is S-shaped and demonstrates the technique of elastic recoil pressure of the lungs measurement (Pst(l)) at 60 and 90% TLC levels and the 70% VC level. Vertical interrupted lines show the values of elastic recoil pressure of the lungs in kilopascals (kPa) at given lung volume levels. The slope of the middle part of the curve presents the value of static lung compliance. Oscillations on the curve are due to heart beats.

changes at static or semistatic (quasi-static) conditions of the lungs during expiration, i.e. from an expiratory pressure-volume (PV) curve of the lungs (see below).

Evaluation of LE in children has so far been based on 'dynamic' lung compliance measurements. On the basis of 'specific' dynamic lung compliance, i.e. dynamic compliance expressed per unit of lung volume (e.g. FRC, TLC, VC), it was assumed that LE in children and adolescents did not change, being the same as in younger adults [30, 86]. The recent data on elastic recoil pressure of the lungs in 6- to 17-year-old children and adolescents [39, 111, 189, 207, 220, 241] have shown a physiological increase in LE suggesting stiffer lungs with growth in the studied age range [207, 220]. In the later age a decrease of LE was found [60, 151, 182].

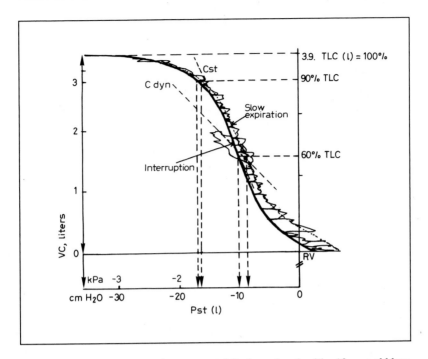

Fig. 8. Expiratory pressure-volume curve of the lungs in a healthy 13-year-old boy, height 154 cm, obtained by the airflow interruption technique. The PV curve at slow expiration is shown. The increasing airflow resistance at lower volumes makes a shift of the slow expiration curve. The measurements of Pst(l) at given percentages of TLC, Cst and Cdyn are also illustrated.

Methods

Indices

The indices of LE measured from expiratory semistatic or static PV curves of the lungs (fig. 7, 8) were: *lung recoil pressure* (Pst (l), Pst, Pst_L), and *static lung compliance* (Cst). During tidal breathing also *dynamic lung compliance* (Cdyn) was measured as another index of LE (fig. 8). However, Cdyn cannot be considered as an adequate index of LE (see below).

Lung compliance (C, static, dynamic), defined as a change of lung volume (Δ V) per unit of transpulmonary pressure (Δ P), was measured within tidal volume range when the static conditions of the lungs were assumed:

$$C = \frac{\Delta V}{\Delta P} = \frac{\Delta ml}{\Delta kPa}.$$

Lung recoil pressure (elastic recoil pressure of the lungs) in vivo is reflected by the magnitude of negative pleural (intrathoracic, intrapleural) pressure acting on the surface of the lungs at different levels of lung expansion under static conditions. Lung recoil pressure represents a difference between pleural (Ppl) and alveolar (Palv) pressures, i.e. the transpulmonary pressure at static conditions of the lungs, when Palv equals zero (i.e. to barometric pressure considered as a zero pressure). At such conditions, i.e. in the absence of airflow, the negative pleural pressure equals Pst(l), and Pst(l) has a negative sign. The evaluation of the elastic properties of the lungs therefore requires the transpulmonary pressure and the corresponding lung volume to be measured simultaneously under static conditions of the lungs. In this publication Pst(l) has been expressed in kilopascals (kPa; SI units), and in cm H_2O (conventional units). In the tables Pst(l) is given with a positive sign in spite of the fact that it was measured from expiratory PV curves recorded with a negative pressure. There is, however, no unanimity in marking Pst(l) from PV curves by positive or negative signs. It seems more logical to record Pst(l) on the left side of the PV diagram, because the negative pressure has been measured. Lung compliance is given in ml per unit of kPa and cmH_2O, respectively.

Technique

The evaluation of LE in older children and adolescents was based on the recordings of the expiratory PV curves of the lungs, obtained as an X-Y plot of transpulmonary pressure changes vs. lung volume changes during expiratory vital capacity (VC) starting from full inspiration to the residual volume level at quasi-static (fig. 7) or static (fig. 8) conditions of the lungs, i.e. during very slow expiration ($\dot{V}$: 0.05–0.02 liters/s) or expiration interrupted (for 0.3 s) with a flow regulator. Transpulmonary pressure was measured as the difference between esophageal and mouth pressures (Ppl-Pao). Esophageal pressure was obtained from an esophageal latex ballon (10 cm long, 3.5 cm perimeter, wall thickness less than 0.1 mm), connected with a 1-meter long polyethylene catether (ID. 1.4 mm) to a differential pressure transducer coupled with an electromanometer and a writing instrument. In the balloon, introduced through a nare after local anesthesia with its tip to the level of the diaphragm dome (calculation of the distance from the nares: 1/5 of body height plus 9 cm) while drinking water, 0.2–0.4 ml of air was left. The latter amount of air was achieved after several coughing maneuvers by the subjects and checked after each PV curve with a 2-ml syringe connected to a three-way stopcock for leakage. The transpulmonary pressure as a difference between esophageal (a substitue of pleural pressure) and mouth (alveolar) pressures, obtained at low expiratory flows and interrupted expiratory flows, was taken as Pst(l). Lung volume (VC) change was measured after electronic integration of the airflow at the mouth with a heated pneumotachograph simultaneously with a change of transpulmonary pressure.

The calibration of a differential pressure transducer for esophageal and mouth pressure measurements (linear within the pressures of 0.1–150 cm $H_2O \doteq 0.01$ to 15 kPa and with symetrical pressure changes) was performed with a water manometer. The calibration of volume was made with a 1-liter syringe and of airflow with a rotameter or a slanting manometer containing a special fluid of lower specific weight than water. The calibration of a pressure signal deflection was 1mm for 0.25 cm H_2O and of a volume signal deflection 1 mm for 25 ml on millimeter paper of an X-Y recorder.

The investigation of LE started after an instruction in the sitting subject with pressure-volume loops recordings. Then the subject was asked to inspire maximally and to

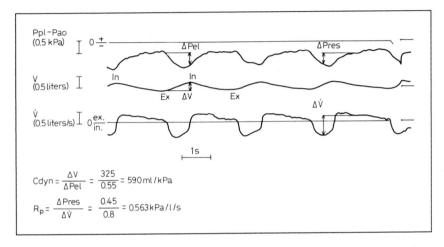

Ppl–Pao
(0.5 kPa)

V
(0.5 liters)

V̇
(0.5 liters/s)

$$Cdyn = \frac{\Delta V}{\Delta Pel} = \frac{325}{0.55} = 590\,ml/kPa$$

$$R_p = \frac{\Delta Pres}{\Delta \dot{V}} = \frac{0.45}{0.8} = 0.563\,kPa/l/s$$

Fig. 9. Separate records of transpulmonary pressure (Ppl–Pao), tidal volume (V) and airflow (V̇) during quiet breathing in a 9-year-old girl, 125 cm tall, with asymptomatic bronchial asthma. The record illustrates dynamic lung compliance (Cdyn) and pulmonary resistance (R_p) measurements. Pres = A change of transpulmonary pressure to the corresponding change of airflow (V̇) for R_P calculation; Pel = a change of transpulmonary pressure to the corresponding change of lung volume (V) for Cdyn calculation.

expire slowly to the residual volume (RV) level. At least 5 deflation PV curves were obtained in each subject and compared by redrawing them on a transparent paper according to the zero pressure end-expiratory resting level, maximal Pst(l) and VC. Thus, a composite deflation PV curve was obtained and used for the analysis, or the best PV curve (with largest VC and Pst(l) at full inspiration) was analyzed. From the deflation (expiratory) PV curves, Pst(l) was measured at several lung volumes, i.e. at 100, 90, 80, 70, 60, 50 and 40% of actual total lung capacity (TLC), and at 25, 30, 40, 50, 60, 70, 80 and 90% of actual vital capacity in healthy subjects as well as in patients. From the nearly straight middle part of the PV curve within the tidal volume range, Cst was obtained as a change of lung volume per unit of pressure (fig. 7, 8).

The slope drawn trough the reversal points of PV loops (fig. 8) gave the Cdyn value. From the separate recordings of transpulmonary pressure, volume and flow, Cdyn was also calculated as a mean from 10 consecutive breaths (fig. 9).

The inspiratory PV curves obtained by the flow interruption technique (fig. 10) made the lung hysteresis assessment possible. The spirometry and the measurements of functional residual capacity (FRC) in a body plethysmograph were carried out also in order for Pst(l) to be determined in the scale of actual TLC, obtained as a sum of FRC plus inspiratory capacity (IC).

In order to get reliable PV curves and from them derived Pst(l) and Cst, the possible methodological errors had to be minimized, i.e. the effects of esophageal elastance (EE), vertical pleural pressure gradient (VPPG) and airflow at slow expiration technique on PV

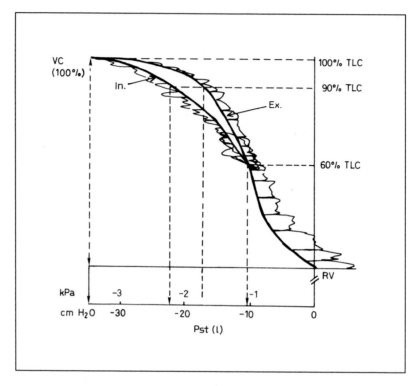

Fig. 10. Inspiratory (In.) and expiratory (Ex.) pressure volume curves of the lungs obtained by the airflow interruption technique illustrating lung hysteresis above FRC level (60% TLC) in the subject, as in figure 8.

curves [220]. The small amount of air, 0.2–0.4 ml, in the esophageal balloon with its tip at the level of the diaphragm dome thus made the errors due to EE and VPPG in obtaining reliable PV curves minimal. However, Pst(l) read off from PV curves, obtained at slow and flow interrupted expiration techniques, differed (fig. 8) if the expiratory flow rate in the slow expiration technique was larger than 0.2 liters/s. The latter difference in Pst(l) measurements appeared mainly below the FRC level, which was due to the pressure required to overcome the increasing pulmonary resistance with decreasing lung volume in the slow expiration technique. The latter difference was small, i.e. less than 1 cm H_2O ($\cong 0.1$ kPa), in healthy subjects at lung volumes larger than 50% of TLC providing the expiratory flow was lower than 0.2 liters/s. The slow expiration technique for obtaining the expiratory PV curves required the expiratory flow to be checked (fig. 11) and the expiratory PV curves with a larger airflow were omitted. The latter error can be more relevant in subjects with airway obstruction (fig. 12).

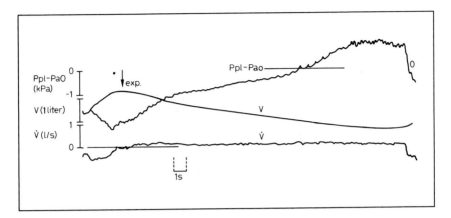

Fig. 11. Time base records of transpulmonary pressure (Ppl–Pao), lung volume (V) and airflow rate (V̇) during slow expiration in a 12-year-old girl, height 141 cm, with cystic fibrosis. Separate records of all three signals on another recorder allow to control the expiratory airflow rate at tracing the pressure-volume curve of the lungs as X-Y plots.

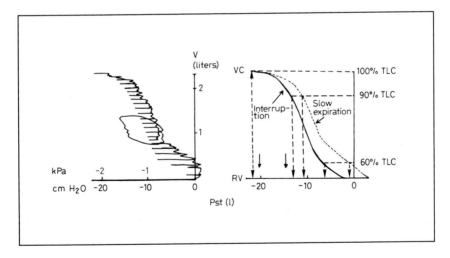

Fig. 12. Expiratory PV curve of the lungs obtained by the airflow interruption technique compared with that obtained during slow expiration in a 16-year-old boy, height 155 cm, with cystic fibrosis. Left panel: Original PV curve. Right panel: The same curves after redrawing. The differences between both curves are more pronounced than in the healthy child (see fig. 8) because of airways obstruction (G_{aw}/TGV: 0.44 liters/s/kPa/liter).

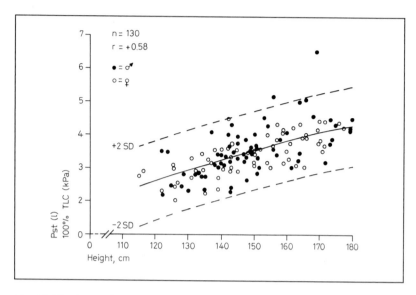

Fig. 13. Elastic recoil pressure of the lungs measured at 100% TLC level (Pst(l) 100% TLC) in relation to body height in healthy boys and girls. For further explanation, see figure 2.

Results

(a) *The indices* assessing LE (obtained from typically S-shaped PV curves) *in 131 healthy children and adolescents* aged 6–17 years are presented in figures 13–20 and tables 89–166.

Elastic recoil pressure of the lungs (Pst(l)) was lower at all lung volume levels measured in smaller children and increased significantly with growth (fig. 13, 14; table 89–136). The relationship between Pst(l) determined at higher lung volume levels and the body height was nonlinear, and at lower lung volume levels it was linear. The slope of the middle part of the average PV curve in younger children (115 cm body height) was steeper than that in older individuals (180 cm body height) (fig. 15).

Static lung compliance (Cst) also increased with increasing body height, age and body surface (fig. 16; table 137–139), and with increasing lung volume (table 140–146). 'Specific' static lung compliance diminished with increasing body height, age and body surface (fig. 17; table 147–155). The smaller the child, the higher was the value of the 'specific' static lung compliance.

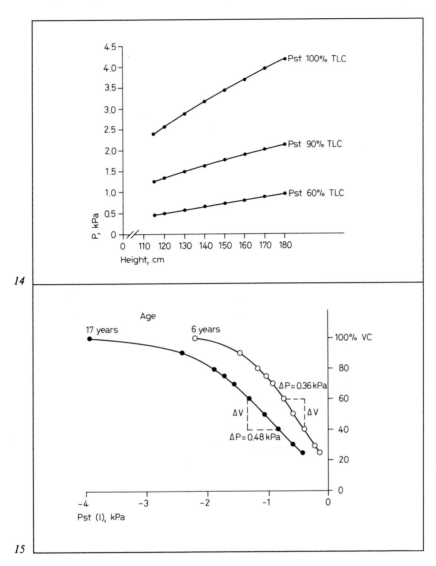

Fig 14. Mean values of elastic recoil pressure of the lungs measured at 100, 90 and 60% total lung capacity in relation to body height in healthy boys and girls. For further explanation, see figure 2.

Fig. 15. Average pressure-volume curve of the lungs in a 6-year-old child and a 17-year-old subject. Elastic recoil pressure of the lungs (Pst(l)) at relatively identical lung volume levels is lower in a younger child than in an older one. The midportion of the pressure-volume curve of the lungs is steeper in a 6-year-old child than a 17-year-old individual. See text for further explanations.

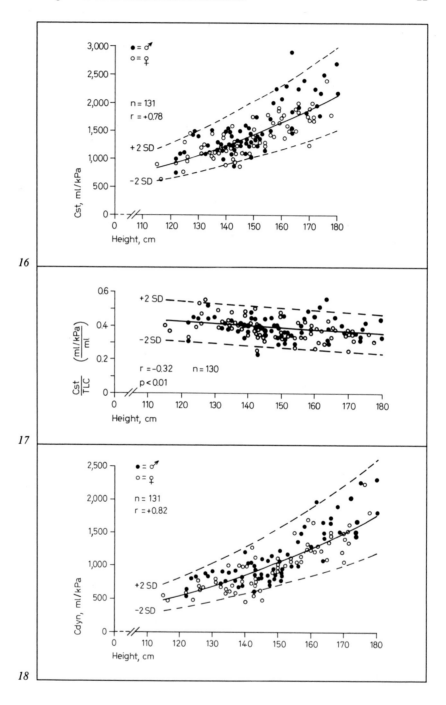

16

17

18

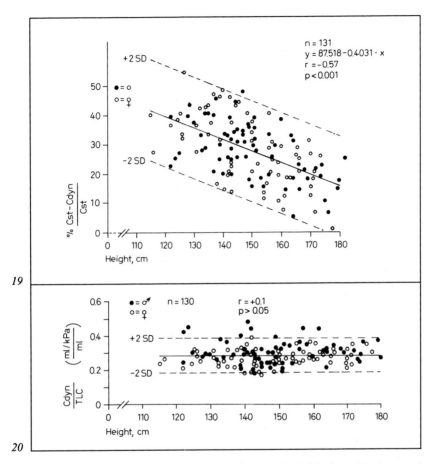

Fig. 16. Static lung compliance (Cst) in relation to body height in healthy boys and girls. For further explanations, see figure 2.

Fig. 17. Static lung compliance expressed per unit of total lung capacity ($\frac{Cst}{TLC}$), i.e. 'specific' static lung compliance, in relation to body height in healthy boys and girls. For further explanations, see figure 2.

Fig. 18. Dynamic lung compliance (Cdyn) in relation to body height in healthy boys and girls. For further explanations, see figure 2.

Fig. 19. Difference between static and dynamic lung compliances expressed as a percentage of static lung compliance (% $\frac{Cst-Cdyn}{Cst}$) in relation to body height in healthy boys and girls. The difference is greater with a decrease in body height. For further explanations, see figure 2. SDy · x = ± 8.8.

Fig. 20. Dynamic lung compliance expressed per unit of total lung capacity, measured in the body plethysmograph ($\frac{Cdyn}{TLC}$), i.e. 'specific' Cdyn, in relation to body height in healthy boys and girls. Mean 'specific' Cdyn value is 0.28 ± 0.050 (SD) ml/kPa/ml. For further explanations, see figure 2.

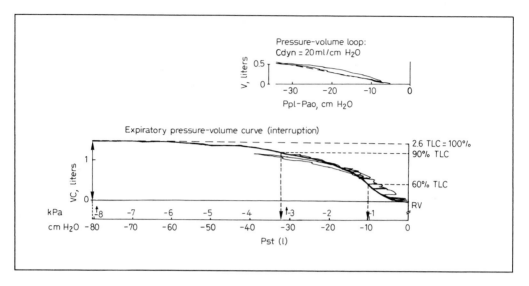

Fig. 21. Pressure-volume loop (upper part) and expiratory pressure-volume curve (lower part) of the lungs in an 18-year-old girl, height 160 cm, with idiopathic pulmonary fibrosis. The PV loop is narrow, sickle-shaped, and elongated. The PV curve is typical by abnormally increased Pst(l) at maximal inspiratory level (100 % TLC) and at 90 % of TLC indicating stiff lungs. VC, Cst and Cdyn are also reduced.

Dynamic lung compliance (Cdyn) increased with increasing body height, age, body surface (fig. 18; table 156–158), and lung volumes (table 159–165). The Cdyn values were lower than those of static lung compliance in all the children studied. In smaller children the latter difference was larger (fig. 19). On average, the difference between the static and dynamic lung compliances was 27 ± 8.8%. 'Specific' dynamic lung compliance was independent of body height (fig. 20; table 166). In our healthy children Cdyn also decreased with increasing breathing frequency.

(b) *Characteristic PV curves of the lungs in lung disease: One type of PV curve with a significantly increased Pst(l) at 100% of TLC (fig. 21), with a reduction of VC and TLC indicated increased retractive forces (stiffness) of the lungs* in almost all the studied patients with idiopathic pulmonary fibrosis (IPF) as an intraparenchymal cause of lung volume restriction. Also, a typical sickle-shaped and narrow PV loop was observed in the majority of the patients with IPF (fig. 21). Similar PV curves were observed in some patients with nonrespiratory malignant tumors after

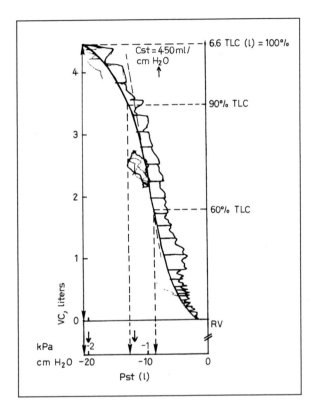

Fig. 22. Expiratory pressure-volume curve (airflow interruption technique) in an asymptomatic asthmatic 19-year-old girl, height 168 cm. The abnormally reduced Pst(l) at 100 and 90% of TLC and increased Cst (4,588 ml/kPa) indicate compliant (emphysematic) lungs.

irradiation and cytostatic therapy, sarcoidosis, as well as in some patients with tetralogy of Fallot (even after corrective heart surgery).

In the patients with abnormalities of the thoracic cage, such as in patients with myositis ossificans or kyphoscoliosis, the lack of an increased Pst(l) at 100% TLC indicated an extraparenchymal cause of lung volume restriction. *Another characteristic type of PV curve with reduced Pst(l), mainly at larger lung volume levels (100% and 90% of TLC), and increased Cst indicated reduced retractive forces of the lungs* (fig. 22). This type of PV curve, observed already in some young asthmatics, suggested lung emphysema. However, not all patients with reduced Pst(l) had an increased Cst, which was therefore considered as a less reliable index for assessing LE abnormalities.

The different courses of the inspiratory and expiratory PV curves (lung hysteresis) in healthy subjects (fig. 10) as well as in patients were observed mainly above the FRC level. Both limbs of the PV curve of the lungs in the same subjects differed mainly within 80–95% of TLC and usually merged at the FRC level.

Discussion

The increase of lung elastic recoil pressure with increasing body height in our studied healthy children and adolescents, and the decrease of the 'specific' static lung compliance with increasing body height, and different slopes of the middle part of the PV curve in subjects with different body height, indicated a physiological change of LE in the period between 6 and 17 years of age [207, 220]. These observations have also been confirmed by others [39, 111, 189, 241].

A simple exponential function, fitted into a static PV curve in our subjects, according to Colebatch et al. [25]:

$$V = A - Be^{-KP},$$

where V is the value of lung volume in liters, P the elastic recoil pressure of the lungs in cm H_2O, and A, B and K are constants – showed, on the basis of the K value, similar developmental LE changes as the Cst/TLC ratio. The K value is the index of compliance in cm H_2O^{-1}, which is independent of lung size and elastic recoil pressure of the lungs at maximum inspiratory level, and expresses the nonlinear course of the PV curve over 50% TLC. Colebatch calculated the K value in a group of our 36 children and adolescents aged 7–16 years and obtained for K value the following equation:

$$K = -3.564 \cdot 10^{-3} \cdot age \text{ (years)} + 0.1564; SD_{yx} = \pm 0.022, r = -0.42.$$

The results indicated a decrease of the K value with age and thus also the same development changes of LE as those observed on the basis of 'specific' static lung compliance. The latter results imply that LE in a smaller child is smaller than in a taller child or an adolescent and that the lungs become more rigid in the course of growth in the studied age range. The above physiological LE changes in childhood and adolescence might be one cause for the more serious respiratory diseases observed in younger children. Reduced LE decreases airways stability and results in an easier airways obstruction. Elastic recoil pressure in a 6 to 8-year-old child is similar to that in a 40 to 50-year-old adult. The question whether the observed changes of LE during childhood and adolescence are mutually counterbalanced with the other parameters of lung mechanical properties during growth remains open.

Dynamic lung compliance did not lead to conclusions concerning the changes of LE with growth. The 'specific' Cdyn value, as a comparable value among children of various body size, did not depend on body height, age or body surface, being similar to those reported in the literature [30, 50, 58, 65, 86].

Cdyn in all the investigated healthy subjects was always smaller than Cst and the difference was greater in smaller and younger children. We conclude, therefore, that the elastic properties of the lungs in children can be correctly assessed solely from the deflation PV curve obtained under static or 'quasi' static conditions in the lungs.

However, in order to make the latter conclusion on the developmental changes in elasticity based on the observations in our group of healthy subjects, the methodological errors which could affect the deflation PV curve, had to be eliminated. Changes of the elastic properties of the esophagus and the adjacent tissues during growth could affect the slope and position of the PV curve. The elasticity of the esophagus and periesophageal structures and its change during the growth of healthy subjects were assessed from esophageal elastance values [98, 121]. For this purpose, in the esophageal balloon alternatively different amounts of air were left and the deflation PV curves were registered. In a group of 53 healthy children and adolescents the esophageal elastance, i.e. the increment of esophageal pressure per 1-milliliter increase of air in the esophagus was roughly the same (0.34 kPa/ml) at higher or lower volume levels within the age range studied (fig. 23), being independent of height, age and body surface. The developmental changes in esophageal elastance could not be a cause of the observed LE changes in our studied subjects.

The study of esophageal elastance showed also the significance of a constant small amount of air in the balloon for lung elastic recoil pressure measurement. If the amount of air in the balloon was larger, the elastance of the esophagus was larger and the curve was shifted towards positivity, and lung elastic recoil pressure values were lower.

Another methodological error, which may affect LE indices could be an inconstant position of the balloon in the esophagus. This is why its

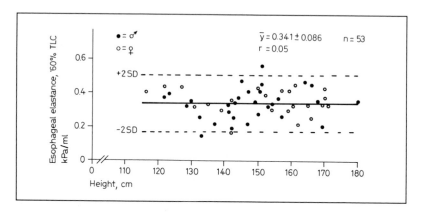

Fig. 23. Esophageal elastance determined at 60% of TLC in relation to body height in boys and girls. $\bar{y}$ = Average value, interrupted lines represent limits for 95% of values of the group.

position was chosen so that its tip was at the level of the diaphragm dome. An esophageal balloon located higher in the esophagus measures a more negative pleural pressure due to the vertical pleural pressure gradient [1, 121, 122]. If a part of the balloon is below the diaphragm, the pressures registered from the esophageal balloon are less negative. The PV curve can thus be shifted more towards negativity or positivity with respect to the pressure axis due to the position of the balloon in the esophagus, as the nose nares–diaphragm dome distance differs during the growth of the children.

In order to assess the developmental changes of the vertical pleural pressure gradient during childhood and adolescence on the PV curves, the PV curves were registered with the esophageal balloon in different positions above the diaphragm and under the diaphragm dome. The vertical pleural pressure gradient per distance of 1 cm along thorax was calculated at 90 and 60% of TLC. Its value was roughly the same at both lung volume levels, i.e. around 0.03 kPa/cm at the higher as well as the lower level. The latter value is similar to that reported in the literature [1, 183] and represents a change in intrathoracic pressure from the top downwards and vice versa on changing the distance by 1 cm. If the tip of the esophageal balloon reached more than 2 cm under the diaphragm dome, the pressure gradient was greater. This finding is another reason for preventing the tip of the esophageal balloon from reaching the abdominal cavity, and for locating the balloon in the thoracic cavity only. The vertical pleural (esophageal) pressure gradient was unchanged in the studied subjects aged 6–17 years. It could not influence, therefore, the values of the LE indices measured.

Another possible inaccuracy in elastic recoil pressure of the lungs and static lung compliance measurements from the PV curve obtained during a very slow expiration may be due to the pressure overcoming the pulmonary resistance during expiration. A shift of the PV curve towards positivity, i.e. towards the zero pressure by a pressure required for overcoming the pulmonary resistance, plays a role only in a more rapid expiration, and not at the rate of 0.05–0.02 liters/s, at which the PV curves were registered (fig. 12). The error was quite negligible, because the pressure inducing the shift of PV curves varied between 0.02 and 0.05 kPa and had no impact on static lung compliance.

The registration of deflation PV curves in children by slow expiration or airflow interruptor methods was more suitable than by the voluntary breath-holding technique at the open glottis. Static lung compliance determined from the PV curve by slow expiration or by the voluntary breath-holding technique showed no difference [220]. The airflow interruptors also give the possibility to obtain PV curves not only during expiration but also during inspiration. Lung hysteresis (fig. 10) can be assessed.

Inspiratory muscle strength was also assessed as another possible error which might affect the features of the PV curve. A larger inspiratory muscle strength can produce a larger lung expansion which may result in higher Pst(l) values in taller children and adolescents. This error affecting the PV curve was assessed by assuming the same elastic recoil pressure at maximal inspiratory level in both the smallest (115 cm body height) and the tallest child (180 cm body height). If the Pst(l) differences were given solely by different inspiratory muscle strength, the PV curves for the tallest and the smallest children would then overlap. However, the PV curves in the tallest children further differed from that in the smallest ones. Also, Pst(l) measured in our 11 healthy children with a body height from 151 to 180 cm from the PV curves with submaximal and maximal PV curves demonstrated that the Pst(l) differences between taller and smaller children were not due to larger inspiratory muscles strength in taller children, but only to different elastic properties of the lungs [217, 220]. Pst(l) measured from the PV curves with both maximal and submaximal pressures in these 11 subjects was similar at larger and lower lung volume levels (90%, 60% TLC, 90%, 50% VC). If the Pst(l) differences between taller and smaller children were merely due to the inspiration maneuver, Pst(l) determined from the submaximal PV curves would be the same in taller children as the

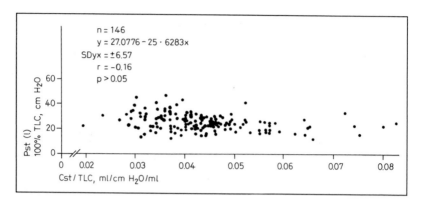

Fig. 24. No relationship of 'specific' static lung compliance (Cst/TLC) to elastic recoil pressure of the lungs obtained at maximal inspiratory level (Pst(l) 100% TLC) in symptom-free asthmatic patients (age 5–25 years) implies the difficulties in predicting the shape of PV curve of the lungs in patients with lung disease by mathematical models.

Pst(l) determined from the maximal PV curves in smaller children, which was not the case in our subjects [220].

An error in Pst(l) measurement can be also made if the Pst(l) is not read off from the expiratory PV curve, which is considered to express LE most properly [182]. For these reason, also lung volume history at the PV curves recording, i.e. whether the transpulmonary pressure was measured solely troughout deflation of the lungs, should be taken into account. The construction of the PV curve of the lungs by the method of 'end-expiratory compliance' obtained during slow tidal breathing at different lung volume levels [96, 189] is rather problematic from the latter aspect. i.e. a changing end-expiratory level and thus uncertain lung volume history, and a lacking transpulmonary pressure at the 100% VC level. Also there are difficulties for a subject to keep breathing stable at different lung volume levels, mainly at larger volumes. Our experience showed the 'end-expiratory compliance' method for obtaining the PV curve of the lungs more difficult in children than recording of PV curve during slow or flow-interrupted expiration of VC after full inspiration, the latter also requiring less time.

Mathematical models developed also for describing the shape of the PV curve of the lungs [25, 61, 96] seem not to be satisfactory, mainly in patients, because Cst expressing the slope of the PV curve does not correlate with the Pst(l) values, e.g. at maximal inspiratory level (100% TLC) (fig. 24).

Conclusions

In a group of 131 healthy children and adolescents aged 6–17 years LE indices, i.e. static and dynamic lung compliance (Cst, Cdyn) and elastic recoil pressure of the lungs [Pst(l)] were determined. Further, the 'specific' static and dynamic lung compliances were calculated. Pst(l) was measured at various lung volume levels from the deflation 'quasi' static pressure-volume curves. Cst and Cdyn increased with an increase of body height, age and body surface. Cdyn was always smaller than Cst. 'Specific' lung compliance which is comparable among children with various body size, as expressed per unit of lung volume was also obtained. 'Specific' Cst decreased with increasing body height, age and body surface. 'Specific' Cdyn was independent of body height, age or body surface. The obtained results imply that LE changes between the ages of 6 and 17 years. Anatomical studies support these conclusions [49, 103]. These conclusions result from Pst(l), 'specific' Cst, and the slope of the middle part of the PV curves of the lungs. A reliable assessment of LE in children and adolescents can be achieved from the expiratory (deflation) PV curve. In order to make LE measurements in children and adolescents helpful and more meaningful for pediatric pulmonologists, it seems that Pst(l) obtained from the expiratory PV curve of the lungs at several (larger and lower) lung volumes (e.g. at 100, 90 and 60% of actual TLC) represents a simple and most informative way in the evaluation of LE in older children and adolescents. Cst, in spite of being measured from the PV curves of the lung, does not provide a satisfactory and complete picture of LE, and is difficult to interpret. Cst is usually measured within the tidal volume range and thus represents a mean value, which can be affected by the abnormalities of LE reflected in the upper or lower parts of the PV curve within the tidal volume range. Cst measured also as a tangent at different lung volume levels from the PV curve can be even more erroneous. Cdyn is an unreliable LE index, especially in smaller children and in patients with airways obstruction because static conditions are not achieved in the lungs at the end of inspiration and expiration. The results on esophageal elastance and the vertical esophageal pleural pressure gradient underlined the importance of a constant small air content (0.2–0.4 ml) in the esophageal balloon and a constant position of the balloon in the esophagus (with its tip at the diaphragm dome level).

Some typical PV curves of the lungs with restrictive and obstructive lung diseases have been illustrated.

III. Airway Patency

A large number of respiratory diseases in children and adolescents have been accompanied by airway patency (caliber) alterations, most frequently by their narrowing (obstruction). *For the assessement of airway obstruction a number of lung function tests are available* [7, 16, 32, 35, 44, 54, 107, 108, 125, 151, 177, 197]. They can be divided into *direct* and *indirect* ones. The widely used tests have been the ventilatory air-flows, measured during quiet breathing and at forced expiration (direct tests). We measured from *direct tests* the following indices: (1) maximum expiratory flow rates from maximum expiratory flow-volume curves at forced expiratory maneuver; (2) lung volumes in relation to time obtained also at forced expiratory maneuver, i.e. dynamic lung volumes; (3) airway resistance and lung (pulmonary) resistance during quiet normal breathing.

From the *indirect tests* of airway patency we measured the indices from multiple-breath nitrogen washout curves of the lungs.

Maximum Expiratory Flow Rates

In recent years, numerous studies have shown the maximum expiratory flow rates (MEF, $\dot{V}_{max}$, FEF) to be advantageous, especially in the detection of initial stages of airways obstruction and they have therefore been widely used in clinical and epidemiological studies [9, 15, 16, 37, 106–108, 114, 115, 142, 151, 159, 176, 185, 204, 206].

Maximum expiratory flow rate (instantaneous) represents the maximum rate of airflow in liters per second obtained during forced expiratory vital capacity maneuver at a defined lung volume level, i.e. at a certain moment of expiration. Maximum expiratory flow rates change along with the changing lung volume. MEF have been measured from the maximum expiratory flow-volume (MEFV) curve, which relates maximum expiratory flow rates and lung volume over the whole forced expiratory vital capacity. The curve has ascendent and descendent parts (fig. 25). The ascendent part

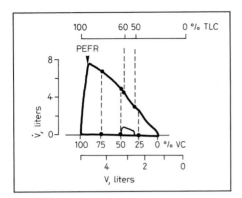

Fig. 25. MEFV curve in a 14-year-old healthy boy, 168 cm tall, illustrating the measurement of expiratory flow rates ($\dot{V}$) at 25, 50 and 75% of VC, and 50 and 60% of TLC. The descendent part of the curve changes from convex to straight and concave shapes in healthy children with somatic growth.

of the curve begins at the maximum inspiratory level (100% VC = 100% TLC) and ends at the moment of attaining the peak expiratory flow rate (PEF, PEFR). From that level, the descendent part of the curve starts and ends at the residual volume level. The descendent part, roughly within the range of 0–80% vital capacity (i.e. after expiring 20% of VC) maintains the same flow-volume relationship during forced expiration in the same individual. Once the subject has attained a certain maximum expiratory effort with limitation of airflow, no further increase of the expiratory muscle effort will change the shape of the descendent part of the flow-volume curve, and thus also the expiratory airflow rate. This part of the curve is therefore called 'effort-independent'. Generally, it is accepted that maximum expiratory flow rates measured at different levels on the descendent part of the MEFV curve (e.g. 50, 60% TLC, 25, 50, 75% VC) are determined only by the mechanical lung properties expressing the patency of the peripheral 'upstream' airways [118]. The descendent part of the MEFV curve, also in children and adolescents, is fairly reproducible, provided the FVC in a series of MEFV curves from a subject is roughly the same (fig. 26). The intraindividual variability of MEFV curves was the least one, if the 'composite' or 'envelope' MEFV curve with the FVC's variability within 5% of the largest FVC was obtained. The intraindividual reproducibility of MEF is poorer when flows are read off only from the MEFV curve with the largest FVC [163, 203].

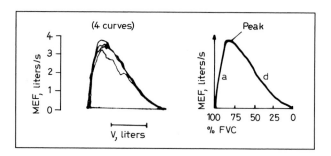

Fig. 26. A series of 4 MEFV curves in a 9-year-old boy, height 136 cm, with cystic fibrosis showing the reproducibility of the terminal portion of the curves, the variability of peak expiratory flow and the gaining of the 'envelope' MEFV curve as a representative one for analysis in a given subject. Left: 4 original curves; right: envelope MEFV curve; a = ascendent part; d = descendent part.

The descendent part of the MEFV curves in its major extent is well reproducible in a given subject provided the expiratory flow is beyond a critical level of effort, i.e. MEF at a given lung volume reached the plateau of maximum expiratory iso-volume-pressure-flow curve and, further, is independent on pleural pressure as an indicator of the expiratory effort. By realizing the fact that the descendent part of the MEFV curve should be considered as a fingerprint of expiratory flow limitation in the lungs for a given subject, the quoted discrepancies in the physiological indices (reference values) measured on the descendent part of the MEFV curves in healthy children and adolescents by different authors might also be diminished. An adequate approach in analyzing MEFV curves for this age range provides 'composite' or 'envelope' MEFV curves [142, 203], taking into account the latter fact. The mechanisms of maximum expiratory flow limitation and their significance for the assessment of the peripheral 'upstream' airway patency can be explained, for example, by combining the theories of Mead et al. [118] and Pride et al. [150].

If the airways are compared with a tube, then a certain rate of gas flow through the tube ($\Delta\dot{V}$) depends on the driving pressure, i.e. on the pressure difference between both ends of the tube (ΔP) and the resistance (R) of the tube of the flowing gas. The resistance is defined by the length of tube, its inner diameter and physical properties of the flowing gas. The whole relationship can be expressed by the following formula:

$$\Delta\dot{V} = \frac{\Delta P}{R}.$$

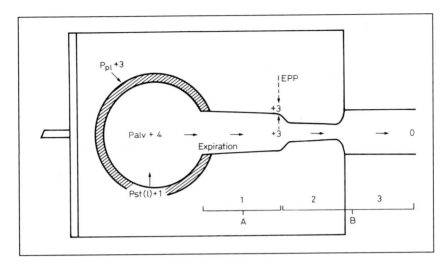

Fig. 27. Schematic illustration of airways during forced expiration maneuver at the moment of maximum expiratory flow rates on the descendent part of MEFV curve. Positive pleural pressure (P_{pl}) makes the central endothoracic airways segment (B2) in a dynamic compression. The peripheral airways segment (A1) is not compressed by the positive pleural pressure, because the pressure at the beginning of the airways (Palv) is higher due the elastic recoil pressure of the lungs (Pst(l)) than that outside of the airways. The pressure in the airways decreases towards the atmosphere until it attains the same value as the pleural pressure (in our case 3.0 kPa). This point is termed the equal pressure point – EPP. The extrathoracic part of the central segment (B3) is not compressed by the positive pleural pressure and may be dilated by the positive intraluminal pressure. The square represents the thorax, the circle the lung alveoli, the tube the airways, and the numbers inside 'alveoli and airways' are pressures. Palv 4.0 kPa was derived as a sum of P_{pl} 3.0 kPa and Pst(l) 1.0 kPa.

A similar situation exists in the airways during tidal breathing, when the pressure at the beginning of the tube is alveolar pressure and that at its end mouth pressure.

At forced expiration maneuver the situation differs from that at tidal breathing (fig. 27). The air-flow through the airways at forced expiration maneuver is modified by the positive pleural pressure compressing the airways from the outside. This pressure acts similarly as in the 'Starling resistor', which consists of a collapsible tube closed inside a chamber and connected by both ends with the outside. The flow through the tube is determined not only by the pressure difference between the beginning and the end of the tube, but mainly by the pressure acting from the outside on the collapsible tube inside the chamber [150].

An analogical situation exists in the lungs at forced expiration. The driving pressure at the beginning of the tube, i.e. of the airways, is the alveolar pressure (Palv), which is the sum of the pleural pressure and the elastic recoil pressure of the lungs (Pst(l)). The lower pressure at the end of the tube (the airways) corresponds to the mouth pressure. The pressure around the collapsible tube equals the pleural pressure. At forced expiration the pleural pressure acting on the external wall of larger airways (trachea, segmental or lobar bronchi) is higher than the pressure inside the airways causing their dynamic compression. The air-flow through the airways under forced expiration conditions is therefore determined by the pressure difference between the alveolar and pleural pressures. This difference corresponds to the elastic recoil pressure of the lungs [Palv – Ppl = Pst(l)], which is the driving pressure for maximum expiratory flow rates [118]. The point, beyond which dynamic compression of the larger airways begins, is called the 'equal pressure point' (EPP). EPP divides the airways into the 'upstream' segment (closer to alveoli, uncompressed, A segment in fig. 27), and the 'downstream' segment (B segment in fig. 27), the intrathoracic part of which is compressed. This implies that the maximum expiratory flow rate (MEF, $\dot{V}_{max}$) determined at a certain lung volume level on the descendent part of the MEFV curve within the range of 0–80% VC is determined by the elastic recoil pressure of the lungs (Pst(l)) and by the resistance of the 'upstream' airway segment (Rus) at a given lung volume level. The relation is expressed by the formula:

$$\dot{V}_{max} = \frac{Pst(l)}{Rus}.$$

In the 'downstream' airway segment (B segment in fig. 27), i.e. from EPP towards the mouth, the driving force for flow is provided by pleural pressure. Maximum expiratory flow rate through this segment is determined by the pleural pressure (Ppl) and the resistance of the 'downstream' segment (Rds);

$$\dot{V}_{max} = \frac{Ppl}{Rds}.$$

Under the conditions of forced expiration the 'upstream' and 'downstream' airway segments are mutually linked up in series, therefore the maximum flow expired through both segments must be identical. How-

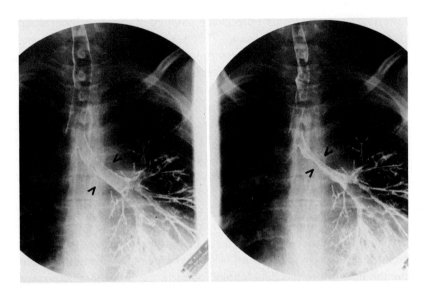

Fig. 28. Functional bronchographic studies in the frontal projections focused on the larger central airways during quiet breathing (left) and during forced expiration or coughing (right) in a 17-year-old girl with repeated bronchitis. During forced expiration the airways became narrowed, especially in the area of the left main bronchus (pointed with arrows). This narrowing is probably located behind the equal pressure point (EPP) and might be a sign of dynamic compression of the central airways, dividing the airways into the peripheral (close to alveoli, upstream) and central (downstream) segments. The narrowing might be also identical with the 'flow-limiting segment'. Bronchographic studies were carried out in a cooperation with the Central X-Ray Department of the University Hospital in Prague, Motol.

ever, the downstream (intrathoracic) segment (B_2 in fig. 27) is compressed by the pleural pressure, whereas the upstream segment is not, and the airway geometry upstream from EPP is fixed. The values of the maximum expiratory flows, determined on the descendent part of the MEFV curve within 0–80% VC range, therefore expresses the patency of the 'upstream' airway segment. *Maximum expiratory flow rates are therefore suitable for the detection of the 'upstream' airways obstruction, i.e. that located between the alveoli and EPP (segmental or lobar bronchi).* Such a dynamic compression of the lobar or segmental bronchi can also be observed at functional bronchography, e.g. during cough, which in fact represents a forced expiration (fig. 28). With a decrease of lung volume, EPP move further upstream, i.e. into the periphery of the lungs. MEF measured, therefore, at lower lung volume levels reflects the patency of more peripheral airways than MEF at larger lung volumes. This can be observed in the patients, e.g. with tracheal stenosis after tracheotomy, in whom first of all MEF at larger lung volumes are reduced, while MEF at lower lung volumes are normal. The data on 'upstream' airway conductance (see below) suggest also in children and adolescents a movement of EPP into the periphery of the lungs with a decrease of lung volume mainly in smaller children [236]. Similar findings were also observed by calculating the conductance of the collapsible flow-limiting S-segment (Gs) [150]. However, measurement of the exact location of EPP was not performed in children and adolescents.

Besides the latter two models analyzing forced expiration, i.e. expiratory flow limitation due to dynamic compression of the airways, there are several other models analyzing forced expiration such as the 'wave speed' concept of Dawson and Elliot [34] on expiratory flow limitation, explaining the flow limitation by a 'choke' point in the intrathoracic airways. Its location is expected to be approximately the same as for EPP. According to the latter concept the magnitude of critical rate of flow depends on cross-sectional area and elastic modulus at the choke point, on gas density and on static recoil pressure of the lungs.

Whatever the mechanism of the limitation of maximum expiratory flow in the lungs is, the descendent part of the MEFV curve in its major extent is well reproducible also in older children and adolescents provided the expiratory flow is beyond the critical level of respiratory muscles effort. In the vast majority of older children and adolescents even with lung disease, reproducible MEFV curves can be obtained. Good instruction and patience of the investigator with a child, and recordings of at least 3 superimposable MEFV curves are a prerequisite for successful and reproducible MEFV curves in children and adolescents.

Besides MEFV curves also MEFV curves with various densities of the expired gas and partial expiratory flow-volume (PEFV) curves can be obtained in this age range (see below) for the refinement of airways obstruction detection.

Methods
Maximum expiratory flow rates were measured from maximum expiratory flow-volume curves (figs. 25, 26). The rate of the expired airflow was measured with a heated pneumotachograph (Fleisch No. 3, 4 or Lilly type) connected to a differential pressure tranducer and with an electromanometer. The lung volume was obtained by electronic integration of the airflow at the mouth. The calibration of air-flow through a pneumota-

chograph was performed with a rotameter delivering the known different rates of airflow or with a slanting manometer. The resistance of pneumotachographs was below 0.5 cm $H_2O/l/s$ ($\cong 0.05$ kPa/l/s). The calibration of the volume integrator was carried out with a 1-liter syringe and a drift of the integrator was less than 2% over an interval of 15 s.

The curves for expiratory flow rates and expired lung volume were also recorded separately as a function of time (see fig. 37).

MEFV curves were displayed on the screen of an oscilloscope and simultaneously registered on a direct writing X-Y recorder within the range of a reliable frequency and amplitude response of the recorder. The volume, i.e. FVC, was recorded on the ordinate and the expiratory flow rate (MEF, $\dot{V}_{max}$) in liters per second was recorded on the abscissa of the MEFV curve. From the MEFV curve peak expiratory flow rate (PEFR, PEF) and maximum expiratory flow rates on the descending part of the curve at 75, 50 and 25% of VC, and further at 60 and 50% of TLC (i.e. at volumes of VC and TLC left in the lungs) were read off (fig. 25). From each subject at least 4–5 MEFV curves were obtained. The technically best curves with FVCs of less then 5% among themselves in a given subject were compared by superimposing them on a transparent paper or by recording them directly (fig. 26) on each other according to the maximal inspiratory level (100% VC), the descendent part of the curve and also end-expiratory resting (FRC) level, if recorded flow-volume loops. Thus, a reproducibility of the MEFV curves was obtained, and a 'composite' or 'envelope' MEFV curve with the largest flow and FVC was chosen as representative for the analysis of MEFs and FVC. From this it follows that by such an approach the MEFV curve with the highest FVC and MEFs in a subject was obtained.

MEF and PEFR, expressed in liters per second, were also expressed per unit of total lung capacity, i.e. in TLC/s. Thus, MEFs and PEFR were corrected for lung size and termed 'specific'. Determination of 'specific' MEF and PEF is very important especially in children and adolescents since, on their basis, it is possible to compare the MEF and PEF values in growing subjects of various age, height and lung size. Lung-size-corrected MEF and PEF are also important in patients with lung disease, in whom the relationship between lung size and other anthropometrical parameters, e.g. body height, surface and age, have been changed by the disease. In a patient with lung fibrosis MEF can be low because the lungs are small and therefore the supply of air for flow is also small.

MEFV curves were also obtained at various densities of the expired gas, i.e. with air and with a mixture of helium and air or oxygen. By superimposing both types of MEFV curves at a point where the descendent parts of both types of the curves coincide, the *volume of isoflow* (V-iso-$\dot{V}$) was measured [37]. The latter index indicates a laminar flow in the upstream airway segment because laminar flow is independent of gas density. V-iso-$\dot{V}$ has been expressed as a percentage of VC and an increase of V-iso-$\dot{V}$ suggests a migration of EPP into the periphery of the lungs at larger lung volumes and expected thus more sensitive to indicate peripheral airways obstruction. The obtained results have been controversial in this respect [53, 227] (see below).

Further, from MEF and elastic recoil pressure values, both measured at identical lung volume levels (i.e. at 25, 50 and 75% VC and 50 and 60% TLC) also the *conductance of the 'upstream' segment of the airways* (Gus) according to Mead et al. [118] was calculated at latter volume levels using the relationship:

$$Gus = \frac{\dot{V}_{max}}{Pst} \text{(1)}$$

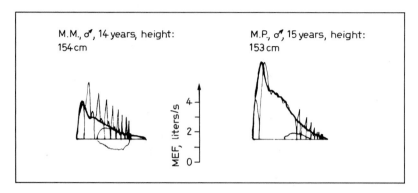

Fig. 29. MEFV curves and superimposed airflows at a series of coughing maneuvers during expiration in patients with cystic fibrosis. 'Spikes' above the descendent part of the curves represent flow transients reflecting the rate of volume displacement of the suddenly narrowed larger intrathoracic airways expanded differently at different lung volume levels. Then the expiratory airflow at coughing coincides with the descendent part of the MEFV curve for a certain period of time as a sign of the flow limitation mechanism of the airways. Finally, the airflow reaches zero at closure of the larynx. The magnitude of flow transients is suitable for an assessment of larger airways rigidity and a coughing maneuver provides valuable information on the airways function.

Gus were further expressed per unit of TLC and corrected in this way for lung size. The dimension of the corrected Gus value is in liters/s/kPa/liter and Gus can be used for the assessment of peripheral airway patency.

Also, *partial expiratory flow-volume (PEFV) curves* were obtained in some patients [14, 161, 193]. Such curves were obtained when a subject started his forced expiration maneuver from a submaximal inspiration, i.e. below the 100% VC (100% TLC) level. In children and adolescents the results on the usefulness of PEFV curves have only very rarely been reported. PEFV curves have been claimed to be more sensitive in the detection of airways obstruction than MEFV curves [161]. *A supramaximal expiratory airflow of the PEFV curves* above the descendent part of the MEFV curves, such as at coughing, can also be useful in the assessment of the collapsibility of the airways (fig. 29). The volume of isoflow and the PEFV curves were recorded with an electronic spirometer (Ohio-Spirometer).

Results and Discussion

Maximum expiratory flow rates ($\dot{V}_{max}$, MEF), read off on the descendent part of maximum expiratory flow-volume curves, and *PEF,* expressed in liters per second, significantly increased with the increase of body height, age and body surface in the studied 111 healthy children and adolescents at all lung volume levels studied (fig. 30, 31; table 167–184). The

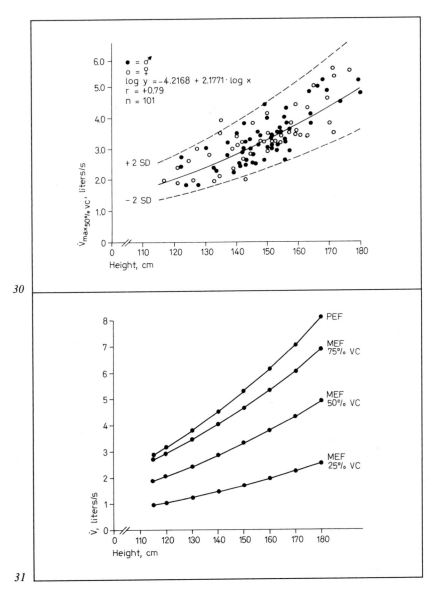

Fig. 30. Maximum expiratory flow rate, measured at 50% of vital capacity level ($\dot{V}_{max\ 50\%\ VC}$) in liters/s, in relation to body height in boys and girls. For further explanations, see figure 2.

Fig. 31. Maximum expiratory flow rates (MEF; $\dot{V}_{max}$) measured at 25, 50 and 75% of VC level and PEF in liters/s, in relation to body height in healthy boys and girls. The data are given as means.

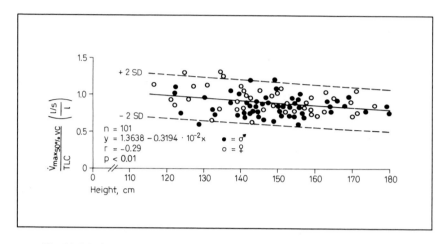

Fig. 32. Maximum expiratory flow rate, measured at 50% of VC and corrected for 1 liter of TLC ($\frac{Vmax\ 50\%\ VC}{TLC}$) in relation to body height in healthy boys and girls. For further explanations, see figure 2.

relationships were nonlinear. No significant differences in MEF have been recorded between boys and girls in spite of the fact that some reference values have been reported separately for both sexes [9, 152, 203, 244]. The MEFV curves in the majority of our healthy children and adolescents had the descendent part straight or convex (fig. 25). PEF was usually obtained after expiring 8–15% of FVC. *'Specific' $\dot{V}_{max}$* were negatively dependent on the body height, age and body surface (fig. 32; table 185–199), moderately descreasing with increasing body height, age and body surface. *'Specific' PEF* was independent of the body height amounting to 1.463 ± (SD) 0.233 liters/s/liter (i.e. TLC/s) on average. The values of *$\dot{V}_{max}$/FVC and PEF/FVC ratios,* i.e. calculated per unit of FVC, significantly decreased also with body height (table 200–205) in healthy children and adolescents. *The conductance of the 'upstream' airway segment* (Gus) corrected for lung size, i.e. the 'specific' Gus values, decreased with increasing body height (fig. 33; table 206–210) and were found higher at lower lung volume levels. A decrease of the ratios $\dot{V}_{max}$/TLC, $\dot{V}_{max}$/FVC and PEF/FVC is due to the fact that the relationships $\dot{V}_{max}$ vs. TLC or vs. FVC, and PEF vs. TLC do not pass the zero origin. A similar situation applies for Gus values. However, the observed developmental changes of the latter ratios result from the physiological data.

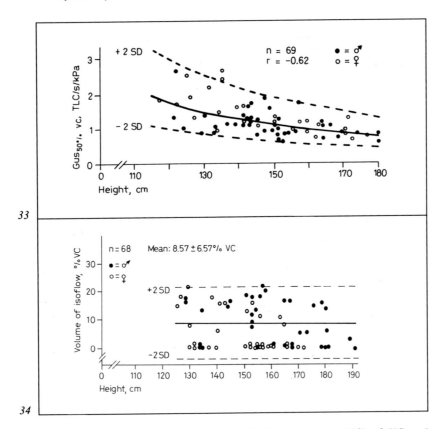

Fig. 33. 'Upstream airway conductance' (Gus) measured at 50% of VC and expressed per 1 liter of TLC, i.e. in a unit of TLC/s/kPa (thus corrected for lung size), in relation to body height in healthy boys and girls. According to this value the 'upstream' airway patency is higher in smaller children than in taller ones and adolescents. For further details, see text.

Fig. 34. 'Volume of isoflow' in relation to body height in healthy subjects 7–25 years old.

The *'volume of isoflow'* (V-iso-V̇) was observed to be independent of body height or age (fig. 34) amounting to 8.6 ± 6.6% VC on average. Fox et al. [53] reported the V-iso-V̇ value to be 5% of VC.

The best correlation of MEF and PEF in liters/s, and Gus in TLC/s/kPa was found with body height in our healthy subjects, resulting also in the smallest coefficient of variation around a power regression. The transformation of x and y variables, i.e. of height and MEF (or PEF), into the decadic logarithmic values, expressed as a power regression equation ($\log y = \log a + b \cdot \log x$), was found to be the best approach for relating both latter variables. By this approach the coefficient of variation around a power regression is the same for the whole span of independent variable, e.g. body height. Thus, the 95% confidence limits bounded the physiological distribution of the data best (fig. 30).

The differences in the latter reference values among authors [152] might thus also be reduced. The linear regression equation computed for MEF and PEF in liters/s on body height [195] gives a relatively large standard deviation from the regression line mainly in smaller children. Similar difficulties can appear also by expressing MEFs or PEF data on body height by a quadratic (parabolic) function.

The published data on MEFs, PEF and the whole MEFV curves in healthy children and adolescents are numerous [9, 39, 47, 65, 85, 92–95, 132, 162, 163, 168, 244] and show large differences between some authors, which is not fully clarified [152].

Multiple regression equations, with independent variables including body height, age, body surface and weight, can hardly be expected to improve the prediction of MEFs and other indices derived from MEFV curves because the strongest correlations of the latter indices were with body height (table 167–184). Also, the standard deviations around multiple regressions might thus be increased and the sensitivity of the functional indices decreased.

A certain minor source of error in reading off MEF from the descendent part of MEF curves in older children and adolescents can be attributed to the MEFV curves obtained with lung volume change measured at the mouth, e.g. by integration of airflow at the mouth. This error in determination of MEFV curves with volume change at the mouth is due to the intrathoracic gas compression during forced expiration, which is not sensed from the volume displacement measured at the mouth. Only the volume change of the thorax during forced expiration measured in a subject in a body plethysmograph includes both the volume displacement at the mouth and the volume change due to intrathoracic gas compression.

The error in reading off MEFs from MEFV curves obtained with lung volume change only at the mouth can be determined by computation of the amount of the compressed gas (V_{comp}) at a defined lung volume level during forced expiration from the rearranged Boyle-Marriotte law:

$$V_{comp} = \frac{TGV \cdot Palv}{P_B - P_{H_2O}}.$$

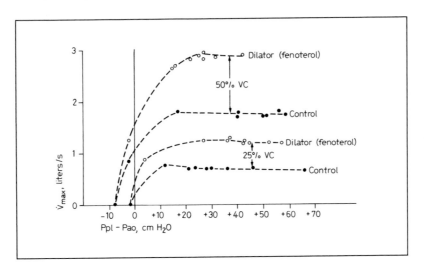

Fig. 35. Isovolume-pressure-flow curves in a 12-year-old girl, height 153 cm, with bronchial asthma obtained at 25 and 50% of VC before and following a bronchodilator with volume change measured at the mouth. These curves provide the possibility of calculating the amount of compressed gas at forced expiration and thus correcting the maximum expiratory flow at given lung volume measured at the mouth. For details, see text. The plateau of the curves represents the airflow limitation at given lung volume.

Palv is alveolar pressure at a certain lung volume of expiration as a sum of elastic recoil pressure of the lungs (Pst(l)) and pleural pressure (Ppl) · P_B – P_{H_2O} is barometric pressure minus water vapor pressure at 37 °C. TGV is the thoracic gas volume exposed to the compression at a certain level of forced expiration and can be obtained as total lung capacity minus the expired volume of air in BTPS conditions. Then at the corrected lung volume level for the amount of intrathoracic compressed gas, MEF can be read off as the corrected one, e.g. the corrected MEF at 25% of VC is obtained at the lung volume (in liters) left in the lungs for 25% VC plus V_{comp} (in liters).

Since Palv varies along the plateau of the iso-volume-pressure-flow (IVPF) curve (fig. 35), then the amount of the compressed gas also varies during forced expiration maneuvers. On the plateau of the IVPF curve Palv can be read off at the initial or final portion of the curve. The computed amount of the compressed gas during forced expiration in a group of our 8 symptom-free asthmatic patients (age: 8–20 years; mean values = FEV_1/FVC: 62%, and sGaw = 0.55 liters/s/kPa/liter), at 25% of VC varied

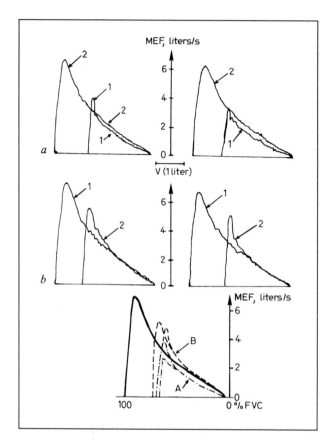

Fig. 36. MEFV and PEFV curves in a 14-year-old girl, height 161 cm, with asymptomatic bronchial asthma showing their different sensitivities in the assessment of airways obstruction dependent on the sequence of curves. *a* PEFV curves were registered as first ones (1) followed by MEFV curves (2). The descendent part of the PEFV curve is more reduced than that of the MEFV curve. *b* The sequence of the curves was changed. MEFV curves were registered as first ones (1) followed by PEFV curves (2). The descendent parts of both types of curves coincide after flow transients disappearing on PEFV curves.

from 20 to 150 ml and at 50% of VC from 40 to 250 ml, depending on Palv read off at the initial or final portion of the plateau of IVPF curves, respectively, before and after a bronchodilator (fenoterol). The correction of MEF for the latter amount of the compressed intrathoracic gas resulted in an error in reading off MEFs (being lower) from MEFV curves with lung volume measured at the mouth to be on average 5% at 25% VC and 8% at

50% VC. Such an error is probably more negligible in healthy older children and adolescents as it was observed for reference values reported in two groups of healthy children and adolescents, from those in one group MEFV curves were obtained with lung volume change at the mouth and in the second group MEFV curves were recorded with lung volume change of the thorax measured in a body plethysmograph [202, 203, 216, 226, 233].

The experience with *PEFV curves* in this period of age for an assessment of airways obstruction is still rare. In adults, PEFV curves have been reported to be superior to MEFV in revealing airways obstruction [14, 161]. We observed PEFV curves to be more sensitive than MEFV curves only in some asthmatic children and adolescents but not in patients with cystic fibrosis.

In some asthmatic children the PEFV curve was reduced in comparison with the MEFV curve, if the PEFV curve was obtained at the first expiratory maneuver followed by the MEFV curve (fig. 36). In reverse order, i.e. if during forced expiration the MEFV curve was obtained as the first one, followed by PEFV curve recording, the difference between MEFV and PEFV curves was not observed.

The descendent part of both types of curves, PEFV and MEFV, coincided after a small overshooting of the descendent part of the MEFV curve by peak flow rate of the PEFV curve, which can be attributed to volume displacement due to bronchial compression (flow transients). It follows from the latter that the order of volume history plays a role for using PEFV curves as a more sensitive index in the detection of airways obstruction. Also, reliable equipment, i.e. a volume integrator, is required. An electronic spirometer for obtaining the PEFV curves ought to be preferred. However, more experience with PEFV curves for airway patency assessment in children and adolescents is necessary.

Dynamic Lung Volumes

Measurements of volumes during a maximum forced expiration represents a widely used and simple approach for the assessment of airway patency. The forced expiratory volume curve (spirogram) shows expired volume as a function of time and characterizes the ability of the respiratory system to move air (gas) rapidly from the lungs. The theoretical background of flow-limiting function of the airways during measurements of

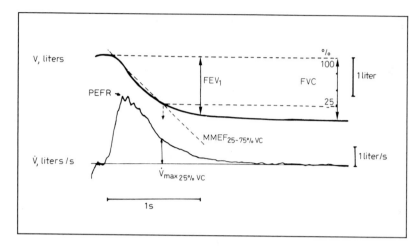

Fig. 37. Separate recordings of lung volume (V – upper curve) and expiratory flow rate ($\dot{V}$ – lower curve) during FVC in a healthy 8-year-old girl, height 131 cm. The measurements of FEV_1, $MMEF_{25-75\%}$, FVC, PEFR and MEFR at 25% of vital capacity ($\dot{V}_{max\,25\%\,VC}$) are shown.

dynamic lung volumes can be applied in a similar manner as for maximum expiratory flow rates measured from MEFV curves (see above).

At forced expiration maneuver, forced expiratory volume (FEV) from the maximal inspiration level at selected time intervals is determined (fig. 37). Most often, the volume of gas expired during the first second (FEV_1) after the start of a forced expiration is determined. Also, the volume of gas expired during two middle quaters of forced expiratory vital capacity (FVC) computed per 1 s is measured as maximum mid-expiratory flow rate ($MMEF_{25-75\%\,VC}$). Contrary to the MEF values, FEV and $MMEF_{25-75\%\,VC}$ represent mean expiratory flow at the defined time intervals. FVC also represents a dynamic lung volume and has to be distinguished from vital capacity obtained during slow expiratory maneuver, at which the complete emptying of the lungs is not limited by time. FEV_1 has very often been expressed as a percentage of FVC ($\%FEV_1/FVC$). However, both the latter indices, i.e. FEV_1 and FVC, reflect the change in airway patency (obstruction) and both can be reduced in obstructive lung discases. As a result, the FEV_1/FVC ratio might not change or it does not change adequately to the extent of the expiratory flow limitation and thus underestimates the degree of airways obstruction. The proportional changes of FEV_1 and FVC have been observed mainly in asthmatic patients during an asthma attack as well as by stimuli-induced bronchoconstriction.

FEV and FVC have been expressed in milliliters or liters, and $MMEF_{25-75\% VC}$ in liters/s. FEV and $MMEF_{25-75\% VC}$ can also be expressed per unit of TLC and thus corrected for lung size such as MEF. Size-corrected FEV and $MMEF_{25-75\% VC}$ are also termed as 'specific' ones.

Other functional indices of airway patency derived from the forced expiratory volume curve have been also reported, such as mean transit time [108, 131]. However, information on the latter in older children and adolescents are only few.

Methods

The forced expiratory volume curves (spirograms) were recorded on a paper of the instrument at the speed of 2–5 cm/s with a heated pneumotachograph after an integration of airflow at the mouth or with a spirometer having a good dynamic (frequency and amplitude) response.

After careful instruction, at least 3–5 forced expiratory spirograms were obtained from each individual. He was asked to take a deep (maximal) inspiration and then to expire completely as fast as possible to the residual volume level.

In children who already had experience (patients) with the forced expiratory maneuver, 3 forced expiratory volume curves (spirograms) were sufficient. However, in an unexperienced child many more attempts had to be made in order to get a reproducible forced expiratory spirogram. From a series of expiratory spirograms, the spirogram with the largest vital capacity and the steepest part of the curve was analyzed. We mostly recorded forced expiratory spirograms simultaneously with the MEFV curves.

Results and Discussion

FVC, FEV_1, $MMEF_{25-75\% VC}$ values (in ml, liters/s) increased with increasing body height in 111 healthy children and adolescents (table 211–231). The values first rise rather moderately, and from 150 cm body height their increase is steeper. The FVC and FEV_1 values in the boys significantly differed from those in the girls, while $MMEF_{25-75\% VC}$ did not. Similar values are reported by Polgar and Weng [149], Hsu et al. [78] and others [9, 23, 63, 69, 81, 83, 144, 152, 166, 194].

The 'specific' $MMEF_{25-75\% VC}$ value, i.e. expressed per unit of TLC and thus corrected for lung size, decreased slightly with an increase of body height (table 232) as well as the ratio $MMEF_{25-75\% VC}/FVC$ (table 233). 'Specific' FEV_1 (i.e. FEV_1/TLC) was independent of body height amounting to 0.623 ± 0.049 (SD) on average in boys and girls together. Similar findings have been reported [65], giving a mean percentage for FEV_1/TLC of 61.6 ± 9.031. *The percentage for FEV_1/FVC was also independent of* body height, age and body surface with a value of 84.47 ± 4.55% on average in boys and girls together. Similar values for the percentage of FEV_1/FVC have been published by others [63, 83, 87, 130, 146, 194] (table 223).

Conclusions

During forced expiration maneuver in 111 healthy children and adolescents, 6–17 years of age, maximum expiratory flow rates ($\dot{V}_{max}$, MEF) at different lung volume levels (25, 50, 75% of vital capacity, and 50, 60% of total lung capacity) were measured. Further, the values of PEF, FEV_1, FVC and $MMEF_{25-75\% VC}$ were determined. All these values assessing airway patency were related to the body height, age and body surface of the subjects. The relationships of the functional values calculated according to body height, age and body surface were expressed in a form of single regression equations with 95% confidence limits. All the values studied increased with increasing body height, age and body surface. The best correlation of the latter indices was with body height. Also the ratios FEV_1/FVC (84.47 ± 4.55%), $MMEF_{25-75\% VC}/FVC$, $\dot{V}_{max}/FVC$ and PEF/FVC were calculated. The $\dot{V}_{max}$, PEF, $MMEF_{25-75\% VC}$ and FEV_1 values were further expressed per unit of TLC and thus corrected for lung size (termed as 'specific'). The 'specific' $\dot{V}_{max}$, $MMEF_{25-75\% VC}$ and 'upstream' airways conductance (Gus) decreased with the body height similarly as $MMEF_{25-75\% VC}/FVC$. The values for 'specific' PEF and 'specific' FEV_1, as well as $\%FEV_1/FVC$ did not depend on body height, age or body surface. A decrease of the 'specific' $\dot{V}_{max}$ and Gus values with an increase in body height, age and body surface suggests that growth of the peripheral airways does not proceed at the same rate (isotropically) as the growth of the lungs (alveoli) in the period between 6 and 17 years of age [236], and that there is a larger airway patency of the more peripheral airways in smaller children than in taller children and adolescents.

Maximum expiratory flow rates measured from MEFV curves on the descendent part of the curve at lower and larger lung volume levels represent important, useful and simple functional parameters for assessing the airway patency (caliber) suitable for the detection of airways obstruction also in children and adolescents. MEFs, first of all at lower lung volumes, have been considered to reflect the early stages of airflow limitation presumably in the 'upstream' (peripheral) airways.

By realizing the regulating function of the airways on maximum expiratory flows at forced expiration, the MEFV curve with a reproducible descendent part were obtained in cooperating older children and adolescents. With equipment similar to that used in adults for this purpose after an appropriate calibration, the comparable MEFV curves in healthy older children and adolescents from different laboratories were obtained. The 'envelope' method of analyzing MEFV curves reduced the intraindividual variability of MEF and made MEF reference values more sensitive in the detection of airways obstruction. No significant differences in MEF were observed between boys and girls.

FEV_1, FVC and $MMEF_{25-75\% VC}$ increased with an increase in body height, age, and body surface but correlated best with body height. There was a significant difference in FVC and FEV_1 between boys and girls but not for $MMEF_{25-75\% VC}$. The difference between FVC and VC (obtained at unlimited duration of expiration), was nonsignificant and only moderate in smaller children. FEV_1 and $MMEF_{25-75\% VC}$ represent also mean expiratory flow rates and therefore include a considerable initial 'effort-dependent' part of forced expiration, mainly FEV_1. They reflect not only airway patency but also the respiratory muscles effort. In the patients the latter dynamic lung volumes were observed to be less discriminative with regard to airways obstruction, and also changed less following bronchodilatation or bronchostriction than, for example, MEF at lower lung volumes [222, 225–227, 234, 237, 238]. The percentage FEV_1/FVC was found to be independent of body height, age, and body surface in our healthy subjects and a value below 75% was considered significantly reduced. The ratio FEV_1/FVC can understimate airways obstruction since both indices may change in proportion.

MEFV curves and forced expiratory spirograms after proper calibration were also recorded graphically. The digital output of the selected indices alone may be misleading in the assessment of airways obstruction without a visual checking of the curves.

Airflow Resistance

The force (pressure) required for a movement of the respiratory system during normal quiet breathing has to overcome elastic, resistive (frictional) and inertial components of the different parts of the respiratory system, i.e. lungs, airways and chest wall. The pressure applied to the respiratory system is a sum of the latter components, which are a function of volume, flow and mass acceleration.

This chapter is focused on the measurement of the resistive properties of the airways and the lungs, i.e. on the resistive pressure to gas (air) flow elicited by airways and lungs, at normal breathing frequencies, in older children and adolescents. The latter measurements became an indispensable part of the assessment of airway patency in subjects of this age range.

The ratio of the resistive pressure change (ΔP) to the corresponding airflow change ($\Delta \dot{V}$) is called airflow resistance (R).

The pressure difference between alveoli and mouth ($\Delta Palv$) as a driving pressure for the corresponding change in flow ($\Delta \dot{V}$) through the airways at normal quiet breathing is defined as 'airway resistance' (Raw):

$$R_{aw} = \frac{\Delta Palv}{\Delta \dot{V}}.$$

The pressure difference between the external surface of the lungs, i.e. pleural (esophageal) pressure, and mouth pressure ($\Delta Ppl - Pao$), as a driving pressure for the corresponding airflow ($\Delta \dot{V}$) in the airways and lung tissue, is defined as 'lung (pulmonary) resistance' (R_L, R_p):

$$R_L = \frac{\Delta Ppl - Pao}{\Delta \dot{V}}.$$

Ppl is pleural pressure and Pao is pressure at the airways opening, i.e. mouth pressure. The part of the pressure difference between alveoli (or pleural pressure) and mouth due to gas inertia may be neglected at normal breathing frequencies and both relationships for R_{aw} and R_L calculations are thus valid. Lung resistance is then a sum of airway resistance and lung tissue resistance ($R_L = R_{aw} + Rti$).

Resistance is expressed in kilopascals per liter per second ($kPa \cdot l^{-1} \cdot s$), or in centimeters of water per liter second ($cm\ H_2O \cdot l^{-1} \cdot s$). Resistance is defined then as a magnitude of driving pressure for an airflow of 1 liter per second.

Airway Resistance

Airway resistance represents a measure of the force (pressure) opposing gas flow in the airways during normal breathing. The magnitude of the latter force is dependent on the geometry of the airways, physical properties of the inspired and expired gas, flow pattern, and rate of gas flow.

R_{aw} has most often been measured in a body plethysmograph during quiet breathing or 'panting', simultaneously with the measurement of functional residual capacity as thoracic gas volume (TGV).

The body plethysmograph is a box with solid rigid walls, in which lung volume changes of the subject during breathing are measured. Two basic types of body plethysmograph are distinguished [20, 43, 44, 116].

(1) Constant-volume body plethysmograph (pressure box, DuBois type). In this type the tested individual breathes inside the plethysmograph and the lung volume changes during breathing are recorded with a pressure transducer as pressure variations inside the plethysmograph and then converted to volume changes. The total volume of air in the plethysmograph does not change during the investigation.

(2) Volume-displacement body plethysmograph (constant-pressure box, Mead type). In this type, lung volume changes during breathing inside the plethysmograph are registered with a spirometer or a pneumotachograph attached to the plethysmograph directly as volume changes. The air volume during breathing is displaced outside the plethysmograph and then back into it. The total volume of air in the plethysmograph varies.

The terms 'constant-volume' and 'constant-pressure' body plethysmographs are incorrect because in both types of plethysmograph volume as well as pressure of air inside varies during the breathing of the subject. Neither of the above-mentioned plethysmographs is ideal.

Principles of R_{aw} Measurement

From the simultaneous recordings of the airflow ($\Delta \dot{V}$) and the driving alveolar pressure ($\Delta Palv$) changes during quiet breathing or 'panting' R_{aw} can be computed. The airflow rate during inspiration and expiration has been measured at the mouth with a pneumotachograph. The principle of $\Delta Palv$ determination at tidal breathing is similar to that of TGV measurement. It is based on the Boyle-Mariotte law on gas in a closed space such as gas in the lungs compressed in expiration and decompressed in inspiration, due to airway resistance. This variation of the lung volume is proportional to the alveolar pressure under isothermic conditions in the lung and is expressed as pressure and volume variations in a body plethysmograph. In a constant-volume plethysmograph the pressure changes, and in a volume-displacement plethysmograph the volume changes are measured. The actual $\Delta Palv$ value depends on TGV, which is exposed to compression and decompression during tidal breathing, as well as on the barometric pressure minus water vapor pressure in the lungs ($P_B - P_{H_2O}$).

The equation for TGV calculation provides the basis for ΔPalv calculation:

$$TGV = \frac{\Delta V}{\Delta Palv} \cdot (P_B - P_{H_2O}).$$

From it the ΔPalv calculation can be derived:

$$\Delta Palv = \frac{\Delta V \cdot (P_B - P_{H_2O})}{TGV}.$$

If ΔPalv is substituted into the equation for the airway resistance calculation, i.e.

$$R_{aw} = \frac{\Delta Palv}{\Delta \dot{V}},$$

then:

$$R_{aw} = \frac{\dfrac{\Delta V \cdot (P_B - P_{H_2O})}{TGV}}{\dfrac{\Delta \dot{V}}{1}}.$$

From it by substituting and rearrangement it follows that:

$$R_{aw} = \frac{\Delta V}{\Delta \dot{V}} \cdot \frac{\Delta Palv}{\Delta V} = \frac{\Delta Palv}{\Delta \dot{V}}.$$

In practice the R_{aw} calculation is required to record the relationships of airflow change on pressure or volume changes in the plethysmograph ($\Delta \dot{V}/\Delta V$), as well as the relationships of alveolar pressure change represented by the mouth pressure on volume (pressure) changes in the plethysmograph ($\Delta Palv/\Delta V$). The $\Delta Palv/\Delta V$ and $\Delta \dot{V}/\Delta V$ relationships can be registered on an X-Y recorder, the former as a straight line, the latter as a slightly S-shaped curve in a normal subject (fig. 38, 39). The slopes of both relationships are measured as angles: tg alpha for $\Delta Palv/\Delta V$ and cotg beta for $\Delta \dot{V}/\Delta V$. The calibration factors for $\Delta Palv$, ΔV, $\Delta \dot{V}$ designated as M as well as the resistance value of the pneumotachograph (Rpn) are included into the final equation for R_{aw} calculation:

$$R_{aw} = \text{tg alpha} \cdot \text{cotg beta} \cdot \text{M-Rpn}.$$

The R_{aw} value is also expressed by its reciprocal airway 'conductance' (G_{aw}), (44):

$$G_{aw} = \frac{1}{R_{aw}}.$$

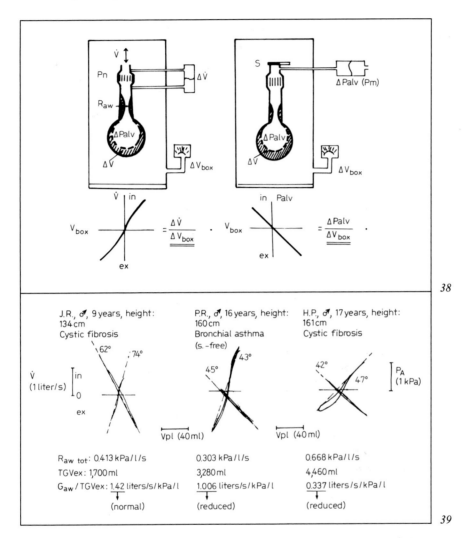

Fig. 38. Schematic illustration of the measurement of thoracic gas volume (TGV – right panel) and airway resistance (R_{aw} – left panel) in a body plethysmograph. Pn = Pneumotachograph; S = shutter. For details, see text.

Fig. 39. A series of various records for R_{aw} and TGV calculations obtained during normal quiet breathing at BTPS conditions in patients. The slopes of the curve (for R_{aw}) and straight line (for TGV) are expressed by angles. TGVex = Thoracic gas volume at resting end-expiratory level (FRC); $R_{aw\,tot}$ = airway resistance measured from the slope passing the points of maximal inspiratory and expiratory pressures of the curve expressing the relationship $\Delta\dot{V}/\Delta Vpl$; G_{aw}/TGVex = specific airway conductance; P_A = alveolar (mouth) pressure; Vpl = volume change in a body plethysmograph.

Airway conductance is also expressed per unit of lung volume, at which level it was measured as 'specific' airway conductance (sG_{aw}). Since G_{aw} is measured mostly at the FRC level obtained as TGV, sG_{aw} is a ratio G_{aw}/TGV. The value of sG_{aw} is expressed in liters/s/kPa/liter (after rearrangement in $s^{-1} \cdot kPa$). The reciprocal of sG_{aw} is 'specific' airway resistance (sR_{aw}), which is a product of R_{aw} and TGV. The dimension of sR_{aw} is kPa/l/s $\cdot$ l (after rearrangement in s $\cdot$ kPa).

In order to obtain a straight line or a slightly S-shaped curve during quiet breathing for the relationship $\Delta \dot{V}/\Delta V$ in healthy subjects as well as in some patients (fig. 39), the inspired and expired gas volume has to be at BTPS conditions. The differences in temperature and humidity of the inspired and expired gas results in volume variations of the chest reflected also by volume variations in a body plethysmograph. Warming and humidifying of the inspired gas results in an increase of gas volume in the chest and, consequently, also in an increase of volume (pressure) in a body plethysmograph while a decrease of expired cooled and less-humid gas results in a lower volume (pressure) change in the plethysmograph. Then the volume variation of the chest is due not only to compression and decompression of alveolar gas proportional to alveolar pressure but also to changes in temperature and humidity of the inspired and expired gas. The result is a loop formation of $\Delta \dot{V}/\Delta V$ (pressure–flow) diagram. The elimination of $\Delta \dot{V}/\Delta V$ looping can be achieved by 'panting' or by connecting the subject to a rebreathing bag with the gas at BTPS conditions. Electronic subtraction of volume signal proportional to temperature and humidity changes from the inspired gas volume signal is controversial for R_{aw} accuracy measurements [245, 246].

The loop formation and S-shaped pressure–flow diagrams can be observed at BTPS conditions in older children and adolescents with various lung diseases (fig. 39). The shape of the latter diagram provides valuable information not reflected by a single R_{aw} figure. The S-shaped $\Delta \dot{V}/\Delta V$ diagram during expiration or even during inspiration indicates gas compression due to airways closure during expiration or inspiration, respectively. Since R_{aw} is measured simultaneously with TGV, some principles of plethysmographic TGV measurement will be mentioned.

The principle of plethysmographic TGV determination is based on the Boyle-Mariotte law of gas stating that the product of pressure (P) and volume (V) of gas at a constant temperature (isothermic conditions) in a closed space is constant ($P \cdot V = k$). From volume and pressure changes of gas (ΔV and ΔP, respectively) in a closed space the volume of gas (V) exposed to volume and pressure variations can be calculated.

Similarly, the intrathoracic gas in a subject breathing against an occlusion (e.g. a shutter) can be estimated when the intrathoracic gas is compressed and decompressed, and the volume (ΔV) and the pressure changes in the thorax as alveolar pressure ($\Delta Palv$) are registered simultaneously.

The original equation expressing Boyle-Mariotte law can be written: $P \cdot V = (P + \Delta Palv) \cdot (V + \Delta V)$. From this equation the TGV calculation can be derived:

$$TGV = \frac{\Delta V}{\Delta Palv} \cdot (P_B - P_{H_2O}),$$

where ΔV and $\Delta Palv$ are volume and pressure changes in the thorax, and $P_B - P_{H_2O}$ is barometric pressure minus the partial water vapor pressure in the lungs. The equation is derived as follows:

$$P_B \cdot V = (P_B + \Delta Palv) \cdot (V + \Delta V),$$

$$P_B \cdot V = P_B \cdot V + \Delta Palv \cdot V + \Delta V \cdot P_B + \Delta Palv \cdot \Delta V,$$

$$\Delta Palv \cdot V = -\Delta V \cdot P_B - \Delta V \cdot \Delta Palv,$$

$$\Delta Palv \cdot V = -\Delta V \cdot (P_B + \Delta Palv).$$

Since $\Delta Palv$ in parentheses is negligible with respect to the barometric pressure (P_B), it thus follows that:

$$\Delta Palv \cdot V = -\Delta V \cdot P_B,$$

then:

$$V = -\frac{\Delta V}{\Delta Palv} \cdot P_B.$$

The negative sign is not significant. From the barometric pressure the partial water vapor pressure (P_{H_2O}) has to be substracted. The water vapor pressure is constant at gas compression and decompression in the lungs because a part of the water vapor is converted during its compression into a liquid state and vice versa. The final formula follows:

$$V \text{ or } TGV = \frac{\Delta V}{\Delta Palv} \cdot (P_B - P_{H_2O}).$$

The lung volume change (ΔV) can be measured as thoracic volume change in a body plethysmograph during occluded breaths. The alveolar pressure change ($\Delta Palv$) during occlusion is measured as a mouth pressure. It is assumed that the pressure in the occluded airways from the alveoli up to an occlusion is the same. Some recent studies [153, 154, 165] have shown a plethysmographic overestimation of TGV in the presence of high airway resistance because alveolar pressure is not reflected properly by mouth pressure during airways occlusion. A phase shift between the thoracic volume change and the alveolar (as a mouth) pressure change results in a loop formation of the ΔV/ΔPalv diagram (fig. 40). The slope of the ΔV/ΔPalv diagram is usually straight. The final calculation requires to be included also the calibration factors (cal.fc.) for volume and pressure changes displayed on an X-Y recorder as well as the volume occupied by the subject in the case of a constant-volume plethysmograph. The modified equation for the TGV calculation is as follows:

$$TGV = \frac{\Delta V}{\Delta Palv} \cdot \frac{\text{calibration factor for V}}{\text{calibration factor for P}} \cdot M \cdot (P_B - P_{H_2O}).$$

M is a correction factor for the volume occupied by the subject's body in a plethysmograph and is calculated from the following formula:

$$M = \frac{Vpl - Vs}{Vpl},$$

Vs is obtained as a product of a subject's body weight and 0.91. Vpl is the volume of a plethysmograph. The slope $\frac{\Delta V}{\Delta Palv}$ is measured as an angle: cotg α. The final formula for TGV calculation:

$$TGV = \text{cotg } \alpha \cdot \frac{\text{cal.fc.V}}{\text{cal.fc.P}} \cdot \frac{Vpl - Vs}{Vpl} \cdot (P_B - P_{H_2O}) - V_D.$$

V_D is a volume of added space by the mouthpiece of the pneumotachograph between the mouth and the shutter.

Method

R_{aw} was measured simultaneously with TGV in children over 5 years of age sitting closed in a body plethysmograph, which was of the same type as for adults. The whole procedure was explained to the child before it entered the plethysmograph. The children were instructed to breath normally and exceptionally to pant for the $\Delta \dot{V}/\Delta V$ diagram at first and then against a closed shutter for the ΔV/ΔPalv diagram. They were told not to blow and to support their cheeks and mouth floor against a closed shutter in order to avoid a looping in the ΔV/ΔPalv diagram, and further, to keep their lips tight around the mouthpiece and not open their mouth against an occluded shutter. A noseclip was also given to the child.

The actual R_{aw} and TGV measurements started usually 2–4 min after the child entered the plethysmograph when a stable temperature was achieved inside. This was indicated by the stable pressure or volume in the body plethysmograph. The stability of the pressure inside the plethysmograph due to heating of air by the subject or to pressure fluctuations of the environment was achieved by the measurement of the pressure in a

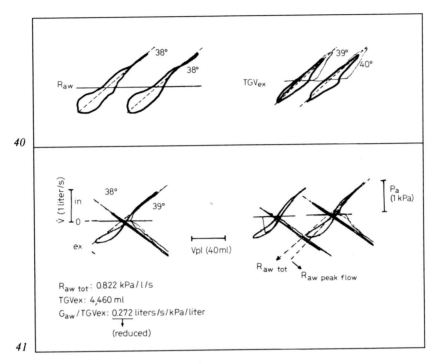

Fig. 40. R_{aw} and TGV recordings in a 16-year-old asthmatic boy, height 163 cm, with a severe airway obstruction (G_{aw}/TGV: 0.098 liters/s/kPa/liter). The records for TGV calculations have a shape of loops in spite of breathing at BTPS conditions.

Fig. 41. A series of R_{aw} and TGV records in an 18-year-old female patient with clinical symptoms of bronchial asthma. The expiratory loops of R_{aw} records result in a calculation of total airway resistance ($R_{aw\ tot}$) or airway resistance at peak flow ($R_{aw\ peak\ flow}$), if the slope of the R_{aw} record was drawn through the points of maximal inspiratory and expiratory pressures or peak flows, respectively. For abbreviations, see figure 39.

plethysmograph with reference to a compensation vessel fitted inside (Siregnost FD 91, Siemens) or outside the plethysmograph (Bodytest, Jaeger).

Communication with the child was via an intercom. The shutter was controlled electrically from the outside. If the temperature was not stable in the plethysmograph and the pressure or volume inside was increasing, the plethysmograph was repeatedly vented to the atmosphere. Then the child with a noseclip took a mouthpiece attached to an assembly with pneumotachograph, shutter, plastic bag with air at BTPS conditions. Mouth pressure was measured via a lateral tap as well as pressure difference in the pneumotachograph by differential pressure transducers.

After several breaths, each of the $\Delta\dot{V}/\Delta V$ diagrams was followed by the $\Delta V/\Delta P$alv diagram of both tracings. At least five technically good diagrams of both types were

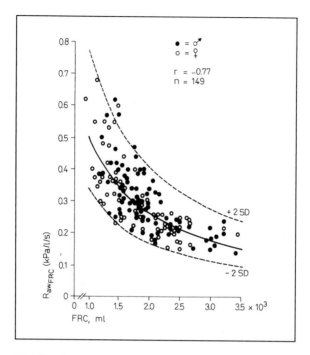

Fig. 42. Airway resistance measured at the level of functional residual capacity ($R_{aw\,FRC}$) in relation to FRC in healthy boys and girls. For further explanations, see figure 2.

obtained in a child. The slopes of both types of diagrams were expressed by angles and for the final R_{aw} and TGV calculations the mean value of 5 reproducible angles was used. Thus, an error due to intraindividual variability of angles was lower than 10%.

In order to know the volume level at which TGV measurements were made, tidal volume was recorded simultaneously besides the system which automatically activated the shutter to occlude the mouth at the end-expiratory or inspiratory resting levels. The selection of angles for TGV measurement was easy because the slopes of the $\Delta V/\Delta Palv$ diagrams were mostly straight except in patients with high R_{aw} (fig. 40). However, the selection of angles for R_{aw} measurement was more difficult because the $\Delta\dot{V}/\Delta V$ diagrams were not only straight but also S-shaped or contained loops (fig. 40, 41). The line drawn through the points of peak inspiratory and expiratory pressures gave resistance refered to as 'total airway resistance' ($R_{aw\,tot}$). The line drawn through the points of peak inspiratory and expiratory flows gave $R_{aw\,peak}$ (fig. 41). The measurement of R_{aw} within the range of 0 to 0.5 liters/s of inspiratory and expiratory flows [44, 45] was quite satisfactory in the subjects in whom the $\Delta\dot{V}/\Delta V$ diagrams were almost straight. In patients with obstructive lung diseases the latter approach resulted in an underestimation of R_{aw} by omitting the abnormalities in the pressure–flow relationship.

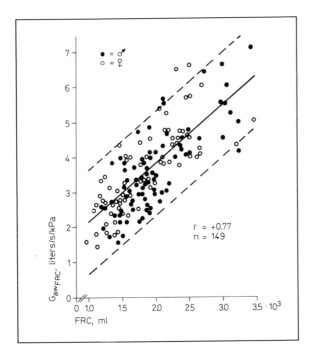

Fig. 43. Airway conductance at the level of functional residual capacity ($G_{aw\,FRC}$) in relation to FRC in healthy boys and girls. For further explanations, see figure 2.

We measured R_{aw} in our subjects during normal breathing, i.e. at the FRC level, as 'total airway resistance' ($R_{aw_{FRC}}$), (fig. 41). R_{aw} and its reversal value G_{aw} at the FRC level were related to body height, age, body surface and to FRC measured as TGV at the end-expiratory resting level (FRC_{box}).

Results and Discussion

In the studied 149 older children and adolescents 6–17 years old, $R_{aw_{FRC}}$ decreased nonlinearly with increasing FRC_{box} values (fig. 42; table 234) and its reciprocal $G_{aw_{FRC}}$ increased linearly with increasing FRC_{box} (fig. 43; table 235). The R_{aw} value decreased with body height, age and body surface (table 236–238), and, conversely, $G_{aw_{FRC}}$ increased in relation to body height, age and body surface (table 239–241). The dependence of $R_{aw_{FRC}}$ and $G_{aw_{FRC}}$ on body height, age and body surface was nonlinear. The latter relationships were best expressed after the logarithmic transformation of both independent and dependent variables as power regression equations. 'Specific' airway conductance (G_{aw}/TGV) was independent of body height, age and body surface in our studied children and adolescents (fig. 44) with an average value amounting to 1.97 ± 0.45 liters/s/kPa/liter. The average value of the G_{awFRC}/TLC$_{box}$ ratio amounted to 0.962 ± 0.198 liters/s/kPa/liter also being independent of body height, age and body surface [223, 226, 236]. Similar values for 'specific' airway conductance have been reported by Baran and Englert [6], i.e. 1.978 ± 0.632, Michaelson et al. [120], i.e. 1.999 ± 0.530, and Weng and Levison [194], i.e. 2.029 ± 0.479 liters/s/kPa/liter for healthy older children and adolescents. No differences for R_{aw}, G_{aw} and sG_{aw} were found between boys and girls.

Since the R_{aw} (or G_{aw}) value has been considered as an index reflecting the patency of larger central airways [105], the increase of G_{aw} (or the decrease of R_{aw}) with growth (body height) suggests an increase in anatomical dimensions of the larger airways with growth. The independence of 'specific' airway conductance on body height, age and body surface suggests that the larger airways grow in proportion to lung alveoli in healthy older children and adolescents. Numerous data on R_{aw}, G_{aw} and TGV have been reported [21, 22, 38, 46, 65, 138, 152, 192].

Body height, age or body surface related R_{aw} (or G_{aw}) reference values cannot, however, be considered appropriate for the assessment of airways obstruction in children and adolescents with lung disease. This is because neither R_{aw} nor G_{aw} alone show at which lung volume level the R_{aw} (or G_{aw}) were measured, and they are both significantly dependent on TGV (fig. 42, 43). The G_{aw} value of 2 liters/s/kPa is normal, for example, for TGV (FRC$_{box}$) = 1 liter, being evidently pathological for TGV = 3 liters (fig. 43). Therefore, R_{aw} or G_{aw} cannot provide adequate information in patients with lung diseases, if the TGV value at the level of which R_{aw} or G_{aw} were measured is not taken into account and R_{aw} or TGV were only compared on the basis of body height, age or body surface with reference values. In patients (e.g. cystic fibrosis, br. asthma, lung fibrosis), lung volumes, i.e. TGV, TLC, are not proportional to body height, age or body surface as in healthy subjects. Only 'specific' G_{aw} or R_{aw} values after being related to body height, age or body surface can be used for the appropriate evaluation of airway patency in patients with lung diseases by this method. The linear relationship of G_{aw} on lung volume is more convenient for the assessment of airways function than the nonlinear R_{aw} relationship on lung volume. With respect to the linear dependence of G_{aw} on FRC$_{box}$, the

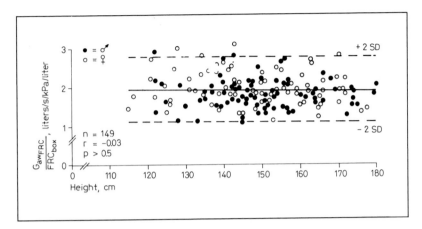

Fig. 44. 'Specific' airway conductance determined at the level of FRC $\left(\frac{G_{aw\,FRC}}{FRC_{box}}\right)$ in relation to body height in healthy boys and girls. For further explanations, see figure 2.

'specific' G_{aw} was not dependent on body height, age or body surface in our healthy older children and adolescents.

The evaluation of airway patency in patients on the basis of G_{aw} value was performed so that the G_{aw} value in a studied subject was compared first with regard to the respective FRC_{box} at the level at which the G_{aw} was measured (fig. 43). Further, the G_{aw} value was converted to 'specific' G_{aw} and then compared with the reference (predicted) value representing only a single number 1.97 ± 0.45 liters/s/kPa/liter. G_{aw} values differing by more than 2 SD from the mean reference value were considered as pathological. A disadvantage of the 'specific' G_{aw} (sR_{aw}) is that a single number can be the same at different slopes expressing the G_{aw}/TGV relationship. 'Specific' G_{aw} remains, however, uninfluenced by an overestimation of TGV in patients with high airway resistance because R_{aw} is underestimated [165]. A simplified method of sR_{aw} measurement has been published [242].

Lung (Pulmonary) Resistance

This measurement provides similar information as airway resistance differing from the latter by addition of lung tissue resistance. Lung resistance (R_L) represents the ratio of the transpulmonary pressure change

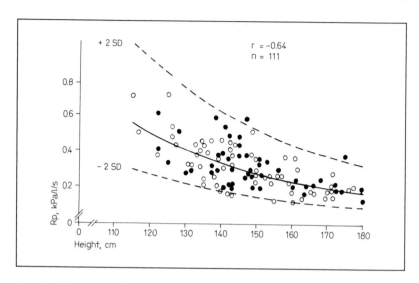

Fig. 45. Pulmonary resistance (Rp) in relation to body height in healthy boys and girls. For further explanations, see figure 2.

(ΔP_{tp}) (a difference between pleural and mouth pressures, $\Delta Ppl - Pao$) to the change in airflow during tidal breathing ($\Delta\dot{V}$). Lung resistance was measured from simultaneous records of transpulmonary pressure and inspiratory-expiratory airflow rate at the mouth during quiet breathing at an isovolume level, i.e. between mid-inspiration and mid-expiration (fig. 9). Transpulmonary pressure was measured as the difference between pressure in the esophageal balloon and mouth pressure. Details on transpulmonary pressure measurements are given in the section dealing with LE. The rate of airflow at the mouth was measured with a heated pneumotachograph (Fleisch No. 2), and the lung volume was obtained by the integration of airflow at the mouth. Pulmonary resistance was measured simultaneously with dynamic lung compliance. The final pulmonary resistance value was calculated as an average value from 10 breathing cycles.

Results and Discussion

The R_L value decreased nonlinearly with increasing body height, age and body surface, similar to the R_{awFRC} value (fig. 45; table 242–244) in the healthy 131 older children and adolescents studied.

Assessment of airway patency by R_L involves the same problems as those related to airway resistance (pp. 62–63). R_L comparison in children on the basis of body height, age or body surface is therefore not correct. Especially in pathological conditions of the lungs, R_L may be measured at different lung volume levels. The evaluation of airways obstruction by R_L related to body height might be misleading. R_L alone, without TGV, is therefore of little value for the evaluation of airway patency.

Determination of the tissue component of pulmonary resistance (R_{ti}) is also of little practical significance. In order to measure lung tissue resistance as a difference between R_L and R_{aw}, it is necessary to measure both R_L and R_{aw} at the same lung volume level and from the same breathing cycle. In our children and adolescents, R_{ti} determined during quiet breathing varied on average between 10.8% (in a child 115 cm tall) and 12.2% (a subject 180 cm tall) of the R_L value. R_{ti} was determined as the difference between R_L and $R_{aw_{in-ex}}$, i.e. R_{aw} measured at mid-tidal volume level (table 245), and expressed as a percentage of R_L. The latter values are lower than those reported by Bachofen [5] giving R_{ti} in the range of from 21 to 34% of R_L in healthy children.

Conclusions

In a body plethysmograph 'airway resistance' ($R_{aw_{FRC}}$), its reciprocal 'airway conductance' ($G_{aw_{FRC}}$), 'specific airway conductance' (sG_{aw}, G_{aw}/TGV) were measured as indices of airway patency in 149 older healthy children and adolescents 6–17 years old during normal breathing. sG_{aw} contains information also on the lung volume at the level at which the airway resistance was measured, which is not the case for 'lung resistance'. Adult types of body plethysmograph were also used for R_{aw}, G_{aw}, sG_{aw} and TGV measurements in children over 5 years of age. R_{aw} at the FRC level decreased while G_{aw} at the FRC level increased with growth (body height, age and body surface), nonlinearly. R_{aw} at the FRC level decreased with an increase of lung volume (FRC), nonlinearly, while G_{aw} at the FRC level increased linearly with an increase of lung volume (FRC). The value of sG_{aw} was independent of height, age and body surface and is suitable for the mutual comparison of R_{aw} or G_{aw} in the studied age range of children and adolescents with different lung size also taking into account the lung volume at which R_{aw} or G_{aw} were measured. The R_{aw} or G_{aw} values unrelated to TGV and only related to height, age or body surface, are not sufficient for assessing airway patency and, consequently, not for comparison of airways obstruction, especially in patients. 'Total airway resistance' calculated from the slope drawn through peak inspiratory and expiratory pressures of the pressure-flow diagram expressed the R_{awFRC} abnormality most adequately.

'Lung (pulmonary) resistance' (R_L) measured in 111 healthy older children and adolescents 6–17 years old decreased also with height, age and body surface. However, the interpretation of R_L for the evaluation of airway patency without knowing the lung volume at which it was measured is difficult and provides similar information as R_{awFRC} related to body height, age and body surface. Lung tissue resistance (R_{ti}) varied on average from 10.8 to 12.2% of lung resistance.

Multiple-Breath Nitrogen Lung Washout Curve

Besides the above-described airway patency indices the multiple-breath lung nitrogen washout curve was also used for this purpose. The tested child breathing oxygen eliminated nitrogen from the lungs. Nitrogen concentration in each expiration was registered continuously with a sensitive nitrogen analyzer (Nitrogen-Analyzer 700, Electro/Med, Houston, Tex.). Simultaneously, lung volume was measured after electronic integration of the airflow at the mouth sensed pneumotachographically (Fleisch No. 2). Both signals were registered on a direct writing recorder (Mingograph-34, Elema Schönander). After attaining a 2% nitrogen concentration in the expired gas, the child performed a forced expiration maneuver for assessing nitrogen residua.

The breathing circuit with a two-way stopcock allowed to breath from its inspiratory branch alternatively air or oxygen from the bag. At the beginning, the studied child was breathing for 1–2 min atmospheric air for an adaptation to the apparatus. Between the mouthpiece and the valve dividing the circuit into inspiratory and expiratory branches, a pneumotachograph for volume registration was included. Into the expiratory branch of the circuit the analyzing chamber of nitrogen analyzer was included. After a period of adaption to the apparatus the child was connected during expiration to the bag with oxygen and the registration of lung nitrogen elimination was started.

Abnormalities of the multiple lung nitrogen washout curve were evaluated according to: (1) time necessary for nitrogen elimination to 2% concentration in the expired gas; (2) oxygen volume required to achieve 2% nitrogen concentration in the expired gas; (3) Becklake index (amount of oxygen necessary for reaching 2% nitrogen concentration in the expired gas per 1 liter of functional residual capacity); and (4) residual nitrogen concentration following forced expiration maneuver when 2% nitrogen concentration in the expired gas was attained.

Results and Discussion

In 86 children and adolescents in the age of 6–17 years and body height 114–182 cm, the above-mentioned four indices characterizing the multiple lung nitrogen washout curve were determined. The results are presented in tables 246–248 demonstrating the dependence of the given parameters on the body height. The time and oxygen volume required for achieving a 2% nitrogen concentration in the expired gas increased with body height. The Becklake index decreased with body height and no residua were found in healthy children and adolescents after reaching 2% nitrogen concentration in the expired gas. Since the time and the amount of oxygen required for reaching 2% nitrogen concentration in the expired gas depend on lung size, the parameters of multiple lung nitrogen washout curve taking into account lung size, as, for example, the Becklake index, ought to be preferred. The course of lung nitrogen elimination depends not only on the airway patency, but also on the elastic properties of the lungs [135]. Hence, this method is less specific for airways obstruction evaluation providing information on a global gas distribution in the lungs. The results obtained are similar to those already published [55, 69, 146, 147, 196, 244].

Conclusions

From the indirect airway patency indices the multiple nitrogen lung washout curve in 86 children and adolescents (6–17 years and 114–182 cm tall) was studied on the basis of four parameters. The latter were related to the body height of the subjects and a linear relation between parameters and body height was obtained.

IV. Work of Breathing

Lung ventilation requires a rhythmical activity of the respiratory muscles. At this activity, a 'work of breathing' is performed. In a patient with a respiratory disease, the respiratory muscles may increase the work of breathing and spend more energy of a patient. The measurement of the work of breathing thus provides useful information on the patient's status. The work which respiratory muscles must exert during breathing, i.e. during lung ventilation, is spent *for overcoming elastic recoil pressure of the lungs and thorax, as well as their dynamic resistances.* The dynamic resistances comprise airway resistance, and, further, the frictional and inertial resistances of the lung tissue and thorax.

The work of breathing has been determined: (1) as the amount of energy required for respiratory muscles activity measured as oxygen consumption, and (2) as the mechanical work performed by the respiratory muscles. If both measurements are carried out simultaneously, the relation of mechanical work to the amount of energy supplied to the respiratory muscles gives *the mechanical efficiency of the respiratory muscles,* i.e. the supplied energy as a mechanical work to the respiratory muscles. For adults it varies from 2 to 25%. Oxygen consumption at rest and at increased ventilation as an excess of oxygen consumption during increased ventilation can be attributed to the metabolic activity of the respiratory muscles [19]. The work of breathing is measured most commonly as mechanical. In physics, the work results from an activity, at which the body is moved by a force along a certain pathway in the direction of the force. The work is defined as a product of force and pathway. During breathing the activity of the respiratory muscles causes a movement of air in the lungs and thus exerts a work. The pressure causing a volume change represents the force and the volume change is an equivalent to the pathway. Calculation of the work breathing (W) of the lungs or the whole respiratory system requires to be determined simultaneously a pressure change causing a volume change of the lungs or the whole respiratory system, i.e. of the lungs and the thorax together. The value of the mechanical work of breathing can be calculated by multiplying the volume (V) and the pressure (P) registered during the breathing cycles (W = P·V). Graphical expression of the mechanical work of breathing is an area delineating the volume and pressure relationship during the breathing cycle. The unit of the work of breathing is joule (J) per 1 liter ventilation or per minute, previously kilopondmeter or gramcentimeter (kpm or gcm). *The work of breathing for lung ventilation can be divided into the work exerted during the movement of the whole respiratory system and the work required for the lungs only.*

Measurement of the work of breathing of the whole respiratory system requires complete relaxation of the subject's respiratory muscles and ventilation with a respirator. The difference between the mouth pressure of the subject and the pressure in the respirator represents the force acting on his respiratory system and the corresponding tidal volume in this passive breathing represents the pathway. *Most commonly the mechanical work of breathing done on the lungs only is measured.* However, this function test is not yet as current as the other lung function tests. The work of breathing of the lungs was usually determined from a pressure-volume loop expressing the relationship of transpulmonary pressure and corresponding tidal volume during a normal breathing cycle.

Within the range of the loop a linear relation of the latter two variables is assumed. The area of the loop represents the part of the work of breathing on the lungs which is required for overcoming dynamic lung resistance (fig. 46). *The dynamic (viscous) work of breathing* is performed during inspiration and expiration (W_{dyn}). The pressure-volume loop also provides a possibility for measuring the *elastic work of breathing* (W_{el}), i.e. the work of the respiratory muscles for overcoming the elastic recoil pressure of the lungs during inspiration. Elastic work of breathing is usually represented by an area of a triangle with perpendiculars erected at the inversion points of tidal volume, i.e. at the end of inspiration and expiration (fig. 46). The sum of the areas corresponding to the elastic and dynamic inspiratory work of the lungs gives *total work of breathing* performed by the respiratory muscles on the lungs during inspiration. The potential elastic energy accumulated at the end of inspiration in the lungs is then a driving force for expiration.

However, correct measurement of the elastic work of breathing also requires a static pressure-volume curve of the thorax in relation to the static pressure-volume curve of the lungs to be registered (Campbell diagram) (fig. 47) [19]. The static pressure-volume curves of the lungs and

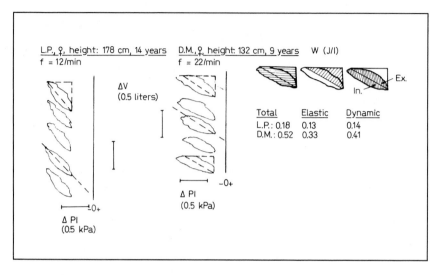

Fig. 46. Pressure-volume loops of the lungs at spontaneous tidal breathing in taller and smaller healthy children illustrating the measurement of total, elastic, and dynamic work of breathing on the lungs by means of a triangle drawn into the loop. The work of breathing and its components are greater in a smaller child. See text for further explanations. Pl = transpulmonary pressure; In = inspirium; Ex = expirium.

thorax have an opposite course crossing themselves at the end-expiratory resting level (functional residual capacity level). The different courses of both curves suggest that the lungs tend to collapse, whereas the thorax tends to expand and occupy a resting level, as, for example, at the pneumothorax, where the pressure difference between the inner and external parts of the lungs in the thorax is zero. Normally, at the FRC level the elastic forces of the lungs and the thorax are balanced and the respiratory muscles are therefore relaxed. As soon as the lung volume increases the elastic recoil pressure of the lungs increases too and the elastic recoil pressure of the thorax decreases. During inspiration the respiratory muscles have to overcome dynamic (nonelastic) pressure as well as elastic recoil pressure of the lungs. A part of the work during inspiration is nevertheless performed by the thorax elasticity alone, as the thorax tends to expand due to its potential energy. The elastic work of breathing during inspiration equals the area bounded by the pressure-volume curves of the lungs and thorax (horizontally hatched area in fig. 47). If the elastic work of breathing

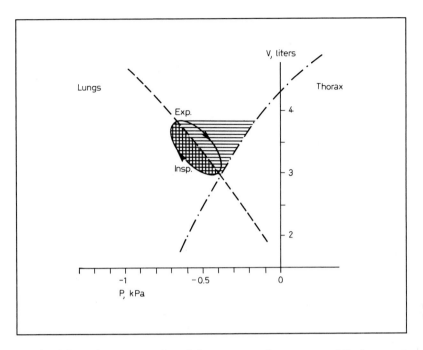

Fig. 47. Schematic representation of the pressure-volume curves of the lungs and thorax (chest wall) and their mutual courses. The curves cross each other at functional residual capacity (end-expiratory resting) level. The horizontally hatched area represents the work of breathing for overcoming the elastic component of the work of breathing on the lungs during quiet inspiration. The horizontally and vertically hatched area corresponds to the work of breathing for overcoming the dynamic (viscous, nonelastic) component of the work of breathing on lungs during quiet inspiration. Further, see text.

is determined from the already-mentioned triangle (fig. 48 – horizontally hatched area), a lesser elastic work of breathing is determined than in reality, because a perpendicular, straight-line-like course of the pressure-volume curve of the thorax is assumed. Consequently, the total work of breathing is also underestimated. Hence, determination of the total and inspiratory work of breathing is correct only providing that the static pressure-volume curve of the thorax was determined [84]. It can be obtained, even in some children, using the relaxation technique for example (fig. 49). In children, determination of the elastic work of breathing, and thus of the total work of breathing, is further complicated by the fact that the slopes of the pressure-volume loop and of the pressure-volume curve of the lungs

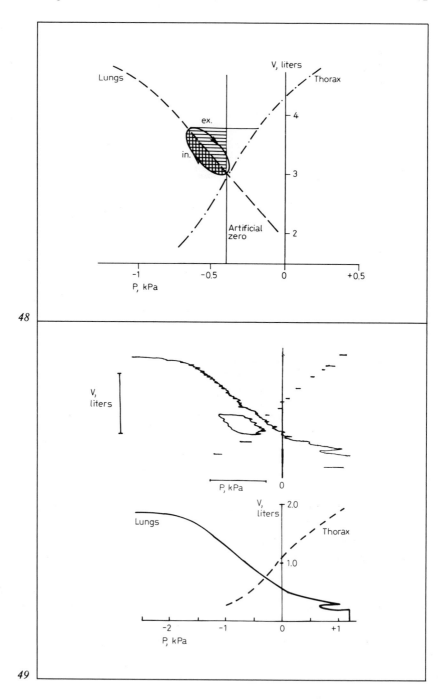

differ at the same volume level. Static and dynamic compliances also differ and the difference is greater the smaller the child.

In this context also the problem of the work of breathing during 'active' expiration has to be clarified. This is considered as part of the viscous work of breathing determined by the area exceeding the vertical zero line in a triangle drawn into the pressure-volume loop. In the method of determining the work of breathing by means of a triangle used so far, the 'active' work of breathing can be seen in obstructive pulmonary diseases (fig. 50); in patients with restrictive lung diseases it practically does not appear (fig. 51). However, according to the Campbell diagram the 'active' work of breathing is represented by the area exceeding the static expiratory pressure-volume curve of the thorax and not only the zero pressure line of the pressure-volume loop (fig. 47, 48). It follows that only a part of the mechanical work on lungs can be determined reliably, i.e. the viscous work of breathing delineated by the area of the transpulmonary pressure-volume loop.

Method

Evaluation of the work of breathing was based on the loops relating transpulmonary pressure and lung volume, and obtained during normal breathing (fig. 46). Transpulmonary pressure was measured as the difference between the pressure in the esophageal balloon and mouth pressure. Lung volume was determined by integration of airflow at the mouth. Details on the method are given in the chapter on 'Lung elasticity'. Transpulmonary pressure was registered on the ordinate simultaneously with tidal volume on the abscissa of an X-Y recorder during quiet breathing. The areas corresponding to the dif-

---

Fig. 48. Schematic representation of the pressure-volume curves of the lungs and thorax (chest wall) with a triangle drawn into the pressure-volume loop of the lungs by constructing a perpendicular at the point of artificial zero. The elastic work of breathing represented by a triangle (horizontally hatched area) is smaller by one-half than as shown in figure 47, further see text and figure 47.

Fig. 49. Pressure-volume curve of the thorax (chest wall) obtained by a relaxation method and of the lungs in a 10-year-old boy, 132 cm tall, with asymptomatic bronchial asthma. The pressure-volume curve of the thorax shows a symmetrical course with that of the lungs but in an opposite direction, and they cross each other roughly at the FRC level, i.e. in the range of the pressure-volume loop. P = pressure; V = volume; further, see text. The curves in the upper part of the figure are original, in the lower part of the figure the same curves are redrawn.

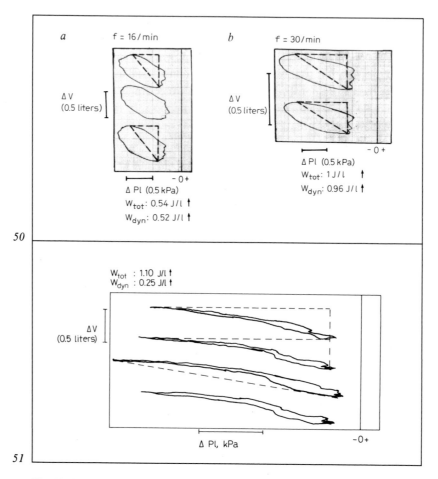

Fig. 50. Pressure-volume loops of the lungs at spontaneous breathing in 2 patients with cystic fibrosis. *a* Twenty-one-year-old patient, height 181 cm. *b* Seven-year-old patient, height 107 cm. The loops are wide. Dynamic work of breathing (i.e. area of the loop) (W_{dyn}) and total work of breathing (W_{tot}) on lungs are increased. f = breathing frequency per minute; ΔPl = a change of transpulmonary pressure; ΔV = a change of lung volume at spontaneous quiet breathing. 'Active' expiratory work of breathing is considered to be a part of the loop area exceeding the vertical arm of the triangle.

Fig. 51. Pressure-volume loops of the lungs at spontaneously breathing in a 17-year-old female patient with idiopathic pulmonary fibrosis (verified by lung biopsy). The loops are narrow sickle-shaped and long. Dynamic work of breathing (i.e. area of the loop) is normal. The hypothenuse of the triangle drawn into the loop is outside of the loop, which makes the measurement of the elastic work problematic. Inspiratory branch of P-V loop might substitute the hypotenuse for calculation of the total work of breathing. For abbreviations, see figure 50.

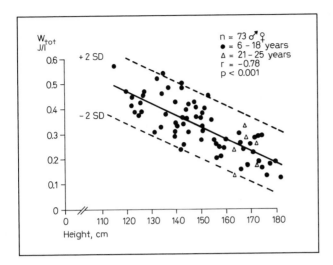

Fig. 52. Total work of breathing on the lungs (W$_{tot}$) in joules per 1 liter of ventilation in relation to body height in healthy boys and girls. Full line represents the mean value, interrupted lines represent the limits for 95% values of the group (± 2 SD from the mean). n = number of subjects; r = correlation coefficient; p = statistical significance of r.

ferent components of the work of breathing of the lungs were determined planimetrically as an average of at least five loops in each subject. The work of breathing and its components were expressed in joules, i.e. J/per 1 liter of ventilation and J/min. The calculation of the work of breathing by planimetry consisted of the following steps. The obtained areas were converted to cm^2 after dividing the numbers measured planimetrically by the calibration factor. The number of cm^2 was converted to gcm and 1 cm^2 equaled 625 gcm. The latter number was computed: $W = P \cdot V$, i.e. $\frac{g}{cm^2} \cdot cm^3 = gcm$; the calibration factors for ΔV 1 cm on paper was 250 ml and for ΔP 1 cm on paper was 2.5 cm H$_2$O. Hence, 1 cm^2 represented the work (W): $250 \times 2.5 = 625$ gcm. Since in the SI system the unit for work is joule (J), 1 gcm $= 9.8066 \times 10^{-5}$ J, or 1 kpm $\cong$ 10 J; therefore, 1 cm^2 on paper equalled 0.0613 J.

Results

The individual values of the work of breathing were related to body height and age. Total work of breathing, as well as its components in J/l, decreased with increasing body height and age (fig. 52–54; table 249–258) (p < 0.001). Work of breathing in J/min related to body height showed a similar dependence, though to a lesser degree (table 259–264) (p < 0.005).

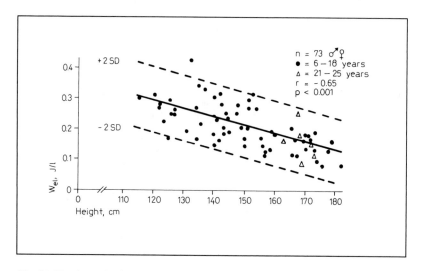

Fig. 53. Elastic work of breathing on the lungs (W_{el}) in joules per 1 liter of ventilation in relation to body height in healthy boys and girls. For further explanations, see figure 52.

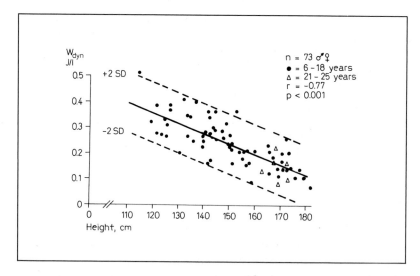

Fig. 54. Dynamic work of breathing on the lungs (W_{dyn}) in joules per 1 liter of ventilation, in relation to body height in healthy boys and girls. For further explanations, see figure 52.

The work of breathing and its components also decreased with advancing age ($p < 0.05 - < 0.001$). The percentage of inspiratory dynamic work of breathing from the total work of breathing decreased with increasing body height, similar to the percentage of the dynamic work of breathing (table 265). The average values of the work of breathing and its components in patients with some respiratory diseases are given in table 266.

Discussion

The values of total mechanical work done on the lungs during quiet breathing in our healthy children, adolescents and young adults are close to those reported in the literature which vary from 0.3 to 0.5 J/l of ventilation [19, 84, 136]. A negative dependence of mechanical work of breathing and its components on height and age implies that a smaller child has to perform for the equal ventilation and per the same unit of time a greater work of breathing than a taller child, adolescent or young adult during quiet breathing. Higher viscous (dynamic) work of breathing in smaller children and its decline during growth show a similar pattern as pulmonary or airway resistance. The viscous work of breathing includes, besides the work exerted on overcoming airway resistance, also the work exerted for overcoming the resistance of lung tissue, which results from the formula: $R_{ti} = R_L - R_{aw}$. Thus, the viscous work of breathing of lung tissue amounts to roughly 11–12% of the viscous (dynamic) work of breathing (see pulmonary resistance). Besides that, the viscous work of breathing includes the work required for overcoming the inertial resistance of the airways and lung tissue ($I_P = I_{aw} + I_{ti}$), which is, however, during quiet breathing, negligible [117]. Higher viscous work of breathing in smaller children results from the narrower anatomical dimensions of the airways. Since pulmonary and airway resistances express the patency of the larger airways [105], W_{dyn} also represents the work exerted on overcoming frictional resistance in this part of the airways. Higher W_{dyn} values per 1 liter of ventilation in smaller children are therefore disadvantageous for them as far as energy requirement is concerned and may have an unfavorable effect, especially on the course of obstructive respiratory diseases.

In this context, it is also important to mention that airway resistance measured at the FRC level during quiet breathing and expressed as 'conductance' per liter of minute ventilation is smaller in a smaller child (for 115 cm: 0.29 liter/s/kPa/liter/min) than in a taller child or an adolescent (for 180 cm: 0.45 liter/s/kPa/liter/min). Airway conductance, as a main component of W_{dyn}, expressed in relation to lung volume (TLC, FRC) as 'specific airway conductance' is nevertheless the same in both smaller and taller children (see chapt. III). In other words, airway patency determined during tidal breathing with respect to lung size is the same in both smaller and taller children. However, airway patency is different with respect to lung ventilation and disadvantageous for smaller children, which is documented also by the higher values of the viscous work of breathing in them (fig. 54).

A decrease in the elastic work of breathing with increasing body height and age as well as a decrease of the total work of breathing is also disadvantageous for the smaller child. However, measurement of the elastic work of breathing contains several difficulties. The first one is that in our group the elastic work of breathing was determined from a triangle, drawn into the pressure-volume loop. By this approach the pressure-volume curve of the thorax, which together with the pressure-volume curve of the lungs delineates the area corresponding to the elastic work of breathing (fig. 47), was not taken into account. The elastic work of breathing measured from a triangle drawn into the pressure-volume loop was thus underestimated. Another problem in the elastic work of breathing measurement was the fact that in our group of healthy subjects dynamic and static lung compliances differed (see chapt. II). The difference was greater the smaller the child, which the Campbell diagram did not assume. Nevertheless, from our data on the elastic work of breathing (W_{el}), the latter work (W_{el}) can be determined with respect to the Campbell diagram providing that, within the range of the tidal volume, the pressure-volume curve of the thorax has a symmetrical course with the pressure-volume curve of the lungs in an opposite direction (fig. 49). The real elastic work of breathing can then equal doublefold the elastic work of breathing determined by means of a triangle minus the work corresponding to a doubled area difference between the static and dynamic lung compliances. A solution of the situation is depicted in figure 55. The pressure-volume curves of the thorax in our healthy subjects as well as in the patients with respiratory diseases (mucoviscidosis, bronchial asthma) demonstrate (fig. 49) that the pressure-volume curve of the thorax really has a symmetrical course in the opposite direction as the pressure-volume curve of the lungs within the range of tidal volume, and static compliance of the thorax within tidal volume range is the same as static compliance of the lungs. Only the slopes of middle parts of the pressure-volume curve of the lungs and the pressure-

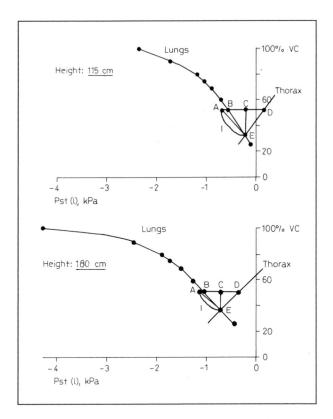

Fig. 55. Schematic illustration of the pressure-volume curve of the lungs and a part of the pressure-volume curve of the thorax including the relative range of tidal volume in healthy subjects 115 and 180 cm tall, respectively. The schema elucidates the calculation of the real elastic work of breathing from the elastic work of breathing obtained by means of a triangle drawn into the pressure-volume (P-V) loop of the lungs. The ACE area represents the actually measured elastic work of breathing as an area of the triangle drawn into the P-V loop. By subtracting the ABE area from the ABCDE area, the real elastic work of breathing bounded by the BCDE area, is obtained. The ABE area represents the amount of the elastic work of breathing given by the difference between the static and dynamic lung compliances. Further, see text.

volume curves of the thorax expressed by the Cst value are decisive in the inspiratory elastic work of breathing assessment. Dynamic lung compliance, does not express the actual elastic properties of the lungs, especially in smaller children (see chapt. II). Elastic work of breathing determined on the basis of dynamic lung compliance does not represent the work exerted on overcoming the elastic recoil pressure of the lung being only as an expression of transpulmonary pressure and lung volume relationship during quiet breathing, which is obviously decisive for lung ventilation.

A more adequate approach to the assessment of the elastic work could be by subtracting the elastic work corresponding to a doublefold difference between static and dynamic lung compliances represented by the ABE area in figure 55 from a doubled value of the elastic work of breathing, which was measured (fig. 53; table 251, 252).

However, after such a correction W_{el} was still higher in a smaller child as compared with a taller subject. Lower elastic recoil pressure of the lungs, higher values of 'specific' static lung compliance and the steeper middle part of the pressure-volume curve of the lungs in smaller children could be expected to lead to lesser elastic work of breathing. We suggest to explain of the greater elastic work of breathing in smaller children by a relatively larger proportion of tidal volume on pressure-volume curves of the lungs and the thorax in comparison with taller children (fig. 55). In a 115-cm tall child the percentage of tidal volume was 20% from VC on average and in a 180-cm tall subject the percentage of tidal volume was 14% from VC on average (see chapt. I). After assuming that the pressure-volume curve of the thorax has a symmetrical, but opposite course to that of the lungs starting at the FRC level, another important fact resulting from the work of breathing measurement can be observed. In a smaller child the pressure-volume curve of the thorax crosses the zero pressure axis, i.e. it reaches a resting position, on average at the volume level of 44% of VC whereas in a taller child the pressure-volume curve of the thorax reaches a resting position at the 65% VC level on average (fig. 55). The course of the pressure-volume curve of the thorax suggests that during inspiration, i.e. up to the point where the pressure-volume curve of the thorax crosses the zero pressure axis (its resting level), the thorax tends to expand. Thus, the elasticity of the thoracic wall helps with the inspiratory respiratory muscles to the inspiration act. As seen from figure 55, a positive participation of the thorax elasticity on the work of breathing in a smaller child is much less as compared with a taller child. In a smaller child the inspiratory muscles are therefore forced to work more during inspiration.

Higher viscous and elastic work of breathing result obviously also in higher total work of breathing in a smaller child (tables 249, 250, 259, 260). The total work of breathing on the lungs corrected ($W_{tot\,cor}$) with respect to the Campbell diagram (fig. 47) can be determined also on the basis of our results, if the inspiratory work (W_{in}) is added to the corrected value of the elastic work of breathing ($W_{el\,cor}$), i.e. $W_{tot\,cor} = W_{el\,cor} + W_{in}$. Corrected W_{el} can be determined so that the W_{el} value given in the tables for a selected height or age is multiplied by a factor of two. From the result obtained, the W_{el} value, corresponding to the doublefold difference between Cst and Cdyn and represented by the area ABE in figure 55, is subtracted. The W_{in} value remains as given in tables 255, 256 and 263, 264.

This approach provides more exact information on the total mechanical work of breathing on the lungs. A smaller child with a higher work of breathing of the lungs has a disadvantage concerning the energy requirements of the inspiratory muscles in comparison with a taller child. Higher values of the work of breathing on the lungs in smaller children might also contribute to more serious courses of respiratory diseases in smaller children.

Conclusions

The principles of the measurement of the mechanical work of breathing on the lungs and its components were described. The problems of the estimation of different components of the work of breathing were pointed out. The determination of the viscous (dynamic) work of breathing, measured from the area delineated by the transpulmonary pressure-volume loop, theoretically makes no difficulties. The measurement of the elastic work of breathing from a triangle drawn into the pressure-volume loop underestimates this component of the work of breathing.

We measured total, dynamic (viscous) and elastic mechanical work of breathing on the lungs in 73 healthy children and adolescents (6–18 years old) and young adults (aged 21–25 years) based on transpulmonary pressure-volume loops. The values of the total work of breathing, its components, expressed per 1 liter of ventilation and per minute, declined with the body height and age of the subjects. A smaller child has to perform a physiologically larger mechanical work of breathing (total, viscous and elastic) than a taller child. After correction of the elastic work of breathing with respect to Campbell diagram, the corrected elastic work of breathing in smaller children still remained higher than in taller children. This is thought to be due to the relatively greater tidal volume in smaller children. For higher values of the total work of breathing on the lungs in smaller children, a higher airway resistance, a relatively greater tidal volume per ventilation unit, and a greater difference between static and dynamic lung compliance are suggested to be responsible. The obtained data on the mechanical work of breathing in the healthy studied subjects allow one to obtain information on the physiological energy requirements of the respiratory muscles during tidal breathing between the ages of 6 and 25 years. Also, a suggestion is given for calculating the real elastic work of breathing based on the values of elastic work of breathing obtained from a triangle drawn into the pressure-volume loop. Examples of the work of breathing on the lungs measured from P–V loops in patients with the various respiratory diseases are also given.

V. Gas Exchange in the Lungs

This process containing oxygen (O_2) supply and carbon dioxide (CO_2) elimination via the lungs proceeds in humans in several stages. Its result is a permanent O_2 supply into the tissues of man and CO_2 elimination from them. In this chapter we report only on some parameters assessing gas exchange in the lungs, i.e. on lung-diffusing capacity, alveolar ventilation, volume of dead space, dead space ventilation, oxygen consumption and CO_2 output. The partial pressures of gases (O_2, CO_2) and acid-base balance values in the arterial blood represent the final result of lung function interaction at all levels as well as of tissue metabolism. The latter parameters can be normal for a long time despite a severe lung function disturbance revealed by other methods of lung function testing. The normal values of blood gases partial pressures and acid-base balance also in the presence of quite disturbed lung function is achieved by compensatory mechanisms of lungs and kidneys. The reference values of the latter parameters in children were published elsewhere and are not given here [32, 58, 82, 87, 186].

Alveolar Ventilation,
Respiratory Functional Dead Space and Its Ventilation,
Oxygen Consumption and Elimination of Carbon Dioxide

Alveolar ventilation represents the volume of gas per unit of time directly participating in the gas exchange between alveoli and lung capillary blood. The volume of airways and alveoli which do not participate in gas exchange, i.e. do not come into contact with the lung capillary blood, is termed the respiratory functional dead space. Its increase in various pulmonary and heart diseases affects adversely gas exchange.

Methods

The calculation of *alveolar ventilation* ($\dot{V}_A$) and *dead space ventilation* ($\dot{V}_D$) was performed on the basis of CO_2 elimination per unit of time, alveolar CO_2 partial pressure and total ventilation per unit of time. $\dot{V}_A$ was calculated according to the formula:

$$\dot{V}_A \text{ (ml)} = \frac{\dot{V}_{CO_2}}{P_{A_{CO_2}}} \times 0.863,$$

where $\dot{V}_{CO_2}$ is the volume of CO_2 in ml per min (STPD), $P_{A_{CO_2}}$ is the alveolar CO_2 partial pressure, 0.863 is the factor converting the volumes to BTPS conditions.

Ventilation of respiratory functional dead space ($\dot{V}_D$) was calculated by subtracting the alveolar ventilation ($\dot{V}_A$) from the total (minute) ventilation ($\dot{V}_E$), i.e. according to the formula:

$$\dot{V}_D = \dot{V}_E - \dot{V}_A,$$

where $\dot{V}_E$ is minute ventilation.

The value of *respiratory functional dead space volume* (V_D) was further obtained by dividing the values of respiratory dead space ventilation by breathing frequency per minute (f), i.e. according to the formula:

$$V_D = \frac{\dot{V}_D}{f}.$$

Oxygen consumption (n'O_2, $\dot{V}_{O_2}$), *carbon dioxide elimination* (n'CO_2, $\dot{V}_{CO_2}$) and *minute ventilation* ($\dot{V}_E$) were determined by collecting the expired gas for 3–4 min into the Douglas bag. The volume of the bag was then measured in a Tissot spirometer and O_2 and CO_2 concentrations in the bag were determined immediately after finishing the collection of gas into the bag with a mass spectrometer (type M3-Varian Mat). The partial pressures of alveolar gases were determined as the end-expiratory phase of alveolar plateau during gas collection into the bag by continual analysis of the expired gas with a mass spectrometer.

The $\dot{V}_A$, V_D, $\dot{V}_D$, $\dot{V}_{O_2}$ and $\dot{V}_{CO_2}$ values obtained by the methods described were determined in 46 healthy children and adolescents from the same group of 56 individuals in whom the lung-diffusing capacity (see below) was measured. Their body height varied between 126 and 178 cm and age from 7 to 17 years (26 boys and 20 girls). The values of the studied parameters of gas exchange were obtained from the same measurement in a recumbent subject, roughly after 10 min of the subject's rest.

Results and Discussion

The values obtained of the studied 5 parameters were correlated with body height, and regression equations were calculated for these relationships. The $\dot{V}_D$, V_D, $\dot{V}_{CO_2}$ and $\dot{V}_{O_2}$ values increased linearly with increasing body height, whereas the $\dot{V}_A$ value increased nonlinearly with height (table 267–271).

These 5 parameters represent supplementary lung function testing and all can be considerably influenced by physical and mental activities of the subjects. The V_D value formed roughly one-third of the tidal volume (V_T). However, the respiratory dead space ventilation value ($\dot{V}_D$) reached 46% of the minute ventilation in a 126-cm tall child and reached 41% of the minute ventilation in a 178-cm tall child. Minute ventilation as a sum of $\dot{V}_A$ and $\dot{V}_D$ (table 267, 268) is close to the minute ventilation obtained in another similar group investigated (table 83–85). Different $\dot{V}_D$ can be caused by different breathing frequencies in smaller and taller children during the study.

Lung-Diffusing Capacity (Transfer Factor)

The lung-diffusing capacity represents a measurement of the transport of gases between the lung alveoli and the lung capillary blood. It depends on many factors, such as the pressure gradient of gases between lung capillary blood and the alveoli, gas solubility in the liquids and tissues, and the given time for the transfer of gases. The transfer is further influenced by a number of other factors, i.e. by properties, permeability and thickness of the alveolocapillary membrane, and its total surface, amount and quality of hemoglobin. This parameter also depends on age, sex, physical activity, gas distribution in the lungs, and lung circulation.

The amount of gas which was transferred from the alveoli into the inside of erythrocytes in lung capillary blood depends therefore on all these variables and does not only reflect a diffusion characteristic of the alveolocapillary membrane. This is why the term 'transfer factor' was introduced for this test [31, 32]. At present, both terms 'lung-diffusing capacity' (D_L) and 'transfer factor' (T_L) have been used. D_L is expressed in a unit of mmol/min/kPa, formerly in ml/min/Torr. In this chapter the term 'lung-diffusing capacity' has been used for this functional parameter.

For the D_L measurement, a gas having a high reaction rate with hemoglobin and a good solubility in the tissue is required, such as oxygen and carbon monoxide (CO). For both CO and O_2, the dilution coefficients are very similar. The most often used methods are with CO, i.e. the 'single breath' and 'steady state' methods [18, 32, 62, 127, 146]. The principle of measuring is analogical in both of them. Lung-diffusing capacity measured with carbon monoxide (D_L) is based on the uptake rate of CO at its known pressure gradient between the alveoli and lung capillary blood. The calculation provides the following equation:

$$DL_{CO} = \frac{\dot{V}_{CO\ or\ n'CO}}{P_{ACO} - P_{VCO}},$$

where $\dot{V}_{CO\ (or\ n'CO)}$ is the amount of CO in mmol or ml per unit of time (uptake rate), P_{ACO} is the alveolar CO partial pressure, P_{VCO} is the CO partial pressure in the lung capillary blood. In smokers this CO partial pressure can be significantly increased, otherwise it is zero [32]. DL_{CO} represents the amount of transferred CO in 1 min from the alveoli to the lung capillary blood at a pressure gradient of 1 kPa (or Torr, mm Hg) between the latter environments.

(1) *Steady state method of DL_{CO} determination* is based on the $\dot{V}_{CO}$ uptake rate measurement as a difference between the amount of inspired CO (calculation: %CO in the inspired mixture × inspired minute volume) and the amount of expired CO (calculation: %CO in the expired mixture × expired minute volume). The subject breathes a gas mixture with 0.01 to 0.06% CO concentration for about 1 min, during which the CO exchange reached a steady state. Further, it is necessary to determine the mean alveolar CO partial pressure. The whole calculation is given by the equation:

$$DL_{CO} = \frac{\dot{V}_{CO}}{\bar{P}_{ACO}}.$$

Determination of the mean CO partial pressure in the alveolar gas ($\bar{P}_{ACO}$) can be performed in two ways: (a) by determination of the functional dead space from analysing the CO_2 partial pressure in the arterial blood according to the Bohr equation. The method assumes equal respiratory functional dead space for CO and CO_2 and requires arterial punction. (b) By withdrawal of the expired gas (15–30 ml) at the end-expiratory level; the composition of the expired gas is assumed to be nearly the same as that of the alveolar gas. $\bar{P}_{ACO}$ represents a sum of small gas amounts from each expiration. The method does not require arterial punction, and has been used in practice [7].

(2) *Single breath method of DL_{CO} determination* was developed by Bohr and introduced by Krogh. The method solved the assessment of the mean alveolar CO partial pressure. At this method the subject inspires from residual volume level up to 100% vital capacity level a mixture containing 0.3% CO, 15% He and 21% O_2, the rest being N_2, and expires after 10 s of holding of breath.

The CO loss from the alveolar gas during the holding of breath is exponential and Krogh expressed it by a differential equation, providing that alveolar CO loss rate equals the rate of CO transport into the lung capillary blood at a given alveolar volume. This is expressed by the following equation:

$$\frac{dF_{ACO}}{dt} = D_{LCO} \times (P_B - P_{H_2O}) \times F_{ACO}.$$

Then D_{LCO} can be expressed at any moment by a modification of the latter equation:

$$D_{LCO} = \frac{dF_{ACO}}{dt} \times \frac{V_A}{(F_{ACO} - F_{\overline{V}}) \times (P_B - P_{H_2O})},$$

where V_A is the alveolar gas volume in ml (STPD), F_{ACO} is the actual CO concentration in the alveolar gas, $F_{\overline{V}}$ is the CO concentration in the mixed lung capillary blood, t = time in minutes, $P_B - P_{H_2O}$ is the gas pressure in the lungs minus the water vapor pressure (i.e. dry gas pressure). For D_{LCO} calculation using this method four basic data must be available, i.e. the amount of CO in the alveolar gas at the start and end of breath holding, time of breath holding and alveolar volume during holding of breath. D_{LCO} calculation is given according to the formula [32]:

$$D_{LCO} = \frac{\text{alveolar volume (STPD)} \times 60}{\text{time (in s) of breath holding} \times (P_B - P_{H_2O})} \times \text{natural logarithm } \frac{F_{ICO}}{F_{ECO}}.$$

F_{ECO}, i.e. the alveolar CO concentration at the end of breath holding, is obtained directly by analysis of the mixture of gas expired into the expiratory bag. The alveolar CO concentration at the start of breath holding (initial alveolar CO concentration, F_{ACO}) is smaller than the concentration of the inspired CO (F_{ICO}). The inspired gas mixture is diluted at the start of breath holding by lung volume change and residual volume, i.e. before the transfer of CO from alveoli into the lung capillary blood starts. The magnitude of the latter dilution can be calculated from the simultaneously measured dilution of an inert gas (helium) insoluble in the blood. F_{ACO} is then calculated as follows:

$$F_{ACO} = F_{ICO} \times \frac{F_{EHe}}{F_{IHe}},$$

where F_{EHe} and F_{IHe} are helium concentrations in the expired (alveolar) and inspired gas mixtures. Instead of the F_{ICO} value, the F_{ACO} value must be substituted into the equation for D_{LCO} calculation. For an easier D_{LCO} value calculation Cotes [32] modified the equation for D_{LCO} in the following way:

$$D_{L_{CO}} = b \times V_A/t \times \log_{10} \frac{F_{I_{CO}} \times F_{E_{He}}}{F_{I_{He}} \times F_{E_{CO}}}.$$

F_I is the gas concentration in the inspired gas. F_E is the gas concentration in the alveolar gas at the end of breath holding (for the latter fraction of gas also a symbol F_A is used), b is a constant (53.6 for $D_{L_{CO}}$ calculation in mmol/min/kPa and 160 in ml/min/Torr), V_A is the effective alveolar volume, t is the breath holding time measured, e.g. from the simultaneous spirographic record. The effective alveolar volume (BTPS) can be obtained by adding up the residual volume and the volume of the inspired gas. Residual volume can be determined by the helium-dilution method or in a body plethysmograph. In a disturbed pulmonary gas distribution the two methods yield different values of alveolar volume, which can result in different $D_{L_{CO}}$ values in the same individual. Calculation of the alveolar volume (V_A) during the test itself can also be performed according to the following formula:

$$V_A = (V_I - V_{ID}) \times \frac{F_{I_{He}}}{F_{E_{He}}},$$

where V_A is the effective alveolar volume, V_I the volume of the inspired gas (BTPS), V_{ID} the volume of the anatomical airway dead space and dead space of the apparatus, $F_{I_{He}}$ and $F_{E_{He}}$ are helium concentrations in the inspired gas and alveolar gas at the end of breath holding, respectively.

Comparison of both methods, i.e. the steady state and single breath methods, revealed certain disadvantages of the former. The $D_{L_{CO}}$ value determined by the 'steady state' method strongly depends on the evenness of gas distribution in the lungs and on the errors due to incorrect withdrawal of the alveolar gas sample at the end-expiratory level when the alveolar gas is 'contaminated' with the gas from the airways not participating in the gas exchange. The CO concentration is then higher and the $D_{L_{CO}}$ lower. $D_{L_{CO}}$ measured by a single breath method requires a more sophisticated apparatus and calculations. Also the breath holding maneuver itself is not a physiological condition during the measurement. The method also requires vital capacity higher than 1 liter and breath holding time of at least 5 s.

Determination of membrane and blood components of the lung-diffusing capacity (D_L) is based on the relationship established by Roughton and Forster [cited in ref. 32]. They divided D_L into membrane and blood components with an assumption that D_L represents the sum of conductances of the membrane and blood components for a given gas. The calculation is given by the following equation:

$$1/D_L = 1/Dm + 1/QVc.$$

D_L is lung diffusing capacity, Dm is its membrane component and QVc is the binding capacity of the erythrocytes present at a given moment in the lung capillary bed. Q represents the amount of absorbed gas, bound by 1 ml of whole blood per 1 min at 0.133 kPa (1 mm Hg) pressure gradient. Vc is the volume of blood in the lung capillaries in ml. The Dm value depends on surface area of the lung alveolocapillary membrane, further on thickness, composition and diffusion coefficient of the tissues of the alveolocapillary membrane. The diffusion coefficient is directly proportional to the solubility of a gas in the alveolocapillary membrane and indirectly proportional to the square of the molecular weight of a given gas. Thus, the D_L value is determined by the diffusing capacity of the alveolocapillary membrane (D_M), the blood volume in the alveolar capillaries (Vc) and the gas (CO)–hemoglobin reaction rate (Q).

The assessment of both D_L components is based on different reaction rate of CO with hemoglobin (Q), which is indirectly dependent on the oxygen partial pressure. The reaction rate of CO with hemoglobin is delayed at higher oxygen concentration in the lung capillary blood. The $D_{L_{CO}}$ value is therefore measured at two conditions, i.e. when a subject is breathing a mixture with two different oxygen concentrations and thus also with different oxygen partial pressures in alveolar gas. The first measurement is with alveolar P_{O_2} at breathing the atmospheric air, the second one with P_{O_2} higher in the alveolar gas than the previous one. Further, the rates CO-hemoglobin reaction (Q) must be obtained. Thus, two values for $D_{L_{CO}}$ and two values for Q are available. Dm and Vc calculation by a graphic solution is easy [32]. Reciprocal D_L values, i.e. $\frac{1}{D_L}$, are related to the reciprocal Q values, i.e. $\frac{1}{Q}$. In this way, a regression-line is obtained. Its slope gives Vc and its intercept Dm values, respectively. Vc and Dm can further be determined by the following calculations:

$$\frac{1}{Vc} = \frac{\dfrac{1}{D_{L_2}} - \dfrac{1}{D_{L_1}}}{\dfrac{1}{Q_2} - \dfrac{1}{Q_1}}; \quad \frac{1}{Dm} = \frac{1}{D_{L_1}} - \frac{\dfrac{1}{D_{L_2}} - \dfrac{1}{D_{L_1}}}{\dfrac{1}{Q_2} - \dfrac{1}{Q_1}} \times \frac{1}{Q_1},$$

where D_{L_1} and D_{L_2} are lung-diffusing capacities determined at normal and higher oxygen partial pressures in the inspired mixtures, Q_1 and Q_2 express the hemoglobin-CO reaction rate at different blood O_2 partial pressures. The $\frac{1}{Q}$ value was calculated according to the following relationship:

$$\frac{1}{Q} = \frac{0.0057 \times PO_2 + 0.33}{\% \text{ blood hemoglobin}}, \text{ (traditional units)},$$

$$\text{i.e. } \frac{1}{Q} = \frac{(1.0 \times 10^{-3} \times PO_2 + 0.134 \times 10^{-3})}{\% \text{ blood hemoglobin}}, \text{ (SI units)}.$$

PO_2 is the oxygen partial pressure in the lung capillary blood, which is lower by roughly 5 Torr (0.67 kPa) than in the alveolar gas. PO_2 calculation is then:

$$PO_2 \text{ (kPa)} = \%O_2 \times \frac{(P_B - 6.27)}{100} - 0.67,$$

or

$$PO_2 \text{ (Torr)} = \%O_2 \times \frac{(P_B - 47)}{100} - 5.$$

Method and Subjects

D_L was measured by the CO single-breath method with an apparatus Resparameter Mk4, Morgan, Ltd., equipped with the analyzers for CO, He and O_2, two inspiratory bags, an open circuit for breathing the gas mixture with high oxygen content and a program controlling the valves which regulated the inspiratory volume, time of breath holding, volume of gas expired from the respiratory dead space, and the volume of the alveolar gas sample. The system further contained two bags for the collection of expired gas as well as a water-sealed spirometer. An automatic electric timer determined the effective time of breath holding.

The subjects were seated comfortably at the apparatus and were instructed about the procedure of the investigation. At first the D_{LCO} measurement started with a higher oxygen content in the circuit, which represented about 5 min breathing of the mixture. Then the subject was asked to expire maximally. At the moment of maximum expiration a preset program was started, in which the inspiratory bag was automatically opened, the timer was also started and the subject inspired maximally, i.e. to his 100% vital capacity level. A red light gave a signal of the time of breath holding. Then the subject expired maximally. During the expiration a part of the expired gas, i.e. its alveolar portion, was collected automatically in the bag. The respiratory dead space volume and amount of alveolar gas sample were also preset according to the size of the subject. After rinsing the apparatus with air and waiting 15 min, the investigation was repeated, this time the inspiratory gas mixture contained the normal oxygen concentration, i.e. atmospheric air. The values obtained were substitued into the equations for the calculation of lung-diffusing capacity and its components. They were as follows: maximum inspiratory volumes for the mixtures with different oxygen concentrations, times of breath-holding for both measurements, CO concentrations during inspiration and expiration (in the alveolar gas) from both measurements with different O_2 contents in the mixtures, and further, He concen-

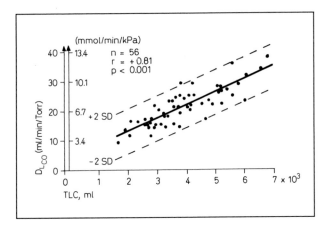

Fig. 56. D_{LCO} in relation to TLC in healthy boys and girls. For further explanations, see figure 52.

trations in both inspiratory mixtures and O_2 concentrations in the alveolar gas. These measurements were performed twice in each individual. Further, the values of barometric pressure, percent of blood hemoglobin and respiratory dead space volume were incorporated into the equations. The volume of the respiratory dead space in the studied subjects was obtained on the basis of their height from the reference values determined in our laboratory. Hemoglobin was measured in each subject on the day of the study. Prior to each D_{LCO} measurement, vital capacity was determined. The cooperation of the children during the investigation was usually very good. The D_{LCO} measurement was successful in the subjects with vital capacity higher than 1,000 ml.

The accuracy of gas analyzers was repeatedly tested using calibration mixtures, which did not significantly differ in different periods of time, and the linearity of the analyzers was stable.

The measurements of D_{LCO}, Dm and Vc were performed in 56 healthy children and adolescents, 5–17 years old, 107–178 cm in body height (36 boys and 20 girls).

Results

The values of D_{LCO} and its components (Dm and Vc) were related to body surface, height, age and total lung capacity. They are given in tables 272–283 and figure 56. Most frequently the best correlation of these values in descending order was observed with TLC, body height, body surface and age. The D_{LCO}, Dm and Vc values increased with the increase of the latter anthropometric parameters and TLC. The D_{LCO}/TLC and Vc/TLC ('specific') values decreased with increasing body height, age and body surface (fig. 57, 58; table 280–283).

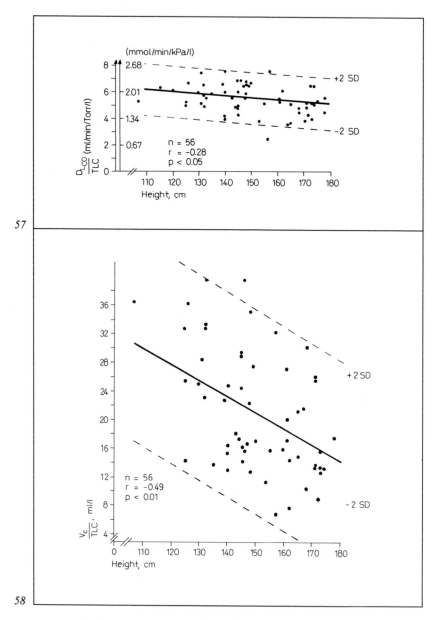

Fig. 57. D$_{LCO}$/TLC in relation to body height in healthy boys and girls. For further explanations, see figure 52 and the text.

Fig. 58. Vc/TLC in relation to body height in healthy boys and girls. For further explanations, see figure 52 and the text.

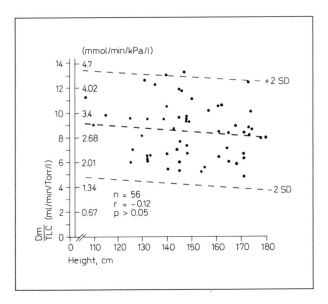

Fig. 59. Dm/TLC in relation to body height in healthy boys and girls. For further explanations, see figure 52 and the text.

The Dm/TLC value did not depend on body height, body surface or age amounting to 2.83 ± (SD) 0.730 mmol/min/kPa/l on average (fig. 59).

Discussion

The D_{LCO}, Dm and Vc values in our group of healthy children and adolescents are close to those reported in the literature [18, 31, 36, 62, 179, 243]. However, the 'specific' values for lung-diffusing capacity and its components, i.e. D_{LCO}/TLC and Dm/TLC, have not been introduced in the practice of lung function testing in children. DeMuth et al. [36] observed an independence of the D_{LCO}/TLC ratio on body height and age, whereas Cotes et al. [31] found a decrease of the Krogh factor ($K_{CO} = D_{LCO}$ expressed per unit of alveolar volume) with body height in children. A decrease of the D_{LCO}/TLC ratio with body height, surface and age gives evidence of a greater alveolar gas exchange per unit of lung size physiologically in the lungs of younger and smaller children than in older children and adolescents. First of all a decrease of the Vc/TLC ratio with body height, surface and age, suggesting a smaller lung capillary blood volume in taller children and adolescents as compared with younger children can be considered as being most responsible for the decrease of $D_{L_{CO}}$/TLC with growth in children. Independence of the Dm/TLC ratio, i.e. the 'specific' membrane component of lung-diffusing capacity (corrected for lung size), on body height, age and body surface further suggests that the alveolo-capillary membrane does not change for a gas transport in the lungs physiologically in the ages from 5 to 17 years or in the range of 107 to 178 cm of body height. A larger alveolar gas exchange in the lungs of smaller children might be related to a larger metabolism in smaller children thus resulting in a larger oxygen supply into their lungs. Larger tidal volume (fig. 5) and minute ventilation per unit of TLC as well as larger conductance of the 'upstream' airway segment (table 206–210; fig. 33) in smaller children lead to similar conclusions as the ratio $D_{L_{CO}}$/TLC. Based on the latter observations, the evaluation of lung-diffusing capacity and its components requires $D_{L_{CO}}$, Dm and Vc to be expressed per unit of TLC, i.e. to correct them for lung size and only then to correlate the latter indices with body height, surface and age. Otherwise, the physiological peculiarities of lung-diffusing capacity during the growth of children are neglected and its decrease or increase can result only from the altered lung size and not from the disorders of gas transport in the lungs. Our results in patients with idiopathic lung fibrosis, in whom the $D_{L_{CO}}$/TLC value indicated a disturbed gas transport in the lungs in 8% only, whereas the $D_{L_{CO}}$ value related to the body surface proved to be pathological in 58% of the same patients [240], confirmed thus the significance of this approach.

Conclusions

In 56 healthy children and adolescents, 5–17 years old, and 107–178 cm tall (36 boys and 20 girls) lung-diffusing capacity ($D_{L_{CO}}$), its membrane (Dm) and capillary Vc) components were investigated by the CO single breath method. The latter functional parameters increased with an increase in body height, surface, age and TLC. $D_{L_{CO}}$ and Vc expressed per unit of TLC, i.e. corrected for lung size, decreased with the growth of the subjects. This suggests a larger alveolar gas exchange in the lungs of smaller children. This was not true for the Dm value expressed per unit of TLC, which indicates a stability of the alveolocapillary membrane for gas exchange during the studied period of growth. For an assessment of the disturbances of gas transport in the lungs in patients based on $D_{L_{CO}}$ and its components measurements, the latter parameters first have to be corrected for lung size, i.e. per unit of TLC.

Summary

In a group of 173 healthy children and adolescents (age 6–18 years) with body height 115–182 cm, static lung volumes, ventilation, indices of lung elasticity and airway patency, and mechanical work of the lungs were studied. In another group of 56 healthy children and adolescents lung-diffusing capacity, alveolar ventilation, respiratory dead space, ventilation of respiratory dead space, oxygen consumption and CO_2 output were also measured. Not all measurements were carried out in all the same subjects. The obtained values, considered as reference values, were related to body height, age and body surface, and also to lung volumes of the studied subjects. For the latter relationships, the regression equations were calculated. The data on volume of isoflow and lung mechanical work were also obtained in 16 healthy subjects 21–25 years of age.

As *static lung volumes*, vital capacity (VC), inspiratory capacity (IC), total lung capacity (TLC), functional residual capacity (FRC), residual volume (RV), inspiratory reserve volume (IRV), expiratory reserve volume (ERV) and tidal volume (V_T) were measured. The latter values were obtained from the spirographic record and FRC measurement in a body plethysmograph and by the helium-dilution method.

As *ventilatory indices,* respiratory frequency (f), minute ventilation (MV), and maximum minute ventilation (MMV) from a spirographic record were obtained.

All static volumes and ventilation indices measured, except respiratory frequency, increased nonlinearly with increasing body height, age and body surface, VC, IC, IRV, FRC and TLC differed significantly between boys and girls, the latter values being higher in boys. A larger proportion of RV and V_T to TLC was revealed in smaller children. Respiratory frequency in the studied age range of subjects was independent of body height, age and body surface, and was on average 20.5 ± 3.7/min.

As indices of *lung elasticity,* elastic recoil pressure of the lung (Pst), static and dynamic lung compliances (Cst and Cdyn) were measured. Cst and Pst were measured from 'quasi' static pressure-volume curves. Cdyn was obtained from the simultaneous recordings of volume, flow and trans-pulmonary pressure during quiet breathing. A difference between Cst and Cdyn was found, which was larger in smaller children. Cst corrected for lung size, i.e. 'specific' Cst, decreased with increasing body height, age and body surface. 'Specific' Cdyn did not change with body height, age and body surface. Pst values, measured at various lung volume levels, increased significantly with increasing body height, age and body surface. The obtained results on lung elasticity suggested a physiological change, i.e. an increase of the elastic properties of the lungs, in the age range from 6 to 17–18 years. From our results in healthy children and adolescents, the previous conclusions on the unchanged lung elasticity in children and adolescents during their growth cannot be confirmed.

The possible methodological errors at lung elasticity assessment in the studied healthy subjects, which might affect the results of lung elasticity indices, were also studied. Four possible methodological errors were investigated, i.e. elasticity of esophagus, vertical intrathoracic pressure gradient, the effect of slow expiration maneuver on 'quasi' static pressure-volume curves, and different inspiratory muscle effort on the shape of pressure-volume curves of the lungs.

Elasticity of the esophagus and periesophageal structures was assessed on the basis of *esophageal elastance*, expressing a pressure change inside the esophagus after its volume change by 1 ml. The mean value of the esophageal elastance in the studied group of healthy subjects was 0.34 kPa/ml. Esophageal elastance was thus excluded as a possible cause of the change of lung elasticity indices observed in our studied healthy subjects.

The effect of the *vertical intrathoracic pressure gradient* on lung elasticity indices was also eliminated because its value did not change with growth of children and adolescents being independent of body height with the value of intrathoracic vertical pressure gradient 0.03 kPa/cm. The latter gradient could not be therefore a cause of the observed increase of the elastic properties of the lung in the studied age range in our healthy children and adolescents.

Also, the *airflow rate*, at which 'quasi' static pressure-volume curves of the lungs were obtained, could not be a cause of the observed increase of lung elasticity in the studied age range. The airflow rate of 0.05–0.2 liters/s could make a mean error in a shift of the pressure-volume curve toward the positivity by 0.028–0.056 kPa in a small child. In a larger subject the latter error is smaller due to a lower pressure for overcoming pulmonary resistance at 'quasi' static pressure-volume curves of the lung recordings. The observed differences in Pst values between larger and smaller children and adolescents are much larger than the observed error due to a low airflow rate at the recording of the pressure-volume curve of the lungs.

By the analysis of the pressure-volume curves of the lungs with maximal and submaximal inspiratory pressures the effects of respirator maneuver with *different inspiratory muscle effort* as another cause on the observed changes in lung elasticity was excluded in the studied healthy subjects aged 6–17 years.

From the indices of *airway patency*, important for the detection of airway obstuction, maximum expiratory flow rates ($\dot{V}_{max}$, MEF) at different lung volume levels, peak expiratory flow rate (PEFR) from maximum expiratory flow-volume (MEFV) curves were measured. Further forced expiratory volume in the first second (FEV_1) and maximum mid-expiratory flow ($MMEF_{25-75\% VC}$) from the forced expiratory volume time curve were obtained. Also, 'upstream' airway conductance (Gus) at various lung volume levels, airway resistance (R_{aw}) and, its reversal, airway conductance (G_{aw}) in a body plethysmograph were measured in the same healthy subjects as the previous lung functional indices. Further, also pulmonary resistance (R_L) at isovolume level (in the middle of tidal volume), nitrogen washout time, nitrogen washout volume and index of Becklake were obtained.

$\dot{V}_{max}$, PEFR, FEV_1, $MMEF_{25-75\% VC}$ and G_{aw} increased nonlinearly with increasing body height, age and body surface. G_{aw} increased linearly with FRC, R_{aw} values decreased with body height, age and body surface as well as with FRC, also nonlinearly. $\dot{V}_{max}$, $MMEF_{25-75\%VC}$, Gus, corrected for lung size, i.e. expressed per liter of TLC in a unit of TLC/s or TLC/s/kPa, decreased with body height, age and body surface. The latter values reflect mainly the patency of the peripheral airways. FEV_1, PEFR and G_{aw}, considered to reflect the patency of the central, larger airways, after correction for lung size by expressing them per liter of TLC, were independent of body height, age and body surface. It follows from the obtained results on airway patency in the studied healthy subjects that the patency of peripheral airways with respect to lung (alveolar) size decreases physiologically with increasing body height, age and body surface, while the patency of central airways with regard to lung size does not change during growth.

During quiet breathing also the *mechanical work of the lungs* and its components were measured, i.e. total work of breathing (W_{tot}), elastic work

(W_{el}), dynamic (viscous) work (W_{dyn}), inspiratory dynamic work (W_{in}), expiratory dynamic work (W_{ex}), and ratio Win/Wtot. The latter functional indices were obtained by the analysis of pressure-volume loops of the lungs with a triangle drawn into the loops. The latter data were obtained not only in children and adolescents but also in 6 healthy subjects 21–25 years of age. All the measured components of lung mechanical work decreased with body height and age. It follows from the obtained results that a smaller child has to perform a larger lung mechanical work at breathing than a taller child or adolescent.

A cause of a larger lung mechanical work in smaller children is due to a larger airway resistance, relatively larger tidal volume with respect to VC and TLC, and a larger difference between static and dynamic lung compliances. The latter factors with reduced elastic properties of the lungs may contribute to a more severe course of respiratory diseases in smaller children.

From the functional parameters assessing *gas exchange* in the lungs, lung-diffusion capacity by a single breath CO method (D_LCO), membrane component (Dm) and pulmonary capillary blood volume (Vc) were measured in 56 healthy children and adolescents (age 5–17 years). The latter indices increased with body height, age, body surface and total lung capacity (TLC), and were also expressed per liter of TLC (corrected for lung size) as 'specific' values, i.e. D_{LCO}/TLC, Dm/TLC and Vc/TLC. The D_{LCO}/TLC and Vc/TLC values decreased with body height, age and body surface suggesting a larger gas exchange in smaller children. The latter observations is in the agreement with a relatively larger tidal volume, minute ventilation and larger peripheral airway patency with respect to lung size in smaller children. The Dm/TLC value being independent of body height, age and body surface suggests the stable properties of alveolocapillary membrane in the age period from 5 to 17 years.

As other indices of gas exchange in the lungs, alveolar ventilation ($\dot{V}_A$), respiratory functional dead space V_D), ventilation of respiratory dead space ($\dot{V}_D$), oxygen consumption and CO_2 output were measured in 46 children and adolescents (age 5–17 years). They increased with increasing body height.

In the studied healthy children and adolescents the obtained data of various functional indices of lung function, given in the tables and figures, are reported in relation to body height, age and body surface. This is to show the functional indices in relation to the most frequently used anthropometrical indices. However, for the assessment of lung function parameters in patients, it is recommended to compare them on the basis of that anthropometrical index with which the lung functional parameter in healthy subjects correlated best and where the variation coefficient was least. It follows from our results of the comparative lung function parameters in patients that body height was the best anthropometrical index with which lung function parameters correlated best and where its variation coefficient was lowest. In this publication lung function parameters also in relation to age and body surface have been included, because we wanted to show the most complete picture and significance of other frequently used anthropometrical indices, on the basis of which lung function parameters have also been predicted. The calculation of a given lung function parameter from the multiple regression equation, which includes height, age and body surface as independent variables, might, however, make the confidence limits for that parameter (dependent variable) wider and thus also less sensitive in detecting functional abnormalities in patients.

References

1 Agostoni, E.: Mechanics of the pleural space. Physiol. Rev. *52:* 57–128 (1972).
2 Ahlström, H.; Jonson, B.: Pulmonary mechanics during the first year of life. Scand. J. resp. Dis. *55:* 141–154 (1974).
3 Avery, M.E.: The lung and its disorders in the newborn infant; 2nd ed. (Saunders, Philadelphia 1968).
4 Auld, P.A.M.; Nelson, N.M.; Cherry, R.B.; Rudolph, A.J.; Smith, C.A.: Measurement of thoracic gas volume in the newborn infant. J. clin. Invest. *42:* 476–483 (1963).
5 Bachofen, H.: Die mechanischen Eigenschaften der Lunge (Huber, Bern 1969).
6 Baran, D.; Englert, M.: La conductance des voies aériennes chez l'enfant et l'adolescent normaux. Bull. Physiopath. resp. *7:* 125–135 (1971).
7 Bates, D.V.; Macklem, P.T.; Christie, R.V.: Respiratory function in disease (Saunders, Philadelphia 1971).
8 Bedell, G.N.; Marschall, E.; DuBois, A.B.; Comroe, J.H., Jr.: Plethysmographic determination of the volume of gas trapped in the lungs. J. clin. Invest. *35:* 664 (1956).
9 Bellon, G.; So, S.; Brun, J.L.; Adeleine, P.; Gilly, R.: Flow-volume curves in children in health and disease. Bull. eur. Physio-path. resp. *18:* 705–715 (1982).
10 Berglund, E.; Birath, G.; Bjure, J.; Grimby, G.; Kjellmer, I.; Sanquist, L.; Söderholm, B.: Spirometric studies in normal subject. I. Forced expirograms in subjects between 7 to 70 years of age. Acta med. scand. *173:* 185–206 (1963).
11 Bernstein, L.; Fragge, R.G.; Gueron, M.; Kreindler, L.; Ghory, J.E.: Pulmonary function in children. I. Determination of norms. J. Allergy *30:* 514–533 (1959).
12 Bjure, J.: Spirometric studies in normal subjects. IV. Ventilatory capacities in healthy children 7 to 17 years of age. Acta paediat., Stockh. *52:* 232–240 (1963).
13 Bohadana, A.B.; Teculescu, D.; Peslin, R.; Jansen da Silva, J.M.; Pino, J.: Comparison of four methods for the total lung capacity measured by body plethysmography. Bull. eur. Physio-path. resp. *16:* 769–776 (1980).
14 Bouhuys, A.; Hunt, V.R.; Kim, B.M.; Zapletal, A.: Maximum expiratory flow rates in induced bronchoconstriction in man. J. clin. Invest. *48:* 1159–1168 (1969).
15 Bouhuys, A.: Pulmonary function measurement in epidemiological studies. Bull. Physio-path. resp. *6:* 561–578 (1970).
16 Bouhuys, A.: Breathing. Physiology, environment and lung disease (Grune & Stratton, New York 1974).
17 Briscoe, W.A.; DuBois, A.B.: The relationship between airway resistance, airway conductance and lung volume in subjects of different age and body size. J. clin. Invest. *37:* 1279–1285 (1958).

18   Bucci, G.; Cook, C.D.; Barrie, H.: Studies of respiratory physiology in children. V. Total diffusion, diffusing capacity of pulmonary membrane, and pulmonary blood volume in normal subjects from 7 to 40 years of age. J. Paediat. *50:* 820–828 (1961).

19   Campbell, E.J.M.: The respiratory muscles and mechanics of breathing, pp. 83–95 (Lloyd-Luke, London 1958).

20   Clément, J.; Woestijne, K.P. van de: Pressure correction in volume and flow displacement body plethysmography. J. appl. Physiol. *27:* 895–897 (1969).

21   Cogswell, J.J.; Hull, D.; Milner, A.D.; Norman, A.P.; Taylor, B.: Lung function in childhood. II. Thoracic gas volumes and helium functional residual capacity measurements in healthy children. Br. J. Dis. Chest *69:* 118–124 (1975).

22   Cogswell, J.J.; Hull, D.; Milner, A.D.; Norman, A.P.; Taylor, B.: Lung function in childhood. III. Measurement of airflow resistance in healthy children. Br. J. Dis. Chest *69:* 177–187 (1975).

23   Cogswell, J.J.; Hull, D.; Milner, A.D.; Norman, A.P.; Taylor, B.: Lung function in childhood. I. The forced expiratory volumes in healthy children using a spirometer and reverse plethysmograph. Br. J. Dis. Chest *69:* 40–50 (1975).

24   Cole, T.J.: Linear and proportional regression models in the prediction of ventilatory function. J.R. Stat. Soc. A. *138:* 297–337 (1975).

25   Colebatch, H.J.H.; Ng, Ck.Y.; Nikov, N.: Use of an exponential function for elastic recoil. J. appl. Physiol. *46:* 387–393 (1979).

26   Comroe, J.H., Jr.; Forster, R.E.; DuBois, A.B.; Briscoe, W.A.; Carlson, E.: The lung; 2nd ed. (Year Book, Chicago 1965).

27   Comroe, J.H., Jr.; Botelho, S.Y.; DuBois, A.B.: Design a body plethysmograph for studying cardiopulmonary physiology. J. appl. Physiol. *14:* 439–444 (1959).

28   Cook, C.D.; Cherry, R.B.; O'Brien, D.; Karlberg, P.; Smith, C.A.: Studies of respiratory physiology in the newborn infant. I. Observations on normal premature and full-term infants. J. clin. Invest. *34:* 975–982 (1955).

29   Cook, C.D.; Hamman, J.F.: Relation of lung volume to height in healthy persons between the ages of 5 and 38 years. J. Pediat. *59:* 710–714 (1961).

30   Cook, C.D.; Helliesen, P.J.; Agathon, S.: Relation between mechanics of respiration, lung size and body size from birth to young adulthood. J. appl. Physiol. *13:* 349–352 (1958).

31   Cotes, J.E.; Dabbs, J.M.; Hall, A.M.; Axford, A.T.; Laurence, K.: Lung volumes, ventilatory capacity, and transfer factor in healthy British boy and girl twins. Thorax *28:* 709–715 (1973).

32   Cotes, J.S.: Lung function; 4th ed. (Blackwell, Oxford 1979).

33   Čopová, M.; Hloušková, Z.; Zapletal, A.: Normal spirometric values in healthy children. Čslká Pediat. *18:* 915–921 (1963).

34   Dawson, S.V.; Elliot, E.A.: Wave-speed limitation on expiratory flow – a unifying concept. J. appl. Physiol. *43:* 498–515 (1977).

35   De Graff, A.C., Jr.; Bouhuys, A.: Mechanics of air flow in airway obstruction. A. Rev. Med. *24:* 111–134 (1973).

36   DeMuth, G.R.; Howatt, W.F.; Hill, B.M.: The growth of lung function. Pediatrics, Springfield *35:* suppl. 1 (1965).

37   Despas, P.J.; Leroux, M.; Macklem, P.: Site of airway obstruction in asthma as determined by measuring maximal expiratory flow breathing air and a helium-oxygen mixture. J. clin. Invest. *51:* 3235–3243 (1972).

38 De Swiniarski, R.; Mataame, M.; Tanche, M.: Plethysmography study and pulmo-
    nary function in well-trained adolescents. Bull. eur. Physio-path. resp. *18:* 39–49
    (1982).

39 DeTroyer, A.; Yernault, J.C.; Englert, M.; Baran, D.; Paiva, M.: Evolution of intra-
    thoracic airway mechanics during lung growth. J. appl. Physiol. *44:* 521–527
    (1978).

40 Dickman, M.L.; Schmidt, C.D.; Garner, R.N.: Spirometric standards for normal
    children and adolescents (ages 5 through 18 years). Am. Rev. resp. Dis. *104:* 680–
    687 (1971).

41 Doershuk, C.F.; Mathews, L.W.: Airway resistance and lung volume in the newborn
    infant. Pediat. Res. *3:* 128–134 (1969).

42 Dolfuss, R.E.; Milic-Emili, J.; Bates, D.V.: Regional ventilation of the lung, studied
    with boluses of 133-xenon. Resp. Physiol. *2:* 234–246 (1967).

43 DuBois, A.B.; Botelho, S.Y.; Bedell, G.N.; Marshall, R.; Comroe, J.H., Jr.: A rapid
    plethysmographic method for measuring thoracic gas volume. A comparison with a
    nitrogen washout method for measuring functional residual capacity in normal sub-
    jects. J. clin. Invest. *35:* 322–326 (1956).

44 DuBois, A.B.; Botelho, S.Y.; Comroe, J.H., Jr.: A new method for measuring airway
    resistance in man using a body plethysmograph. Values in normal subject and in
    patients with respiratory disease. J. clin. Invest. *35:* 327–335 (1956).

45 DuBois, A.B.; Woestijne, K.P. van de: Body plethysmography. Prog. resp. Res.,
    vol. 4 (Karger, Basel 1969).

46 Düggelin, S.; Bühlmann, A.A.: Lungenvolumina und Atemwegwiderstände bei
    gesunden Zürcher Schulkindern – Normalwerte. Helv. paediat. Acta *35:* 21–30
    (1980).

47 Dugdale, A.E.; Moeri, M.: Normal values of forced vital capacity (FVC), forced
    expiratory volume (FEV$_1$) and peak flow rate (PFR) in children. Archs Dis. Childh.
    43: 229 (1968).

48 Dunnil, M.S.: Postnatal growth of the lung. Thorax *17:* 329–333 (1962).

49 Emery, J.: The anatomy of the developing lung (Heineman, London 1969).

50 Engström, I.; Karlberg, P.; Swarts, C.: Respiratory studies in children. IX. Relation-
    ships between mechanical properties of the lungs, lung volumes and ventilatory
    capacity in healthy children 7–15 years of age. Acta paediat. *51:* 68–80 (1962).

51 Engström, I.: Respiratory studies in children. XI. Mechanics of breathing lung vol-
    umes and ventilatory capacity in asthmatic children from attack to symptom-free
    status. Acta paediat., suppl. 155 (1964).

52 Engström, I.; Karlberg, P.; Kraepelien, S.: Respiratory studies in children. I. Lung
    volumes in healthy children, 6–14 years of age. Acta paediat., Stockh. *45:* 277–294
    (1965).

53 Fox, W.W.; Bureau, M.A.; Tausig, L.A.; Martin, R.R.; Beaudry, P.H.: Helium flow-
    volume curves in the detection of early small airway disease. Pediatrics, Springfield
    54: 293–299 (1979).

54 Fry, D.L.; Hyatt, R.E.: Pulmonary mechanics. A unified analysis of the relationship
    between pressure, volume and gas flow in the lungs of normal and diseased human
    subjects. Am. J. Med. *29:* 672–689 (1960).

55 Gandevia, B.: Normal standards for single breath tests of ventilatory capacity in
    healthy children. Archs Dis. Childh. *35:* 236–239 (1960).

56   Gaultier, C.; Zinman, R.: Maximal static pressures in healthy children. Resp. Physiol. *51:* 45–61 (1983).

57   Gaultier, C.; Girard, F.: Croissance pulmonaire normale et pathologiques: relations structure-function. Bull. eur. Physio-path. resp. *16:* 791–842 (1980).

58   Gaultier, C.: Physiology of respiration. Applications of functional exploration of the lungs in infants and children; in Gerbeaux, Couvreur, Tournier, Pediatric respiratory disease (Wiley, New York 1982).

59   Geubelle, F.; Breny, H.: Volumes pulmonaires de filles et garçons sains, âgés de 5 à 16 ans. Poumon Cœur *25:* 1051–1064 (1969).

60   Gibson, G.J.; Pride, N.B.: Lung distensibility. The static pressure-volume curve of the lungs and its use in clinical assessment. Br. J. Dis. Chest *70:* 143–184 (1976).

61   Gibson, G.J.; Pride, N.B.; Davis, J.; Schroter, R.C.: Exponential description of the static pressure-volume curve of normal and diseased lungs. Am. Rev. resp. Dis. *120:* 799–811 (1979).

62   Giammona, S.T.; Daly, W.J.: Pulmonary diffusing capacity in normal children, ages 4 to 13. Am. J. Dis. Child. *110:* 144–152 (1965).

63   Giammona, S.T.: Evaluation of pulmonary function in children. Pediat. Clins N. Am. *18:* 285–303 (1971).

64   Godfrey, S.; Kamburoff, P.L.; Nairn, J.L.: Spirometry, lung volumes and airway resistance in normal children ages 5 to 18 years. Br. J. Dis. Chest *64:* 15–24 (1970).

65   Haluszka, J.: Application of the whole body plethysmography in examination of respiratory system in children. Predicted values, interrelations, methodical suggestions (Rabka, 1976).

66   Hart, M.C.; Orzalesi, M.M.; Cook, C.D.: Relation between anatomic respiratory dead space and body size and lung volume. J. appl. Physiol. *18:* 519–522 (1963).

67   Helliesen, P.J.; Cook, C.D.; Friedlander, L.; Agathon, S.: Studies of respiratory physiology in children. I. Mechanics of respiration and lung volumes in 85 normal children 5 to 17 years of age. Pediatrics, Springfield *22:* 80–93 (1958).

68   Herdegen, L.; Janoušková, A.; Böswart, J.; Štěbetáková, L.: Normal lung volumes in children. Čslká Pediat. *18:* 972–978 (1963).

69   Herdegen, L.; Böswart, J.; Janoušková, A.: Intrapulmonal gas mixing in children. Čslká Pediat. *18:* 964–971 (1962).

70   Hjalmarson, O.: Mechanics of breathing in newborn infants with pulmonary disease. Acta paediat. scand., suppl. 247 (1974).

71   Hloušková, Z.; Zapletal, A.; Šamánek, M.; Ruth, C.: Clinical status and lung function development in patients with lung resection in childhood. Čslká Pediat. *28:* 517–519 (1973).

72   Houštěk, J.; Čopová, M.; Zapletal, A.; Tomášová, H.; Šamánek, M.: Alpha-1 antitrypsin deficiency in a child with chronic lung disease. Chest *64:* 773–776 (1973).

73   Houštěk, J.; Zapletal, A.: Respiratory disease in children (Avicenum, Praha 1973).

74   Houštěk, J.; Hloušková, Z.; Zapletal, A.: Diffuse interstitial lung fibrosis. Adv. Pediat. *4:* 153–198 (1975).

75   Hrubá, B.; Šamánek, M.; Tůma, S.: Radiocirculography in congenital heart disease in children with intracardiac shunts. Pediat. Radiol. *1:* 47–52 (1973).

76 Hrubá, B.; Šamánek, M.; Zapletal, A.: Hemodynamics in interstitial lung fibrosis studied by radiocirculography. Čslká Pediat. *29:* 361–363 (1974).

77 Hötter, G.J.: Lungenfunktion unter besonderer Berücksichtigung des wachsenden Organismus (Steinkopff, Darmstadt 1977).

78 Hsu, H.K.; Jenkins, D.E.; et al.: Ventilatory function of normal children and young adults. Mexican American, white, and black. I. Spirometry. J. Pediat. *95:* 14–25 (1979).

79 Hyatt, R.E.; Schilder, D.P.; Fry, D.L.: Relationship between maximum expiratory flow and degrees of lung inflation. J. appl. Physiol. *16:* 331–333 (1958).

80 Hyatt, R.E.; Okeson, G.C.; Rodarte, J.R.: Influence of expiratory flow limitation on the pattern of lung emptying in normal man. J. appl. Physiol. *35:* 411–419 (1973).

81 Cherniack, R.M.: Ventilatory function in normal children. Can. med. Ass. J. *87:* 80 (1962).

82 Cherniack, R.M.; Cherniack, L.; Naimark, A.: Respiration in health and in disease; 2nd ed. (Saunders, Philadelphia 1972).

83 Janoušková, A.; Herdegen, L.; Štěbetáková, L.: Forced expiratory maneuver in children – Evaluation. Čslká Pediat. *18:* 979–987 (1963).

84 Jonson, B.; Olsson, L.G.: Measurement of the work of breathing to overcome pulmonary viscous resistance. Scand. J. Lab. Invest. *28:* 135–140 (1971).

85 Juhl, B.: Pulmonary investigations on 1011 school children using Wright's peak flow meter. Scand. J. clin. Lab. Invest. *25:* 355–361 (1970).

86 Kamel, M.; Weng, T.R.; Featherby, E.A.; Jackman, W.S.; Levison, H.: Relationship of mechanics of ventilation to lung volume in children and young adults. Scand. J. resp. Dis. *50:* 125–134 (1969).

87 Kendig, E.L., Jr.: Disorders of the respiratory tract in children (Saunders, Philadelphia 1977).

88 Keogh, B.A.; Crystal, R.G.: Pulmonary function testing in interstitial pulmonary disease. Chest *78:* 856–865 (1980).

89 Kjellman, B.: Regional lung function studied with 133 Xe and external detectors (radiospirometry) in children without cardiopulmonary disease. Acta paediat. scand. *57:* 527–533 (1968).

90 Kjellman, B.: Ventilatory efficiency, capacity and lung volumes in healthy children. Scand. J. clin. Lab. Invest. *28:* 19–29 (1969).

91 Klaus, M.; Tooley, W.H.; Weaver, K.H.; Clements, J.A.: Lung volume in the newborn infant. Pediatrics, Springfield *30:* 111–116 (1962).

92 Knudson, R.J.; Burrows, B.: Early detection of obstructive lung disease. Med. Clins N. Am. *57:* 681–690 (1973).

93 Knudson, R.J.; Slatin, R.C.; Lebowitz, M.D.; Burrows, B.: The maximal expiratory flow-volume curve. Normal standards, variability and effects of age. Am. Rev. resp. Dis. *113:* 587–600 (1976).

94 Knudson, R.J.; Clark, D.F.; Kennedy, T.C.; Knudson, D.E.: Effect of aging alone on mechanical properties of the normal adult lung. J. appl. Physiol. *43:* 1054–1062 (1977).

95 Knudson, R.J.; Lebowitz, M.D.; Holberg, C.J.; Burrows, B.: Changes in the normal maximal expiratory flow-volume curve with growth and aging. Am. Rev. resp. Dis. *127:* 725–734 (1983).

96   Kraemer, R.; Wiese, G.; Bachmann, D.; Geubelle, F.: Determination of end-expira-
     tory compliance in asthmatic children by means of an exponential function. Prog.
     resp. Res., vol. 17, pp. 100–106 (Karger, Basel 1981).
97   Krieger, I.: Thoracic gas volume in infancy. Am. J. Dis. Child. *11:* 399 (1966).
98   Krueger, J.J.; Bain, T.; Petterson, J.J., Jr.: Elevation gradient of intrathoracic pres-
     sure. J. appl. Physiol. *16:* 465–468 (1961).
99   Kureš, H.: Lung elasticity determination as a diagnostic aid. Čslká Pediat. *20:* 239–
     242 (1965).
100 Kureš, H.: Development of airway resistance. Čslká Pediat. *27:* 274–276 (1972).
101 Kureš, H.: An additive method for airway resistance measurement. Acta Paediat.
     scand. *63:* 351–356 (1974).
102 Lindell, S.E.: Regional lung function and closing volume. Scand. J. resp. Dis., suppl.
     85 (1974).
103 Loosli, C.G.; Potter, E.L.: Pre- and postnatal development of the respiratory portion
     of the human lung. With special reference to the elastic fibers. Am. Rev. resp. Dis.
     80: suppl., p. 1 (1959).
104 Lyons, H.A.; Tanner, R.W.: Total lung volume and its subdivisions in children.
     Normal standards. J. appl. Physiol. *17:* 601–604 (1962).
105 Macklem, P.T.; Mead, J.: Resistance of central and peripheral airways measured by
     a retrograde catheter. J. appl. Physiol. *22:* 295–301 (1967).
106 Macklem, P.T.: Obstruction in small airways. A challenge to medicine. Am. J. Med.
     52: 721–724 (1972).
107 Macklem, P.T.: Workshop on screening programs for early diagnosis of airway
     obstruction. Am. Rev. resp. Dis. *109:* 567–571 (1974).
108 Macklem, P.T.; Permutt, S.: The lung in the transition between health and disease;
     1st ed. (Marcel Dekker, New York 1979).
109 Máček, M.; Vávra, J.: Cardiopulmonary and metabolic changes during exercise in
     children 6–14 years old. J. appl. Physiol. *30:* 202–204 (1971).
110 Mansell, A.; Dubrawski, C.; Levison, H.; Bryan, C.A.; Crosier, D.N.: Lung elastic
     recoil in cystic fibrosis. Am. Rev. resp. Dis. *109:* 190–197 (1974).
111 Mansell, A.L.; Bryan, A.C.; Levison, H.: Relationship of lung recoil to lung volume
     and maximum expiratory flow in normal children. J. appl. Physiol. *42:* 817–823
     (1977).
112 Mansell, A.L.; Bryan, A.C.; Lewison, H.: Airway closure in children. J. appl. Physiol.
     33: 711–714 (1972).
113 Matthys, H.; Keller, R.; Herzog, H.: Plethysmographic assessment of trapped air in
     man. Respiration *27:* 447–461 (1970).
114 McFaden, E.R., Jr.; Linden, D.A.: A reduction in maximum midexpiratory flow
     rate. A spirometric manifestation of small airway disease. Am. J. Med. *52:* 725–737
     (1972).
115 McFaden, E.R., Jr.; Ingram, R.H.: Peripheral airway obstruction. J. Am. med. Ass.
     235: 259–260 (1976).
116 Mead, J.: Volume displacement body plethysmograph for respiratory measurements
     in human subjects. J. appl. Physiol. *15:* 736–740 (1960).
117 Mead, J.: Mechanical properties of lungs. Physiol. Rev. *41:* 281–330 (1961).
118 Mead, J.; Turner, J.M.; Macklem, P.T.; Little, J.B.: Significance of the relationship
     between lung recoil and maximum expiratory flow. J. appl. Physiol. *22:* 95–108
     (1967).

119 Mellins, R.B.; Levine, O.R.; Ingram, R.H., Jr.; Fishman, A.P.: Obstructive disease of the airways in cystic fibrosis. Pediatrics, Springfield *41:* 560–573 (1968).

120 Michaelson, E.D.; Watson, H.; Silva, G.; Zapata, A.; Sefarini-Michaelson, S.M.; Sackner, M.A.: Pulmonary function in normal children. Bull. eur. Physio-path. resp. *14:* 525–550 (1978).

121 Milic-Emili, J.; Mead, J.; Turner, J.M.; Glauser, E.M.: Improved technique for estimating pleural pressure from esophageal balloons. J. appl. Physiol. *19:* 207–211 (1964).

122 Milic-Emili, J.; Mead, J.; Turner, J.M.: Topography of esophageal pressure as a function of posture in man. J. appl. Physiol. *19:* 212–216 (1964).

123 Milic-Emili, J.; Henderson, A.M.; Dolovich, B.; Trop, D.; Kaneko, K.: Regional distribution of inspired gas in the lung. J. appl. Physiol. *21:* 749–759 (1966).

124 Murray, A.B.; Cook, C.D.: Measurement of peak expiratory flow rates in 220 normal children from 4.5 to 18.5 years of age. J. Pediat. *62:* 186–189 (1963).

125 Muysers, K.; Smidt, U.: Respirations-Massenspektrometrie (Schattauer, Stuttgart 1960).

126 Nairn, J.R.; Bennet, A.J.; Andrew, J.D.; MacArthur, P.: A study of respiratory function in normal school children. Archs Dis. Childh. *36:* 253–258 (1961).

127 Navrátil, M.; Kadlec, K.; Daum, S.: Pathophysiology of respiration (SZN, Praha 1966).

128 Neergaard, K.; Wirz, K.: Über eine Methode zur Messung der Lungenelastizität am lebenden Menschen, insbesondere beim Emphysem. Z. klin. Med. *105:* 35–50 (1927).

129 Neergaard, K.; Wirz, K.: Die Messung der Strömungswiderstände in den Atemwegen des Menschen, insbesondere beim Asthma und Emphysem. Z. klin. Med. *105:* 51–82 (1927).

130 Neijens, H.J.; Wesselius, T.; Kerrebijn, K.F.: Exercise-induced bronchoconstriction as an expression of bronchial hyperreactivity. A study of its mechanism in children. Thorax *36:* 517–522 (1981).

131 Neuburger, N.; Levison, H.; Bryan, A.C.; Kruger, K.: Transit time analysis of the forced expiratory spirogram in growth. J. appl. Physiol. *40:* 329–332 (1976).

132 Neukirch, E.; Korobaeff, M.; Perdrizet, S.: Courbe débit-volume chez des enfants et des adolescents sains de 10 à 19 ans. Bull. eur. Physio-path. resp. *18:* 725–741 (1982).

133 Nolte, D.: Der bronchiale Strömungswiderstand im Kindesalter. Klin. Wschr. *46:* 783–786 (1968).

134 Nolte, D.: Zur Altersabhängigkeit des bronchialen Strömungswiderstandes und des intrathorakalen Gasvolumens. Beitr. klin. Erfol. Tuberk. Lungenkr. *139:* 80–89 (1969).

135 Otis, A.B.; McKerrow, C.B.; Barlett, R.A.; Mead, J.; McIlroy, M.B.; Silverstone, N.J.; Radford, E.P., Jr.: Mechanical factors in distribution of pulmonary ventilation. J. appl. Physiol. *8:* 427–443 (1956).

136 Otis, A.: The work of breathing. Physiol. Rev. *34:* 449–458 (1954).

137 Palka, M.J.: Spirometric predicted values for teenage boys. Relation to body composition and exercise performance. Bull. eur. Physio-path. resp. *18:* 59–64 (1982).

138 Paul, T.; Zapletal, A.; Šamánek, M.: Volume of 'trapped air' in obstructive lung diseases. Studia pneumol. phthisiol. czech. *32:* 11–16 (1972).

139 Paul, T.; Zapletal, A.; Šamánek, M.; Čopová, M.: Physical working capacity and work of breathing in idiopathic interstitial lung fibrosis. Čslká Pediat. *29:* 366–368 (1974).

140 Paul, T.; Zapletal, A.; Šamánek, M.; Špičák, V.; Čopová, M.: Physical fitness and effect of physical work on airway function. Čslká Pediat. *30:* 463–468 (1975).

141 Paul, T.; Šamánek, M.; Zapletal, A.: Gas exchange in patients after lung resection for bronchiectasis. Studia pneumol. phthisiol. czech. *37:* 556–558 (1977).

142 Peslin, R.; Bohadana, A.; Hannhart, B.; Jardin, P.: Comparison of various methods for reading maximal expiratory flow-volume curves. Am. Rev. resp. Dis. *119:* 831–838 (1979).

143 Phelan, P.D.; Williams, H.E.: Ventilatory studies in healthy infants. Pediat. Res. *3:* 425–432 (1969).

144 Pimmel, R.L.; Millner, T.K.; Fouke, J.M.; Eyles, J.G.: Time-constant histograms from the forced expired volume signal. J. appl. Physiol. *51:* 1581–1593 (1981).

145 Pistelli, G.; Paci, A.; Dalle Luche, A.; Giuntini, C.: Pulmonary volumes in children. II. Normal values in female children 6 to 15 years old. Bull. eur. Physio-path. resp. *14:* 513–523 (1978).

146 Polgar, G.; Promadhat, V.: Pulmonary function testing in children. Techniques and standards (Saunders, Philadelphia 1971).

147 Polgar, G.: Practical pulmonary physiology. Pediat. Clins N. Am. *20:* 303–322 (1973).

148 Polgar, G.: Airway resistance in the newborn infant. J. Pediat. *59:* 915–921 (1961).

149 Polgar, G.; Weng, I.R.: The functional development of the respiratory system. Am. Rev. resp. Dis. *120:* 625–695 (1979).

150 Pride, N.B.; Permutt, S.; Riley, R.L.; Bromberger-Barnea, B.: Determinants of maximal expiratory flow from the lungs. J. appl. Physiol. *23:* 646–662 (1967).

151 Quanjer, P.H.: Standardized lung function testing. Bull. eur. Physio-path. resp., suppl. 5 (1983).

152 Quanjer, P.H.; Polgar, G.; Wise, M.; Karlberg, J.; Borsboom, G.: Compilation of reference values for lung function measurements in children (Leiden 1983).

153 Rodenstein, D.O.; Stanescu, D.C.; Francis, C.: Demonstration of failure of body plethysmography in airway obstruction. J. appl. Physiol. *52:* 949–954 (1982).

154 Rodenstein, D.O.; Stanescu, D.C.: Frequency dependence of plethysmographic volume in healthy and asthmatic subjects. J. appl. Physiol. *54:* 159–169 (1983).

155 Rohrer, F.: Der Strömungswiderstand in den menschlichen Atemwegen und der Einfluss der unregelmässigen Verzweigung des Bronchialsystems auf den Atmungsverlauf verschiedener Lungenbezirke. Arch. ges. Physiol. *162:* 225–299 (1915).

156 Ruth, C.; Šamánek, M.: Distribution of pulmonary blood flow in idiopathic interstitial lung fibrosis. Čslká Pediat. *29:* 363–366 (1974).

157 Ruth, C.; Šamánek, M.: Lung scintigraphy significance after lung resection in children and adolescents. Studia pneumol. phthisiol. czech. *38:* 33–35 (1978).

158 Salazar, E.; Knowles, J.H.: An analysis of pressure-volume characteristics of the lungs. J. appl. Physiol. *19:* 97–104 (1964).

159 Seely, J.E.; Zuskin, E.; Bouhuys, A.: Cigarette smoking: Objective evidence for lung damage in teenagers. Science *173:* 741–743 (1971).

160 Seliger, V.: Physical fitness of Czechoslovak children at 12–15 years of age. Acta Univ. Carol. Gymn. *5:* 1–69 (1970).

161 Schachter, E.N.; Kreisman, H.; Littner, M.; Beck, G.J.: Airway response to exercise in mild asthmatics. Ann. Allergy clin. Immunol. *61:* 390–398 (1978).

162 Schoenberg, J.B.; Beck, G.J.; Bouhuys, A.: Growth and decay of pulmonary function in healthy blacks and whites. Resp. Physiol. *33:* 367–393 (1978).

163 Schrader, P.C.; Quanjer, P.H.; Zomeren, B.C. van; De Groodt, E.G.; Wever, A.M.J.; Wise, M.E.: Selection of variables from maximum expiratory flow-volume curves. Bull. eur. Physio-path. resp. *19:* 43–49 (1983).

164 Snedecor, G.W.; Cochran, G.W.: Statistical methods (Iowa State University Press, Ames 1967).

165 Stanescu, D.C.; Rodenstein, D.O.; Cauberghs, M.; Woestijne, K.P. van de: Failure of body plethysmography in bronchial asthma. J. appl. Physiol. *52:* 939–948 (1982).

166 Strang, L.B.: The ventilatory capacity of normal children. Thorax *14:* 305–310 (1959).

167 Suchý, J.: Developmental anthropology of inhabitants in ČSR, pp. 115–119 (Charles University, Praha 1972).

168 Svenonius, E.; Kautto, R.; Arborelius, M., Jr.: Flow-volume measurements with a spirometer. Results from healthy children. Lung *157:* 201–208 (1980).

169 Šamánek, M.; Paul, T.; Ruth, C.; Tůma, S.; Zapletal, A.: Regional lung function in children. Čslká Pediat. *28:* 535–539 (1973).

170 Šamánek, M.; Ruth, C.; Zapletal, A.; Paul, T.: Regional ventilation in patients with idiopathic interstitial lung fibrosis. Čslká Pediat. *29:* 373–375 (1974).

171 Šamánek, M.; Zapletal, A.; Mišúr, M.; Ruth, C.: Differences between static and dynamic lung compliance in healthy children. Bull. Physio-path. resp. *7:* 815–816 (1971).

172 Šamánek, M.; Ruth, C.: Indications of radioisotopes studies in respiratory and cardiovascular diseases. Čslká Pediat. *29:* 267–272 (1974).

173 Šamánek, M.: Local regulations of lung ventilation and perfusion. Čas. Lék. Čes. *105:* 1303–1307 (1966).

174 Šamánek, M.; Ruth, C.; Hloušková, Z.: Regional lung function after lung resection in childhood. Studia pneumol. phthisiol. czech. *38:* 29–32 (1978).

175 Šamánek, M.; Ruth, C.: Lung perfusion scintigraphy (Avicenum, Praha 1979).

176 Tattersall, S.F.; Benson, M.K.; Hunter, D.; Mansel, A.; Pride, N.B.; Fletcher, C.M.: The use and tests of peripheral lung function for predicting future disability from airway flow obstruction in middle-aged smokers. Am. Rev. resp. Dis. *118:* 1035–1050 (1978).

177 Taussig, L.M.; Chernick, V.M.D.; Wood, R.M.D.; Farrell, P.M.D.; Mellins, R.B.: Standardization of lung function testing in children. J. Pediat. *97:* 668–676 (1980).

178 Thiemann, H.H.: Normwerte der Lungenfunktionsdiagnostik im Kindesalter. Z. Erkrank. Atm.-Org. *145:* 249–257 (1976).

179 Tlustý, L.; Hloušková, Z.; Daum, S.: Normal values of lung diffusing capacity in children and adolescents. Čslká Pediat. *26:* 474–477 (1971).

180 Todisco, T.; Grassi, V.; Dottorini, M.; Sorbini, C.A.: Reference values for flow-volume curves during forced vital capacity breathing in male children and young adults. Respiration *39:* 1–7 (1980).

181 Tůma, S.; Šamánek, M.; Pražský, F.; Čopová, M.; Zapletal, A.: Pulmonary blood bed in idiopathic interstitial lung fibrosis. Čslká Pediat. *29:* 369–372 (1974).

182 Turner, J.M.; Mead, J.; Wohl, M.E.: Elasticity of human lungs in relation to age. J. appl. Physiol. *25:* 664–671 (1968).

183 Van de Woestijne, K.P.; Trop, D.; Clément, J.: Influence of the mediastinum on the measurement of esophageal pressure and lung compliance in man. Pflügers Arch. ges. Physiol. *323:* 323–341 (1971).

184 Van de Woestijne, K.P.; Zapletal, A.: The maximum expiratory flow-volume curve: peak flow and effort independent portion; in Bouhuys, Airway dynamics, vol. 11, pp. 61–72 (Thomas, Springfield 1970).

185 Van de Woestijne, K.P.: Spécificité des tests proposés pour le dépistage de la maladie des petites voies aériennes. Bull. eur. Physio-path. resp. *12:* 477–486 (1967).

186 Vávrová, V.; Mrzena, B.; Vokáč, Z.: pH, PCO_2 et composants nonrespiratoire de l'équilibre acido-basique de sang cutané artérialisé chez 97 enfants sains, âgés de 3 mois à 15 ans. Poumon Cœur *25:* 1121–1126 (1969).

187 Vojtek, V.; Koďousek, R.; Šerý, Z.; Berková, I.; Vortel, V.; Fingerland, A.; Hájek, V.; Kučera, K.; Dvořák, J.: Primary disseminated adiaspiromycosis of lungs caused by *Emmonsia crescens.* Studia pneumol. phthisiol. czech. *30:* 97–98 (1970).

188 Vokáč, Z.; Vávrová, V.: Blood gases as a criterion of respiratory disorders. Čslká Pediat. *19:* 961–972 (1964).

189 Von der Hardt, H.; Logvinoff, M.M.; Dickreiter, J.; Geubelle, F.: Static recoil of the lungs and static compliance in healthy children. Respiration *32:* 325–339 (1975).

190 Von der Hardt, H.; Nowak-Beneke, R.: Lung volumes in healthy boys and girls, 6–15 years of age. Lung *154:* 51–63 (1976).

191 Weibel, E.R.: Morphometry of the human lung (Springer, Berlin 1963).

192 Weinrich, R.; Wuthe, H.; Weinrich, C.; Müller, E.; Vogel, J.: Referenzwerte respiratorischer Funktionsparameter im Kindesalter. IV. Bodyplethysmographische Referenzwerte. Dt. GesundhWes. *33:* 1887–1892 (1978).

193 Wellmann, J.J.; Brown, R.; Ingram, R.H., Jr.; Mead, J.; McFaden, E.R., Jr.: Effect of volume history on successive partial expiratory flow-volume maneuvers. J. appl. Physiol. *41:* 153–158 (1976).

194 Weng, T.R.; Levison, H.: Standards of pulmonary function in children. Am. Rev. resp. Dis. *99:* 879–894 (1969).

195 Wiesemann, H.; Hardt, H. von der: Reliability of flow-volume measurements in children. Respiration *41:* 181–187 (1981).

196 Williams, H.E.; Phelan, P.D.: Respiratory illness in children (Blackwell, Oxford 1975).

197 Woolcock, A.J.; Vincent, N.J.; Macklem, P.T.: Frequency dependence of compliance as a test for obstruction in the small airways. J. clin. Invest. *48:* 1097–1106 (1969).

198 Worth, H.; Smidt, U.: Phase II of expiratory curves of respiratory and inert gases in normal and in patients with emphysema. Bull. eur. Physio-path. resp. *18:* 247–253 (1982).

199 Wu, B.; Motoyama, E.K.; Leuchtenberg, N. de; Zapletal, A.; Cook, C.D.: Peripheral airway obstruction in children with heart disease. Am. Pediat. Soc. 80th Meet. Proc., 1970, p. 153.

200 Wuthe, H.; Petro, W.; Müller, E.; Wotzka, G.; Vogel, J.: Referenzwerte respiratorischer Funktionsparameter im Kindesalter. I. Referenzwerte des Closing volume und Slope-Index. Dt. GesundhWes. *32:* 1136–1142 (1977).

201 Wuthe, H.; Pechmann, H.; Müller, E.; Vogel, J.: Referenzwerte respiratorischer Funktionsparameter im Kindesalter. VIII. Referenzwerte für den oszillatorischen Atemtraktwiderstand. Dt. GesundhWest *35:* 592–595 (1980).

202 Zapletal, A.; Motoyama, E.K.; Woestijne, K.P. van de; Gibson, L.E.; Bouhuys, A.: Use of the body plethysmography in children. Prog. resp. Res. *4:* 228–235 (1969).

203 Zapletal, A.; Motoyama, E.K.; Woestijne, K.P. van de; Hunt, V.R.; Bouhuys, A.: Maximum expiratory flow-volume curves and airway conductance in children and adolescents. J. appl. Physiol. *26:* 308–316 (1969).

204 Zapletal, A.; Motoyama, E.K.; Woestijne, K.P. van de; Bouhuys, A.: Maximum expiratory flows in healthy children and cystic fibrosis. Vnitřní lék. *16:* 323–336 (1970).

205 Zapletal, A.: Dynamic and static lung compliance in children with chronic respiratory disease. Prog. resp. Res. *6:* 533–539 (1971).

206 Zapletal, A.; Motoyama, E.K.; Gibson, L.E.; Bouhuys, A.: Pulmonary mechanics in asthma and cystic fibrosis. Pediatrics, Springfield *48:* 64–72 (1971).

207 Zapletal, A.; Mišúr, M.; Šamánek, M.: Static recoil pressure of the lungs in children. Bull. Physio-path. resp. *7:* 139–143 (1971).

208 Zapletal, A.; Paul, T.; Janoušková, A.; Šamánek, M.; Vojtek, V.: Pulmonary function tests in a child with disseminated adiaspiromycosis of the lungs caused by the fungus *Emmonsia crescens.* Acta Univ. Palack. Olomouc. Facult. Med. Tom. *63:* 31–42 (1972).

209 Zapletal, A.; Šamánek, M.; Paul, T.: Lung elasticity indices in healthy children and adolescents. Čslká Pediat. *27:* 276–281 (1972).

210 Zapletal, A.; Paul, T.; Čopová, M.; Vávrová, V.; Šamánek, M.: Lung recoil pressure and maximum expiratory flows in children with lung obstruction. Studia pneumol. phthisiol. czech. *32:* 4–10 (1972).

211 Zapletal, A.; Šamánek, M.; Tůma, S.; Ruth, C.; Paul, T.: Assessment of airway function in children. Bull. Physio-path. resp. *8:* 535–543 (1972).

212 Zapletal, A.; Šamánek, M.: Pulmonary elasticity during growth and aging. Bull. Physio-path. resp. *9:* 1231–1233 (1973).

213 Zapletal, A.: Work of breathing. Vnitřní lék. *19:* 561–573 (1973).

214 Zapletal, A.; Jech, J.; Paul, T.; Šamánek, M.: Pulmonary function studies in children living in an air-polluted area. Am. Rev. resp. Dis. *107:* 400–409 (1973).

215 Zapletal, A.; Paul, T.; Šamánek, M.; Čopová, M.; Suková, B.: Significance of lung mechanics and volumes in idiopathic interstitial lung fibrosis. Čslká Pediat. *29:* 375–381 (1974).

216 Zapletal, A.; Šamánek, M.: Maximum expiratory flows and forced expiratory volumes. Normal values in children and adolescents. Čas. Lék. česk. *113:* 1225–1232 (1974).

217 Zapletal, A.; Šamánek, M.: Lung elasticity in healthy children and in children with lung disease. Proc. XIVth Int. Congr. Pediatrics, Buenos Aires 1974, vol. 11, pp. 131–133.

218 Zapletal, A.: Airway mechanics, airway resistance and mechanisms of airway obstruction in children. Proc. XIVth Int. Congr. Pediatrics, Buenos Aires 1974, vol. 11, pp. 134–136.

219 Zapletal, A.; Šamánek, M.; Rakowská, S.; Čopová, M.; Suková, B.: Airway function after inhalation of bronchodilators. Čas. Lék. Česk. *114:* 644–650 (1975).

220 Zapletal, A.; Paul, T.; Šamánek, M.: Pulmonary elasticity in children and adolescents. J. appl. Physiol. *40:* 953–961 (1976).

221 Zapletal, A.; Paul, T.; Šamánek, M.: Normal values of static lung volumes and ventilation in children and adolescents. Čslká Pediat. *31:* 532–539 (1976).

222 Zapletal, A.; Šamánek, M.; Paul, T.; Hloušková, Z.: Airway patency, lung elasticity and volumes in patients after lung resection for bronchiectasis in childhood. Studia pneumol. phthisiol. czech. *37:* 550–553 (1977).

223 Zapletal, A.; Šamánek, M.: Airway and pulmonary resistance in children and adolescents. Normal values significance in airway obstruction assessment. Čslká Pediat. *32:* 513–522 (1977).

224 Zapletal, A.; Šamánek, M.; Hloušková, Z.; Špičák, V.; Čopová, M.: Variability of airway obstruction in asthmatics assessed by methods of lung function testing. Čslká Pediat. *32:* 406–413 (1977).

225 Zapletal, A.; Jech, J.; Kašpar, J.; Šamánek, M.: Flow-volume curves as a method for detecting airway obstruction in children from an air-polluted area. Bull. eur. Physiopath. resp. *13:* 803–812 (1977).

226 Zapletal, A.; Paul, T.: Šamánek, M.: Die Bedeutung heutiger Methoden der Lungenfunktionsdiagnostik zur Feststellung einer Obstruktion der Atemwege bei Kindern und Jugendlichen. Z. Erkrank. Atm.-Org. *149:* 343–371 (1977).

227 Zapletal, A.; Šamánek, M.: Volume of isoflow in the detection of airway obstruction and abnormalities of lung elasticity in man. Bull. eur. Physio-path. resp. *14:* 265–277 (1978).

228 Zapletal, A.; Houštěk, J.; Šamánek, M.; Vávrová, V.; Šrajer, V.: Lung function abnormalities in cystic fibrosis and changes during growth. Bull. eur. Physio-path. resp. *15:* 575–592 (1979).

229 Zapletal, A.; Paul, T.; Šamánek, M.: Contemporary possibilities of airway obstruction assessment by methods of lung function testing. Čslká Pediat. *38:* 449–456 (1978).

230 Zapletal, A.; Paul, T.; Šamánek, M.: Lung function investigation by body plethysmography; in Houštěk, Studěnikin, Actual problems in pediatrics (Avicenum, Praha 1980).

231 Zapletal, A.; Šamánek, M.: Lung elasticity in physiology and pathology in childhood; in Houštěk, Studěnikin, Actual problems in pediatrics (Avicenum, Praha 1980).

232 Zapletal, A.; Paul, T.; Vislocký, I.; Šamánek, M.: Functional manifestations of restrictive lung processes. Studia pneumol. phthisiol. czech. *41:* 86–94 (1981).

233 Zapletal, A.: Small airway function in children and adolescents in health and disease. Prog. resp. Res. *17:* 52–67 (1981).

234 Zapletal, A.; Zbojan, J.; Filipská, A.; Šamánek, M.; Špičák, V.: Effect of long-acting bronchodilators and repeated dosage on airway patency in asthmatic children assessed by 'flow-volume' curves. Čslká Pediat. *36:* 626–634 (1981).

235 Zapletal, A.; Vávrová, V.; Štefanová, J.; Hořák, J.; Šamánek, M.: Lung function studies in assessment of chest physiotherapy and mucolytic therapy in cystic fibrosis. Čslká Pediat. *38:* 519–524 (1983).
236 Zapletal, A.; Šamánek, M.; Paul, T.: Upstream and total airway conductance in children and adolescents. Bull. eur. Physio-path. resp. *18:* 31–37 (1982).
237 Zapletal, A.; Hloušková, Z.; Šamánek, M.: Lung function in patients with repeated bronchitis from childhood. Čslká Pediat. *31:* 665–671 (1976).
238 Zapletal, A.; Štefanová, J.; Hořák, J.; Vávrová, V.; Šamánek, M.: Chest physiotherapy and airway obstruction in patients with cystic fibrosis. A negative report. Eur. J. resp. Dis. *64:* 426–433 (1983).
239 Zapletal, A.; Šamánek, M.: Lung elasticity in children and adolescents with lung disease. Mod. Probl. Pediat., vol. 21, pp. 27–44 (Karger, Basel 1982).
240 Zapletal, A.; Houštěk, J.; Šamánek, M.; Čopová, M.; Paul, T.: Lung function in children and adolescents with idiopathic interstitial pulmonary fibrosis. Pediat. Pulmonol. *1:* 154–166 (1985).
241 Baran, D.; Yernault, J.C.; Paiva, M.; Englert, M.: Static mechanical lung properties in healthy children. Scand. J. resp. Dis. *57:* 139–147 (1976).
242 Dab, I.; Alexander, F.: A simplified approach to the measurement of specific airway resistance. Pediat. Res. *10:* 996–999 (1976).
243 Haluszka, J.; Branski, H.: Die Beurteilung des Gasaustausches in der Lunge bei Kindern. Z. Erkrank. Atm.-Org. *157:* 297–303 (1981).
244 Solymar, L.; Aronsson, P.H.; Bake, B.; Bjure, J.: Nitrogen single breath test, flow-volume curves and spirometry in healthy children, 7–18 years of age. Eur. J. resp. Dis. *61:* 275–286 (1980).
245 Jaeger, M.J.; Otis, A.B.: Measurement of airway resistance with a volume displacement body plethysmograph. J. appl. Physiol. *19:* 813–820 (1964).
246 Jaeger, M.J.; Bouhuys, A.: Loop formation in pressure vs. flow diagrams obtained by body plethysmographic techniques. Prog. Resp. Res. *4:* 116–130 (1969).

Addendum

Explanations to Tables

Abbreviations:

SD y·x; SD log y·x = Standard deviation of y value on x value from the regression line or curve.

SD = Standard deviation from the mean.

n = Number of subjects studied.

r = Correlation coefficient between functional and somatometric parameters.

Small differences for the same reference functional values given in the columns of tables and those computed according to the regression equations are due to the smaller decimal numbers given in the regression equations and standard deviations in tables.

Contents to Tables

I. Static Lung Volumes and Lung Ventilation
   Tables 1–88 114

II. Lung Elasticity
   Tables 89–166 148

III. Airway Patency
   Tables 167–248 173

IV. Work of Breathing
   Tables 249–266 205

V. Gas Exchange in the Lungs
   Tables 267–283 210

Table 1. Vital capacity (VC) in relation to body height in boys and girls

Height cm	VC, ml		
	mean	lower limits	upper limits
115	1,385	1,157	1,658
116	1,418	1,185	1,698
118	1,486	1,241	1,779
120	1,556	1,300	1,862
122	1,627	1,359	1,948
124	1,701	1,421	2,036
126	1,777	1,484	2,127
128	1,855	1,549	2,220
130	1,935	1,616	2,316
132	2,017	1,685	2,414
134	2,101	1,755	2,515
136	2,188	1,828	2,619
138	2,277	1,902	2,725
140	2,368	1,978	2,834
142	2,461	2,056	2,946
144	2,556	2,136	3,060
146	2,654	2,218	3,177
148	2,755	2,301	3,297
150	2,857	2,387	3,420
152	2,962	2,475	3,546
154	3,070	2,564	3,674
156	3,179	2,656	3,806
158	3,292	2,750	3,940
160	3,406	2,846	4,077
162	3,524	2,944	4,218
164	3,643	3,044	4,361
166	3,766	3,146	4,507
168	3,891	3,251	4,657
170	4,018	3,357	4,810
172	4,148	3,466	4,965
174	4,281	3,577	5,124
176	4,416	3,690	5,286
178	4,554	3,805	5,451
180	4,695	3,923	5,620

Formula: log y = a + b·log x;
y = VC (ml); x = body height (cm);
log VC (ml) = – 2.4716 + 2.7240·log height (cm);
SD log y·x = ± 0.0395; n = 173; r = + 0.94.

Table 2. Vital capacity (VC) in relation to age in boys and girls

Age years	VC, ml		
	mean	lower limits	upper limits
6	1,397	1,027	1,901
7	1,656	1,217	2,253
8	1,919	1,410	2,610
9	2,185	1,606	2,972
10	2,454	1,803	3,338
11	2,725	2,003	3,708
12	3,000	2,205	4,081
13	3,276	2,408	4,458
14	3,555	2,613	4,837
15	3,836	2,820	5,220
16	4,119	3,027	5,604
17	4,404	3,237	5,992

Formula: log y = a + b·log x;
y = VC (ml); x = age (years);
log VC (ml) = 2.2877 + 1.1021·log age (years);
SD log y·x = ± 0.0677; n = 173; r = + 0.82.

Table 3. Vital capacity (VC) in relation to body surface in boys and girls

Body surface m²	VC, ml		
	mean	lower limits	upper limits
0.6	1,030	828	1,281
0.7	1,261	1,014	1,568
0.8	1,501	1,207	1,867
0.9	1,752	1,409	2,178
1.0	2,011	1,617	2,500
1.1	2,278	1,832	2,832
1.2	2,552	2,053	3,174
1.3	2,834	2,279	3,524
1.4	3,123	2,511	3,883
1.5	3,418	2,749	4,250
1.6	3,719	2,991	4,635
1.7	4,026	3,238	5,006
1.8	4,339	3,489	5,395
1.9	4,657	3,745	5,791
2.0	4,980	4,005	6,193

Formula: log y = a + b·log x;
y = VC (ml); x = body surface (m²);
log VC (ml) = 3.3034 + 1.3084·log body surface (m²);
SD log y·x = ± 0.0479; n = 173; r = + 0.91.

Table 4. Vital capacity (VC) in relation to body height in boys

Height cm	VC, ml		
	mean	lower limits	upper limits
115	1,418	1,238	1,623
116	1,452	1,269	1,662
118	1,523	1,330	1,743
120	1,596	1,394	1,827
122	1,671	1,460	1,912
124	1,748	1,527	2,001
126	1,828	1,597	2,092
128	1,909	1,668	2,186
130	1,994	1,742	2,282
132	2,080	1,817	2,381
134	2,169	1,895	2,482
136	2,260	1,974	2,587
138	2,354	1,056	2,694
140	2,450	2,140	2,804
142	2,548	2,226	2,917
144	2,649	2,315	3,032
146	2,753	2,405	3,151
148	2,859	2,498	3,273
150	2,968	2,593	3,397
152	3,079	2,690	3,524
154	3,193	2,790	3,655
156	3,310	2,892	3,788
158	3,429	2,996	3,925
160	3,551	3,102	4,065
162	3,676	3,211	4,207
164	3,803	3,323	4,353
166	3,934	3,437	4,503
168	4,067	3,553	4,655
170	4,203	3,672	4,811
172	4,342	3,793	4,970
174	4,484	3,917	5,132
176	4,629	4,044	5,298
178	4,776	4,173	5,467
180	4,927	4,304	5,639

Formula: log y = a + b·log x;
y = VC (ml); x = body height (cm);
log VC (ml) = −2.5768 + 2.7799·log height (cm);
SD log y·x = ±0.0294; n = 86; r = +0.96.

Table 5. Vital capacity (VC) in relation to age in boys

Age years	VC, ml		
	mean	lower limits	upper limits
6	1,462	1,087	1,965
7	1,728	1,285	2,324
8	1,999	1,486	2,688
9	2,272	1,689	3,055
10	2,548	1,895	3,426
11	2,826	2,102	3,800
12	3,107	2,310	4,178
13	3,389	2,521	4,558
14	3,674	2,732	4,940
15	3,960	2,945	5,325
16	4,248	3,159	5,713
17	4,538	3,375	6,102

Formula: log y = a + b·log x;
y = VC (ml); x = age (years);
log VC (ml) = 2.3186 + 1.0876·log age (years);
SD log y·x = ±0.0646; n = 86; r = +0.82.

Table 6. Vital capacity (VC) in relation to body surface in boys

Body surface m²	VC, ml		
	mean	lower limits	upper limits
0.6	1,055	859	1,297
0.7	1,297	1,055	1,594
0.8	1,551	1,262	1,906
0.9	1,815	1,477	2,231
1.0	2,090	1,701	2,569
1.1	2,374	1,932	2,918
1.2	2,667	2,170	3,278
1.3	2,969	2,415	3,649
1.4	3,278	2,667	4,029
1.5	3,595	2,925	4,418
1.6	3,919	3,189	4,816
1.7	4,250	3,458	5,223
1.8	4,587	3,733	5,638
1.9	4,931	4,012	6,061
2.0	5,282	4,297	6,491

Formula: log y = a + b·log x;
y = VC (ml); x = body surface (m²);
log VC (ml) = 3.3202 + 1.3370 log body surface (m²);
SD log y·x = ±0.0450; n = 86; r = +0.91.

Table 7. Vital capacity (VC) in relation to body height in girls

Height cm	VC, ml		
	mean	lower limits	upper limits
115	1,365	1,128	1,651
116	1,396	1,154	1,689
118	1,461	1,207	1,767
120	1,527	1,262	1,847
122	1,595	1,318	1,930
124	1,665	1,376	2,014
126	1,736	1,435	2,101
128	1,810	1,496	2,190
130	1,886	1,559	2,281
132	1,963	1,623	2,375
134	2,043	1,688	2,471
136	2,124	1,756	2,569
138	2,207	1,824	2,670
140	2,293	1,895	2,774
142	2,380	1,967	2,879
144	2,469	2,041	2,987
146	2,561	2,117	3,098
148	2,654	2,194	3,211
150	2,750	2,273	3,327
152	2,848	2,354	3,445
154	2,948	2,436	3,566
156	3,050	2,521	3,689
158	3,154	2,607	3,815
160	3,260	2,695	3,944
162	3,369	2,784	4,075
164	3,479	2,876	4,209
166	3,592	2,969	4,346
168	3,708	3,065	4,485
170	3,825	3,162	4,628
172	3,945	3,261	4,772
174	4,067	3,362	4,920
176	4,191	3,465	5,071
178	4,318	3,569	5,224
180	4,447	3,676	5,380

Formula: $\log y = a + b \cdot \log x$;
$y = VC$ (ml); x = body height (cm);
$\log VC$ (ml) $= -2.2970 + 2.6361 \cdot \log x$;
SD $\log y \cdot x = \pm 0.0415$; $n = 87$; $r = +0.94$.

Table 8. Vital capacity (VC) in relation to age in girls

Age years	VC, ml		
	mean	lower limits	upper limits
6	1,360	996	1,856
7	1,608	1,176	2,195
8	1,860	1,363	2,539
9	2,115	1,550	2,886
10	2,372	1,738	3,237
11	2,632	1,928	3,591
12	2,893	2,120	3,948
13	3,157	2,313	4,308
14	3,422	2,508	4,670
15	3,690	2,704	5,035
16	3,958	2,901	5,402
17	4,228	3,099	5,770

Formula: $\log y = a + b \cdot \log x$;
$y = VC$ (ml); x = age (year);
$\log VC$ (ml) $= 2.2860 + 1.0892 \cdot \log$ age (years);
SD $\log y \cdot x = \pm 0.0678$; $n = 87$; $r = +0.83$.

Table 9. Vital capacity (VC) in relation to body surface in girls

Body surface m²	VC, ml		
	mean	lower limits	upper limits
0.6	1,010	831	1,227
0.7	1,229	1,011	1,494
0.8	1,457	1,199	1,771
0.9	1,694	1,394	2,058
1.0	1,937	1,594	2,354
1.1	2,188	1,801	2,659
1.2	2,445	2,012	2,971
1.3	2,708	2,228	3,290
1.4	2,976	2,449	3,616
1.5	3,250	2,675	3,949
1.6	3,529	2,904	4,288
1.7	3,812	3,138	4,632
1.8	4,101	3,375	4,983
1.9	4,394	3,616	5,339
2.0	4,691	3,860	5,700

Formula: $\log y = a + b \cdot \log x$;
$y = VC$ (ml); x = body surface (m²);
$\log VC$ (ml) $= 3.2873 + 1.2754 \cdot \log$ body surface (m²);
SD $\log y \cdot x = \pm 0.0425$; $n = 87$; $r = +0.93$.

Table 10. Total lung capacity measured in a body plethysmograph (TLC_{box}) in relation to body height in boys and girls

Height cm	TLC$_{box}$ ml		
	mean	lower limits	upper limits
115	1,909	1,637	2,227
116	1,953	1,674	2,278
118	2,041	1,750	2,380
120	2,132	1,827	2,486
122	2,225	1,907	2,595
124	2,320	1,989	2,706
126	2,418	2,073	2,820
128	2,519	2,159	2,938
130	2,622	2,248	3,058
132	2,727	2,338	3,181
134	2,835	2,431	3,307
136	2,946	2,526	3,436
138	3,060	2,623	3,569
140	3,176	2,723	3,704
142	3,294	2,824	3,842
144	3,415	2,928	3,984
146	3,539	3,035	4,128
148	3,666	3,143	4,276
150	3,796	3,254	4,427
152	3,928	3,368	4,581
154	4,063	3,483	4,739
156	4,201	3,602	4,900
158	4,341	3,722	5,064
160	4,485	3,845	5,231
162	4,631	3,971	5,402
164	4,781	4,099	5,576
166	4,933	4,229	5,754
168	5,088	4,362	5,934
170	5,246	4,498	6,119
172	5,407	4,636	6,307
174	5,571	4,777	6,498
176	5,738	4,920	6,693
178	5,909	5,066	6,891
180	6,082	5,214	7,093

Formula: $\log y = a + b \cdot \log x$;
$y = TLC_{box}$ (ml); x = body height (cm);
$\log TLC_{box}$ (ml) = $-2.0467 + 2.5853 \cdot \log$ height (cm);
SD $\log y \cdot x = \pm 0.0338$; $n = 154$; $r = +0.96$.

Table 11. Total lung capacity measured in a body plethysmograph (TLC_{box}) in relation to age in boys and girls

Age years	TLC$_{box}$ ml		
	mean	lower limits	upper limits
6	1,941	1,469	2,566
7	2,281	1,726	3,015
8	2,623	1,985	3,467
9	2,968	2,245	3,923
10	3,314	2,507	4,380
11	3,662	2,771	4,840
12	4,011	3,035	5,301
13	4,362	3,300	5,765
14	4,714	3,566	6,230
15	5,067	3,834	6,697
16	5,421	4,102	7,165
17	5,776	4,371	7,635

Formula: $\log y = a + b \cdot \log x$;
$y = TLC_{box}$ (ml); x = age (years);
$\log TLC_{box}$ (ml) = $2.4734 + 1.0469 \cdot \log$ age (years);
SD $\log y \cdot x = \pm 0.0613$; $n = 154$; $r = +0.84$.

Table 12. Total lung capacity measured in a body plethysmograph (TLC_{box}) in relation to body surface in boys and girls

Body surface m^2	TLC$_{box}$ ml		
	mean	lower limits	upper limits
0.6	1,465	1,191	1,801
0.7	1,769	1,439	2,175
0.8	2,083	1,694	2,562
0.9	2,406	1,957	2,959
1.0	2,738	2,226	3,366
1.1	3,076	2,502	3,783
1.2	3,422	2,783	4,208
1.3	3,775	3,070	4,641
1.4	4,133	3,361	5,082
1.5	4,497	3,657	5,530
1.6	4,867	3,958	5,985
1.7	5,242	4,263	6,446
1.8	5,622	4,572	6,913
1.9	6,007	4,885	7,386
2.0	6,396	5,201	7,864

Formula: $\log y = a + b \cdot \log x$;
$y = TLC_{box}$ (ml); x = body surface (cm^2);
$\log TLC_{box}$ (ml) = $3.4374 + 1.2240 \cdot \log$ body surface (m^2);
SD $\log y \cdot x = \pm 0.0454$; $n = 154$; $r = +0.92$.

Table 13. Total lung capacity measured in a body plethysmograph (TLC_{box}) in relation to body height in boys

Height cm	TLC$_{box}$, ml		
	mean	lower limits	upper limits
115	1,966	1,732	2,232
116	2,011	1,771	2,283
118	2,101	1,851	2,385
120	2,194	1,932	2,490
122	2,289	2,016	2,599
124	2,387	2,102	2,709
126	2,487	2,109	2,823
128	2,589	2,281	2,940
130	2,695	2,374	3,059
132	2,803	2,469	3,182
134	2,913	2,566	3,307
136	3,026	2,666	3,436
138	3,142	2,767	3,567
140	3,260	2,872	3,701
142	3,381	2,978	3,839
144	3,505	3,087	3,979
146	3,631	3,199	4,123
148	3,761	3,313	4,269
150	3,893	3,429	4,419
152	4,028	3,548	4,572
154	4,165	3,669	4,729
156	4,306	3,793	4,888
158	4,449	3,919	5,051
160	4,595	4,048	5,217
162	4,744	4,179	5,386
164	4,896	4,313	5,558
166	5,051	4,449	5,734
168	5,209	4,587	5,914
170	5,370	4,730	6,096
172	5,534	4,874	6,282
174	5,701	5,021	6,472
176	5,870	5,171	6,665
178	6,043	5,323	6,861
180	6,220	5,468	7,061

Formula: $\log y = a + b \cdot \log x$;
$y = TLC_{box}$ (ml); x = body height (cm);
$\log TLC_{box}$ (ml) = $-2.0018 + 2.5698 \cdot \log$ height (cm);
SD $\log y \cdot x = \pm 0.0276$; n = 82; r = +0.96.

Table 14. Total lung capacity measured in a body plethysmograph (TLC_{box}) in relation to age in boys

Age years	TLC$_{box}$, ml		
	mean	lower limits	upper limits
6	2,017	1,542	2,638
7	2,359	1,804	3,086
8	2,703	2,066	3,535
9	3,046	2,329	3,984
10	3,391	2,593	4,435
11	3,736	2,857	4,886
12	4,082	3,121	5,338
13	4,428	3,386	5,791
14	4,775	3,651	6,244
15	5,122	3,916	6,698
16	5,469	4,182	7,152
17	5,817	4,448	7,607

Formula: $\log y = a + b \cdot \log x$;
$y = TLC_{box}$ (ml); x = age (years);
$\log TLC_{box}$ (ml) = $2.5136 + 1.0167 \cdot \log$ age (years);
SD $\log y \cdot x = \pm 0.0585$; n = 82; r = +0.83.

Table 15. Total lung capacity measured in a body plethysmograph (TLC_{box}) relation to body surface in boys

Body surface m^2	TLC$_{box}$, ml		
	mean	lower limits	upper limits
0.6	1,497	1,244	1,803
0.7	1,813	1,506	2,182
0.8	2,139	1,777	2,575
0.9	2,475	2,056	2,980
1.0	2,821	2,343	3,396
1.1	3,175	2,637	3,822
1.2	3,536	2,937	4,258
1.3	3,905	3,244	4,702
1.4	4,281	3,556	5,154
1.5	4,664	3,874	5,615
1.6	5,052	4,196	6,082
1.7	5,447	4,524	6,557
1.8	5,846	4,856	7,039
1.9	6,252	5,193	7,527
2.0	6,662	5,534	8,021

Formula: $\log y = a + b \cdot \log x$;
$y = TLC_{box}$ (ml); x = body surface (m^2);
$\log TLC_{box}$ (ml) = $3.4504 + 1.2397 \cdot \log$ body surface (m^2);
SD $\log y \cdot x = \pm 0.0404$; n = 82; r = +0.92.

Table 16. Total lung capacity measured in a body plethysmograph (TLC$_{box}$) in relation to body height in girls

Height cm	TLC$_{box}$, ml mean	lower limits	upper limits
115	1,860	1,575	2,196
116	1,902	1,611	2,245
118	1,987	1,683	2,346
120	2,075	1,758	2,450
122	2,166	1,834	2,556
124	2,258	1,913	2,666
126	2,353	1,993	2,778
128	2,451	2,076	2,893
130	2,551	2,161	3,011
132	2,653	2,247	3,132
134	2,758	2,336	3,255
136	2,865	2,427	3,382
138	2,975	2,520	3,512
140	3,087	2,615	3,644
142	3,202	2,712	3,780
144	3,319	2,812	3,918
146	3,439	2,914	4,060
148	3,562	3,017	4,205
150	3,687	3,124	4,353
152	3,815	3,232	4,504
154	3,946	3,343	4,658
156	4,079	3,456	4,816
158	4,216	3,571	4,976
160	4,354	3,689	5,140
162	4,496	3,809	5,307
164	4,640	3,931	5,478
166	4,787	4,055	5,651
168	4,937	4,183	5,828
170	5,090	4,312	6,009
172	5,247	4,444	6,193
174	5,405	4,578	6,380
176	5,566	4,715	6,570
178	5,730	4,854	6,765
180	5,898	4,996	6,962

Formula: log y = a + b·log x;
y = TLC$_{box}$ (ml); x = body height (cm);
log TLC$_{box}$ (ml) = −2.0377 + 2.5755·log height (cm);
SD log y·x = ±0.0361; n = 72; r = +0.96.

Table 17. Total lung capacity measured in a body plethysmograph (TLC$_{box}$) in relation to age in girls

Age years	TLC$_{box}$, ml mean	lower limits	upper limits
6	1,886	1,408	2,527
7	2,220	1,657	2,975
8	2,558	1,909	3,427
9	2,897	2,162	3,882
10	3,239	2,417	4,340
11	3,583	2,674	4,801
12	3,929	2,932	5,264
13	4,276	3,191	5,729
14	4,625	3,452	6,197
15	4,975	3,713	6,666
16	5,327	3,976	7,138
17	5,680	4,239	7,611

Formula: log y = a + b·log x;
y = TLC$_{box}$ (ml); x = age (years);
log TLC$_{box}$ (ml) = 2.4520 + 1.0584·log age (years);
SD log y·x = ±0.0637; n = 72; r = +0.84.

Table 18. Total lung capacity measured in a body plethysmograph (TLC$_{box}$) in relation to body surface in girls

Body surface m^2	TLC$_{box}$, ml mean	lower limits	upper limits
0.6	1,425	1,157	1,756
0.7	1,718	1,394	2,116
0.8	2,019	1,639	2,487
0.9	2,328	1,889	2,867
1.0	2,644	2,146	3,257
1.1	2,967	2,408	3,655
1.2	3,296	2,676	4,060
1.3	3,631	2,947	4,473
1.4	3,971	3,224	4,892
1.5	4,317	3,504	5,318
1.6	4,667	3,789	5,749
1.7	5,022	4,077	6,186
1.8	5,381	4,368	6,629
1.9	5,745	4,664	7,077
2.0	6,112	4,962	7,530

Formula: log y = a + b·log x;
y = TLC$_{box}$ (ml); x = body surface (m^2);
log TLC$_{box}$ (ml) = 3.4223 + 1.2089·log body surface (m^2);
SD log y·x = ±0.0454; n = 72; r = +0.93.

Table 19. Functional residual capacity measured in a body plethysmograph (FRC_{box}) in relation to body height in boys and girls

Height cm	FRC_{box}, ml		
	mean	lower limits	upper limits
115	923	745	1,143
116	944	762	1,169
118	988	797	1,223
120	1,032	833	1,279
122	1,079	871	1,336
124	1,126	909	1,395
126	1,175	948	1,455
128	1,225	988	1,517
130	1,276	1,030	1,581
132	1,328	1,072	1,646
134	1,382	1,116	1,712
136	1,438	1,160	1,781
138	1,494	1,206	1,851
140	1,552	1,253	1,923
142	1,611	1,301	1,996
144	1,672	1,350	2,071
146	1,734	1,400	2,148
148	1,798	1,451	2,227
150	1,863	1,504	2,307
152	1,929	1,557	2,390
154	1,997	1,612	2,474
156	2,066	1,668	2,560
158	2,137	1,725	2,647
160	2,209	1,783	2,737
162	2,283	1,843	2,828
164	2,358	1,904	2,921
166	2,435	1,966	3,017
168	2,513	2,029	3,114
170	2,593	2,093	3,213
172	2,675	2,159	3,313
174	2,758	2,226	3,416
176	2,842	2,295	3,521
178	2,929	2,364	3,628
180	3,016	2,435	3,737

Formula: $\log y = a + b \cdot \log x$;
$y = FRC_{box}$ (ml); x = body height (cm);
$\log FRC_{box}$ (ml) = $-2.4820 + 2.6434 \cdot \log$ height (cm);
SD $\log y \cdot x = \pm 0.0470$; n = 154; r = +0.92.

Table 20. Functional residual capacity measured in a body plethysmograph (FRC_{box}) in relation to age in boys and girls

Age years	FRC_{box}, ml		
	mean	lower limits	upper limits
6	936	681	1,287
7	1,105	804	1,519
8	1,275	928	1,754
9	1,447	1,053	1,990
10	1,621	1,179	2,228
11	1,795	1,306	2,468
12	1,971	1,434	2,710
13	2,148	1,563	2,953
14	2,326	1,692	3,198
15	2,505	1,822	3,444
16	2,685	1,953	3,691
17	2,865	2,084	3,939

Formula: $\log y = a + b \cdot \log x$;
$y = FRC_{box}$ (ml); x = age (years);
$\log FRC_{box}$ (ml) = $2.1363 + 1.0734 \cdot \log$ age (years);
SD $\log y \cdot x = \pm 0.0699$; n = 154; r = +0.82.

Table 21. Functional residual capacity measured in a body plethysmograph (FRC_{box}) in relation to body surface in boys and girls

Body surface m^2	FRC_{box}, ml		
	mean	lower limits	upper limits
0.6	723	545	957
0.7	872	658	1,154
0.8	1,025	774	1,358
0.9	1,183	894	1,567
1.0	1,345	1,016	1,782
1.1	1,511	1,141	2,001
1.2	1,680	1,268	2,224
1.3	1,851	1,398	2,452
1.4	2,026	1,530	2,683
1.5	2,203	1,664	2,918
1.6	2,383	1,800	3,156
1.7	2,566	1,937	3,398
1.8	2,751	2,077	3,643
1.9	2,936	2,218	3,890
2.0	3,127	2,361	4,141

Formula: $\log y = a + b \cdot \log x$;
$y = FRC_{box}$ (ml); x = body surface (m^2);
$\log FRC_{box}$ (ml) = $3.1290 + 1.2163 \cdot \log$ body surface (m^2);
SD $\log y \cdot x = \pm 0.0617$; n = 154; r = +0.86.

Table 22. Functional residual capacity measured in a body plethysmograph (FRC_{box}) in relation to body height in boys

Height cm	FRC_{box}, ml		
	mean	lower limits	upper limits
115	941	790	1,121
116	963	809	1,148
118	1,008	846	1,201
120	1,054	885	1,256
122	1,101	925	1,312
124	1,150	965	1,370
126	1,200	1,007	1,429
128	1,251	1,050	1,490
130	1,303	1,094	1,553
132	1,357	1,140	1,617
134	1,413	1,186	1,683
136	1,469	1,233	1,750
138	1,527	1,282	1,819
140	1,587	1,332	1,890
142	1,648	1,383	1,962
144	1,710	1,435	2,037
146	1,774	1,489	2,113
148	1,839	1,544	2,190
150	1,905	1,600	2,270
152	1,974	1,657	2,351
154	2,043	1,715	2,434
156	2,114	1,775	2,518
158	2,187	1,836	2,605
160	2,261	1,898	2,693
162	2,337	1,962	2,784
164	2,414	2,027	2,876
166	2,493	2,093	2,970
168	2,574	2,161	3,066
170	2,656	2,230	3,163
172	2,739	2,300	3,263
174	2,825	2,372	3,365
176	2,912	2,445	3,468
178	3,000	2,519	3,574
180	3,091	2,595	3,681

Formula: $\log y = a + b \cdot \log x$;
$y = FRC_{box}$ (ml); x = body height (cm);
$\log FRC_{box}$ (ml) $= -2.4915 + 2.6523 \cdot \log$ height (cm);
SD $\log y \cdot x = \pm 0.0381$; $n = 82$; $r = +0.94$.

Table 23. Functional residual capacity measured in a body plethysmograph (FRC_{box}) in relation to age in boys

Age years	FRC_{box}, ml		
	mean	lower limits	upper limits
6	960	715	1,290
7	1,131	842	1,519
8	1,303	970	1,750
9	1,476	1,099	1,982
10	1,650	1,229	2,216
11	1,826	1,360	2,452
12	2,002	1,491	2,689
13	2,197	1,623	2,927
14	2,357	1,755	3,166
15	2,536	1,888	3,406
16	2,716	2,022	3,647
17	2,896	2,156	3,889

Formula: $\log y = a + b \cdot \log x$;
$y = FRC_{box}$ (ml); x = age (years);
$\log FRC_{box}$ (ml) $= 2.1584 + 1.0592 \cdot \log$ age (years);
SD $\log y \cdot x = \pm 0.0643$; $n = 82$; $r = +0.82$.

Table 24. Functional residual capacity measured in a body plethysmograph (FRC_{box}) in relation to body surface in boys

Body surface m^2	FRC_{box}, ml		
	mean	lower limits	upper limits
0.6	719	568	910
0.7	874	691	1,106
0.8	1,035	818	1,309
0.9	1,201	949	1,520
1.0	1,372	1,084	1,736
1.1	1,548	1,223	1,958
1.2	1,728	1,365	2,186
1.3	1,912	1,511	2,419
1.4	2,099	1,659	2,656
1.5	2,290	1,810	2,898
1.6	2,485	1,964	3,144
1.7	2,683	2,120	3,395
1.8	2,884	2,279	3,649
1.9	3,088	2,440	3,907
2.0	3,295	2,604	4,169

Formula: $\log y = a + b \cdot \log x$;
$y = FRC_{box}$ (ml); x = body surface (m^2);
$\log FRC_{box}$ (ml) $= 3.1375 + 1.2635 \cdot \log$ body surface (m^2);
SD $\log y \cdot x = \pm 0.0513$; $n = 82$; $r = +0.89$.

Table 25. Functional residual capacity measured in a body plethysmograph (FRC_{box}) in relation to body height in girls

Height cm	FRC_{box}, ml		
	mean	lower limits	upper limits
115	906	707	1,160
116	926	723	1,186
118	969	756	1,241
120	1,012	790	1,296
122	1,057	825	1,354
124	1,103	861	1,412
126	1,150	898	1,473
128	1,198	936	1,535
130	1,248	974	1,598
132	1,299	1,014	1,663
134	1,351	1,055	1,730
136	1,404	1,097	1,799
138	1,459	1,139	1,869
140	1,515	1,183	1,940
142	1,572	1,228	2,014
144	1,631	1,273	2,089
146	1,691	1,320	2,165
148	1,752	1,368	2,244
150	1,815	1,417	2,324
152	1,879	1,467	2,406
154	1,944	1,518	2,489
156	2,011	1,570	2,575
158	2,079	1,623	2,662
160	2,148	1,677	2,751
162	2,219	1,733	2,842
164	2,292	1,789	2,935
166	2,365	1,847	3,029
168	2,441	1,906	3,126
170	2,517	1,966	3,224
172	2,596	2,027	3,324
174	2,675	2,089	3,426
176	2,756	2,152	3,530
178	2,839	2,217	3,636
180	2,923	2,283	3,744

Formula: $\log y = a + b \cdot \log x$;
$y = FRC_{box}$ (ml); x = body height (cm);
$\log FRC_{box}$ (ml) = $-2.4314 + 2.6149 \cdot \log$ height (cm);
SD $\log y \cdot x = \pm 0.0538$; n = 72; r = +0.91.

Table 26. Functional residual capacity measured in a body plethysmograph (FRC_{box}) in relation to age in girls

Age years	FRC_{box}, ml		
	mean	lower limits	upper limits
6	919	648	1,303
7	1,085	765	1,538
8	1,252	883	1,775
9	1,421	1,002	2,014
10	1,591	1,122	2,255
11	1,762	1,243	2,498
12	1,935	1,365	2,643
13	2,109	1,488	2,989
14	2,283	1,611	3,236
15	2,459	1,735	3,485
16	2,635	1,859	3,735
17	2,812	1,984	3,986

Formula: $\log y = a + b \cdot \log x$;
$y = FRC_{box}$ (ml); x = age (years);
$\log FRC_{box}$ (ml) = $2.1285 + 1.0732 \cdot \log$ age (years);
SD $\log y \cdot x = \pm 0.0759$; n = 72; r = +0.81.

Table 27. Functional residual capacity measured in a body plethysmograph (FRC_{box}) in relation to body surface in girls

Body surface m²	FRC_{box}, ml		
	mean	lower limits	upper limits
0.6	718	523	987
0.7	861	627	1,183
0.8	1,008	734	1,384
0.9	1,158	843	1,590
1.0	1,311	955	1,800
1.1	1,466	1,068	2,014
1.2	1,625	1,183	2,231
1.3	1,785	1,300	2,451
1.4	1,948	1,419	2,674
1.5	2,113	1,539	2,901
1.6	2,279	1,660	3,130
1.7	2,448	1,783	3,361
1.8	2,618	1,907	3,595
1.9	2,790	2,032	3,831
2.0	2,964	2,159	4,069

Formula: $\log y = a + b \cdot \log x$;
$y = FRC_{box}$ (ml); x = body surface (m²);
$\log FRC_{box}$ (ml) = $3.1177 + 1.1766 \cdot \log$ body surface (m²);
SD $\log y \cdot x = \pm 0.0690$; n = 72; r = +0.85.

Table 28. Residual volume measured in a body plethysmograph (RV_{box}) in relation to body height in boys and girls

Height cm	RV_{box}, ml		
	mean	lower limits	upper limits
115	519	356	758
116	529	362	772
118	549	376	801
120	569	390	830
122	589	404	860
124	610	418	890
126	631	432	921
128	653	447	952
130	674	462	984
132	697	477	1,017
134	720	493	1,050
136	743	509	1,084
138	766	525	1,118
140	790	541	1,153
142	814	558	1,188
144	839	575	1,224
146	864	592	1,261
148	889	609	1,298
150	915	627	1,335
152	941	645	1,374
154	968	663	1,412
156	995	682	1,452
158	1,022	701	1,492
160	1,050	720	1,532
162	1,078	739	1,574
164	1,107	759	1,615
166	1,136	779	1,658
168	1,165	799	1,700
170	1,195	819	1,744
172	1,225	840	1,788
174	1,256	861	1,833
176	1,287	882	1,878
178	1,318	904	1,924
180	1,350	925	1,970

Formula: $\log y = a + b \cdot \log x$;
$y = RV_{box}$ (ml); x = body height (cm);
$\log RV_{box}$ (ml) = $-1.6765 + 2.1314 \cdot \log$ height (cm);
SD $\log y \cdot x = \pm 0.0830$; n = 154; r = +0.73.

Table 29. Residual volume measured in a body plethysmograph (RV_{box}) in relation to age in boys and girls

Age years	RV_{box}, ml		
	mean	lower limits	upper limits
6	524	344	798
7	599	393	913
8	673	442	1,026
9	746	489	1,137
10	818	537	1,246
11	888	583	1,354
12	958	629	1,460
13	1,028	674	1,566
14	1,096	719	1,670
15	1,164	764	1,773
16	1,231	808	1,876
17	1,298	852	1,978

Formula: $\log y = a + b \cdot \log x$;
$y = RV_{box}$ (ml); x = age (years);
$\log RV_{box}$ (ml) = $2.0422 + 0.8705 \cdot \log$ age (years);
SD $\log y \cdot x = \pm 0.0925$; n = 154; r = +0.65.

Table 30. Residual volume measured in a body plethysmograph (RV_{box}) in relation to body surface in boys and girls

Body surface m²	RV_{box}, ml		
	mean	lower limits	upper limits
0.6	423	283	632
0.7	493	330	736
0.8	563	377	841
0.9	632	423	945
1.0	702	470	1,049
1.1	772	517	1,153
1.2	841	563	1,257
1.3	911	610	1,361
1.4	980	656	1,464
1.5	1,050	703	1,568
1.6	1,119	749	1,672
1.7	1,188	795	1,775
1.8	1,258	842	1,879
1.9	1,327	888	1,982
2.0	1,396	935	2,086

Formula: $\log y = a + b \cdot \log x$;
$y = RV_{box}$ (ml); x = body surface (m²);
$\log RV_{box}$ (ml) = $2.8467 + 0.9912 \cdot \log$ body surface (m²);
SD $\log y \cdot x = \pm 0.0881$; n = 154; r = +0.69.

Table 31. Residual volume measured in a body plethysmograph (RV$_{box}$) in relation to body height in boys

Height cm	RV$_{box}$, ml		
	mean	lower limits	upper limits
115	538	366	791
116	547	373	804
118	566	385	831
120	585	398	859
122	604	411	887
124	623	424	915
126	643	438	944
128	663	451	974
130	683	465	1,003
132	704	479	1,034
134	725	493	1,064
136	746	508	1,095
138	767	522	1,127
140	789	537	1,159
142	811	552	1,191
144	834	567	1,224
146	856	583	1,257
148	879	599	1,291
150	902	614	1,325
152	926	630	1,360
154	950	647	1,395
156	974	663	1,430
158	998	680	1,466
160	1,023	696	1,502
162	1,048	713	1,539
164	1,073	731	1,576
166	1,099	748	1,614
168	1,125	766	1,652
170	1,151	784	1,690
172	1,177	802	1,729
174	1,204	820	1,768
176	1,231	838	1,808
178	1,258	857	1,848
180	1,286	876	1,889

Formula: log y = a + b·log x;
y = RV$_{box}$ (ml); x = body height (cm);
log RV$_{box}$ (ml) = −1.2720 + 1.9427·log height (cm);
SD log y·x = ±0.0838; n = 82; r = +0.68.

Table 32. Residual volume measured in a body plethysmograph (RV$_{box}$) in relation to body height in girls

Height cm	RV$_{box}$, ml		
	mean	lower limits	upper limits
115	504	346	735
116	515	353	750
118	535	367	780
120	556	382	811
122	578	397	843
124	600	412	875
126	623	427	908
128	646	443	941
130	669	459	976
132	693	476	1,011
134	718	493	1,046
136	743	510	1,083
138	768	527	1,120
140	794	545	1,158
142	821	563	1,196
144	848	582	1,235
146	875	600	1,275
148	903	620	1,316
150	931	639	1,357
152	960	659	1,399
154	990	679	1,442
156	1,020	700	1,485
158	1,050	720	1,530
160	1,081	742	1,575
162	1,112	763	1,621
164	1,144	785	1,668
166	1,177	807	1,715
168	1,210	830	1,763
170	1,243	853	1,812
172	1,277	876	1,861
174	1,312	900	1,912
176	1,347	924	1,963
178	1,382	949	2,014
180	1,418	973	2,067

Formula: log y = a + b·log x;
y = RV$_{box}$ (ml); x = body height (cm);
log RV$_{box}$ (ml) = −2.0493 + 2.3062·log height (cm);
SD log y·x = ±0.0819; n = 72; r = +0.78.

Table 33. Inspiratory capacity (IC) in relation to body height in boys and girls

Height cm	IC, ml		
	mean	lower limits	upper limits
115	971	772	1,220
116	992	790	1,247
118	1,037	825	1,303
120	1,082	861	1,360
122	1,129	898	1,418
124	1,177	936	1,478
126	1,226	975	1,540
128	1,276	1,015	1,603
130	1,327	1,056	1,668
132	1,380	1,098	1,734
134	1,434	1,141	1,802
136	1,489	1,185	1,871
138	1,546	1,230	1,943
140	1,604	1,276	2,015
142	1,663	1,323	2,089
144	1,723	1,371	2,165
146	1,785	1,421	2,243
148	1,848	1,471	2,322
150	1,913	1,522	2,403
152	1,978	1,574	2,486
154	2,045	1,628	2,570
156	2,114	1,682	2,656
158	2,184	1,738	2,744
160	2,255	1,795	2,834
162	2,328	1,852	2,925
164	2,402	1,911	3,018
166	2,477	1,971	3,113
168	2,554	2,033	3,209
170	2,632	2,095	3,308
172	2,712	2,159	3,408
174	2,793	2,223	3,510
176	2,876	2,289	3,614
178	2,960	2,356	3,720
180	3,046	2,424	3,827

Formula: $\log y = a + b \cdot \log x$;
$y = IC$ (ml); x = body height (cm);
$\log IC$ (ml) = $-2.2711 + 2.5517 \cdot \log$ height (cm);
SD $\log y \cdot x = \pm 0.0502$; $n = 172$; $r = +0.90$.

Table 34. Inspiratory capacity (IC) in relation to age in boys and girls

Age years	IC, ml		
	mean	lower limits	upper limits
6	987	707	1,378
7	1,155	827	1,612
8	1,323	947	1,848
9	1,492	1,068	2,083
10	1,661	1,189	2,319
11	1,830	1,311	2,556
12	2,000	1,432	2,793
13	2,170	1,554	3,030
14	2,340	1,676	3,268
15	2,511	1,798	3,506
16	2,681	1,920	3,744
17	2,852	2,042	3,982

Formula: $\log y = a + b \cdot \log x$;
$y = IC$ (ml); x = age (years);
$\log IC$ (ml) = $2.2017 + 1.0187 \cdot \log$ age (years);
SD $\log y \cdot x = \pm 0.0734$; $n = 172$; $r = +0.80$.

Table 35. Inspiratory capacity (IC) in relation to body surface in boys and girls

Body surface m²	IC, ml		
	mean	lower limits	upper limits
0.6	724	569	922
0.7	878	689	1,117
0.8	1,037	814	1,320
0.9	1,201	943	1,528
1.0	1,369	1,075	1,743
1.1	1,542	1,211	1,963
1.2	1,718	1,350	2,188
1.3	1,899	1,492	2,417
1.4	2,083	1,636	2,651
1.5	2,270	1,783	2,889
1.6	2,460	1,932	3,131
1.7	2,653	2,084	3,377
1.8	2,849	2,238	3,626
1.9	3,047	2,394	3,879
2.0	3,249	2,552	4,135

Formula: $\log y = a + b \cdot \log x$;
$y = IC$ (ml); x = body surface (m²);
$\log IC$ (ml) = $3.1365 + 1.2463 \cdot \log$ body surface (m²);
SD $\log y \cdot x = \pm 0.0530$; $n = 172$; $r = +0.89$.

Table 36. Inspiratory capacity (IC) in relation to body height in boys

Height cm	IC, ml		
	mean	lower limits	upper limits
115	1,017	860	1,202
116	1,039	879	1,229
118	1,084	917	1,283
120	1,131	956	1,338
122	1,179	997	1,394
124	1,228	1,038	1,452
126	1,278	1,081	1,511
128	1,329	1,124	1,572
130	1,382	1,169	1,634
132	1,436	1,214	1,698
134	1,491	1,261	1,763
136	1,547	1,308	1,830
138	1,605	1,357	1,898
140	1,664	1,407	1,967
142	1,724	1,458	2,039
144	1,785	1,509	2,111
146	1,848	1,563	2,185
148	1,912	1,617	2,261
150	1,977	1,672	2,338
152	2,044	1,728	2,417
154	2,112	1,786	2,497
156	2,181	1,844	2,579
158	2,252	1,904	2,663
160	2,324	1,965	2,748
162	2,397	2,027	2,835
164	2,472	2,090	2,923
166	2,548	2,155	3,013
168	2,626	2,220	3,105
170	2,704	2,287	3,198
172	2,785	2,355	3,293
174	2,867	2,424	3,390
176	2,950	2,494	3,488
178	3,034	2,566	3,588
180	3,120	2,639	3,690

Formula: log y = a + b·log x;
y = IC (ml); x = body height (cm);
log IC (ml) = −2.14866 + 2.50211·log height (cm);
SD log y·x = ±0.03660; n = 85; r = +0.93.

Table 37. Inspiratory capacity (IC) in relation to body height in girls

Height cm	IC, ml		
	mean	lower limits	upper limits
115	939	721	1,222
116	960	738	1,250
118	1,003	770	1,305
120	1,047	804	1,363
122	1,092	839	1,421
124	1,138	875	1,482
126	1,196	911	1,543
128	1,234	948	1,607
130	1,284	987	1,672
132	1,335	1,026	1,738
134	1,388	1,066	1,806
136	1,441	1,107	1,876
138	1,496	1,149	1,947
140	1,552	1,192	2,020
142	1,609	1,236	2,095
144	1,668	1,281	2,171
146	1,728	1,327	2,249
148	1,789	1,374	2,328
150	1,851	1,422	2,409
152	1,915	1,471	2,492
154	1,980	1,521	2,577
156	2,046	1,572	2,663
158	2,114	1,624	2,751
160	2,183	1,677	2,841
162	2,253	1,731	2,933
164	2,325	1,786	3,026
166	2,398	1,842	3,121
168	2,472	1,900	3,218
170	2,548	1,958	3,317
172	2,626	2,017	3,417
174	2,704	2,078	3,520
176	2,784	2,139	3,624
178	2,866	2,202	3,730
180	2,949	2,266	3,838

Formula: log y = a + b·log x;
y = IC (ml); x = body height (cm);
log IC (ml) = −2.28904 + 2.55347·log height (cm);
SD log y·x = ±0.05757; n = 87; r = +0.88.

Table 38. Inspiratory reserve volume (IRV) in relation to body height in boys and girls

Height cm	IRV, ml		
	mean	lower limits	upper limits
115	667	474	939
116	683	485	961
118	715	508	1,007
120	749	532	1,054
122	783	557	1,103
124	819	582	1,153
126	855	608	1,204
128	893	634	1,257
130	932	662	1,311
132	971	690	1,367
134	1,012	719	1,424
136	1,053	748	1,483
138	1,096	779	1,543
140	1,140	810	1,605
142	1,185	842	1,668
144	1,231	875	1,733
146	1,278	908	1,799
148	1,326	942	1,867
150	1,376	978	1,936
152	1,426	1,014	2,008
154	1,478	1,050	2,080
156	1,531	1,088	2,155
158	1,585	1,126	2,231
160	1,641	1,166	2,309
162	1,697	1,206	2,388
164	1,755	1,247	2,470
166	1,814	1,289	2,552
168	1,874	1,331	2,637
170	1,935	1,375	2,724
172	1,998	1,420	2,812
174	2,062	1,465	2,902
176	2,127	1,511	2,994
178	2,194	1,559	3,087
180	2,261	1,607	3,183

Formula: $\log y = a + b \cdot \log x$;
y = IRV (ml); x = body height (cm);
$\log$ IRV (ml) = $-2.7899 + 2.7244 \cdot \log$ height (cm);
SD $\log y \cdot x = \pm 0.0751$; n = 159; r = +0.83.

Table 39. Inspiratory reserve volume (IRV) in relation to age in boys and girls

Age years	IRV, ml		
	mean	lower limits	upper limits
6	697	445	1,090
7	819	524	1,281
8	942	602	1,473
9	1,065	681	1,666
10	1,189	760	1,860
11	1,314	840	2,055
12	1,439	920	2,250
13	1,568	1,001	2,447
14	1,691	1,081	2,644
15	1,817	1,162	2,842
16	1,944	1,243	3,040
17	2,072	1,325	3,239

Formula: $\log y = a + b \cdot \log x$;
y = IRV (ml); x = age (years);
$\log$ IRV (ml) = $2.0297 + 1.0456 \cdot \log$ age (years);
SD $\log y \cdot x = \pm 0.0982$; n = 159; r = +0.69.

Table 40. Inspiratory reserve volume (IRV) in relation to body surface in boys and girls

Body surface m^2	IRV, ml		
	mean	lower limits	upper limits
0.6	480	339	683
0.7	592	418	838
0.8	708	500	1,003
0.9	831	587	1,176
1.0	958	676	1,356
1.1	1,089	769	1,542
1.2	1,225	865	1,734
1.3	1,364	964	1,932
1.4	1,508	1,065	2,135
1.5	1,655	1,169	2,343
1.6	1,806	1,275	2,556
1.7	1,959	1,384	2,774
1.8	2,117	1,495	2,996
1.9	2,277	1,608	3,223
2.0	2,440	1,723	3,454

Formula: $\log y = a + b \cdot \log x$;
y = IRV (ml); x = body surface (m^2);
$\log$ IRV (ml) = $2.9813 + 1.3489 \cdot \log$ body surface (m^2);
SD $\log y \cdot x = \pm 0.0764$; n = 159; r = +0.83.

Table 41. Inspiratory reserve volume (IRV) in relation to body height in boys

Height cm	IRV, ml mean	lower limits	upper limits
115	701	509	966
116	718	521	989
118	753	546	1,037
120	788	572	1,086
122	824	598	1,136
124	862	626	1,188
126	901	654	1,241
128	940	682	1,296
130	981	712	1,352
132	1,023	742	1,410
134	1,066	774	1,469
136	1,110	806	1,530
138	1,156	839	1,592
140	1,202	872	1,656
142	1,250	907	1,722
144	1,298	942	1,789
146	1,348	979	1,858
148	1,400	1,016	1,928
150	1,452	1,054	2,001
152	1,506	1,093	2,074
154	1,561	1,133	2,150
156	1,617	1,173	2,227
158	1,674	1,215	2,306
160	1,733	1,258	2,387
162	1,793	1,301	2,470
164	1,854	1,346	2,554
166	1,917	1,391	2,641
168	1,980	1,437	2,729
170	2,046	1,485	2,818
172	2,112	1,533	2,910
174	2,180	1,582	3,004
176	2,250	1,633	3,099
178	2,320	1,684	3,197
180	2,392	1,735	3,301

Formula: log y = a + b·log x;
y = IRV (ml); x = body height (cm);
log IRV (ml) = −2.79590 + 2.73794·log height (cm);
SD log y·x = ±0.069875; n = 80; r = +0.84.

Table 42. Inspiratory reserve volume (IRV) in relation to body height in girls

Height cm	IRV, ml mean	lower limits	upper limits
115	640	457	897
116	655	467	918
118	686	489	961
120	717	512	1,005
122	750	535	1,051
124	783	558	1,097
126	817	583	1,145
128	852	608	1,194
130	887	634	1,245
132	925	660	1,297
134	963	687	1,350
136	1,002	715	1,404
138	1,042	743	1,460
140	1,083	773	1,517
142	1,125	802	1,576
144	1,167	833	1,636
146	1,211	864	1,698
148	1,256	896	1,760
150	1,302	929	1,825
152	1,349	962	1,890
154	1,397	997	1,958
156	1,446	1,032	2,026
158	1,496	1,067	2,096
160	1,547	1,104	2,168
162	1,599	1,141	2,241
164	1,653	1,179	2,316
166	1,707	1,218	2,392
168	1,762	1,258	2,470
170	1,819	1,298	2,549
172	1,877	1,339	2,630
174	1,936	1,381	2,713
176	1,996	1,424	2,797
178	2,057	1,468	2,883
180	2,120	1,511	2,975

Formula: log y = a + b·log x;
y = IRV (ml); x = body height (cm);
log IRV (ml) = −2.69813 + 2.67126·log height (cm);
SD log y·x = ±0.07359; n = 79; r = +0.84.

Table 43. Expiratory reserve volume (ERV) in relation to body height in boys and girls

Height cm	ERV, ml		
	mean	lower limits	upper limits
115	437	310	616
116	448	318	632
118	471	334	663
120	494	350	696
122	518	367	730
124	543	385	765
126	568	403	801
128	595	422	838
130	622	441	876
132	649	461	915
134	678	481	956
136	708	502	997
138	738	523	1,040
140	769	546	1,084
142	801	568	1,129
144	834	592	1,175
146	867	615	1,222
148	902	640	1,271
150	937	665	1,321
152	974	691	1,372
154	1,011	717	1,425
156	1,049	744	1,478
158	1,088	772	1,533
160	1,128	800	1,590
162	1,169	830	1,648
164	1,211	859	1,707
166	1,254	890	1,767
168	1,298	921	1,829
170	1,342	953	1,892
172	1,388	985	1,956
174	1,435	1,018	2,022
176	1,483	1,052	2,090
178	1,532	1,087	2,159
180	1,582	1,122	2,229

Formula: log y = a + b·log x;
y = ERV (ml); x = body height (cm);
log ERV (ml) = −3.2703 + 2.8686·log height (cm);
SD log y·x = ±0.0754; n = 159; r = +0.84.

Table 44. Expiratory reserve volume (ERV) in relation to age in boys and girls

Age years	ERV, ml		
	mean	lower limits	upper limits
6	446	287	692
7	532	342	826
8	620	399	962
9	709	457	1,101
10	800	515	1,242
11	892	575	1,386
12	986	635	1,531
13	1,081	696	1,678
14	1,176	757	1,827
15	1,273	820	1,977
16	1,371	883	2,128
17	1,469	946	2,281

Formula: log y = a + b·log x;
y = ERV (ml); x = age (years);
log ERV (ml) = 1.7583 + 1.1449·log age (years);
SD log y·x = ±0.0967; n = 159; r = +0.73.

Table 45. Expiratory reserve volume (ERV) in relation to body surface in boys and girls

Body surface m²	ERV, ml		
	mean	lower limits	upper limits
0.6	330	222	489
0.7	405	273	601
0.8	484	327	718
0.9	567	383	841
1.0	653	441	968
1.1	742	501	1,100
1.2	834	562	1,235
1.3	928	626	1,375
1.4	1,024	691	1,518
1.5	1,124	758	1,665
1.6	1,225	826	1,815
1.7	1,328	896	1,968
1.8	1,434	968	2,125
1.9	1,541	1,040	2,284
2.0	1,651	1,114	2,446

Formula: log y = a + b·log x;
y = ERV (ml); x = body surface (m²);
log ERV (ml) = 2.8152 + 1.3373·log body surface (m²);
SD log y·x = ±0.0864; n = 159; r = +0.79.

Table 46. Expiratory reserve volume (ERV) in relation to body height in boys

Height cm	ERV, ml		
	mean	lower limits	upper limits
115	426	307	592
116	438	315	608
118	462	332	642
120	487	350	676
122	513	369	712
124	539	388	749
126	567	408	788
128	596	429	828
130	625	450	869
132	656	472	911
134	688	495	955
136	720	518	1,009
138	754	543	1,047
140	789	568	1,095
142	824	593	1,145
144	861	620	1,196
146	899	647	1,249
148	938	675	1,303
150	978	704	1,359
152	1,020	734	1,417
154	1,062	765	1,476
156	1,106	796	1,536
158	1,151	829	1,599
160	1,197	862	1,663
162	1,245	896	1,729
164	1,293	931	1,797
166	1,343	967	1,866
168	1,394	1,004	1,937
170	1,447	1,042	2,010
172	1,501	1,080	2,085
174	1,556	1,120	2,162
176	1,613	1,161	2,240
178	1,671	1,203	2,321
180	1,731	1,244	2,407

Formula: $\log y = a + b \cdot \log x$;
y = ERV (ml); x = body height (cm);
$\log ERV (ml) = -3.81064 + 3.12550 \cdot \log$ height (cm);
SD $\log y \cdot x = \pm 0.07165$; n = 80; r = +0.86.

Table 47. Expiratory reserve volume (ERV) in relation to body height in girls

Height cm	ERV, ml		
	mean	lower limits	upper limits
115	447	318	628
116	457	325	642
118	478	340	672
120	499	355	702
122	522	371	733
124	544	387	765
126	568	404	798
128	591	421	831
130	616	438	866
132	641	456	901
134	667	474	937
136	693	493	974
138	720	512	1,012
140	748	532	1,051
142	776	552	1,091
144	805	573	1,132
146	835	594	1,173
148	865	615	1,216
150	896	637	1,259
152	928	660	1,304
154	960	683	1,349
156	993	706	1,395
158	1,026	730	1,443
160	1,061	755	1,491
162	1,096	780	1,540
164	1,132	805	1,591
166	1,168	831	1,642
168	1,205	858	1,694
170	1,243	885	1,747
172	1,282	912	1,802
174	1,321	940	1,857
176	1,361	969	1,914
178	1,402	998	1,971
180	1,444	1,027	2,033

Formula: $\log y = a + b \cdot \log x$;
y = ERV (ml); x = body height (cm);
$\log ERV (ml) = -2.74162 + 2.61668 \cdot \log$ height (cm);
SD $\log y \cdot x = \pm 0.07421$; n = 79; r = +0.83.

Table 48. Percentage of residual volume from total lung capacity measured in a body plethysmograph $\left(\% \frac{RV}{TLC} \text{ box}\right)$ in relation to body height in boys and girls

Height cm	% $\frac{RV}{TLC}$ box		
	mean	lower limits	upper limits
115	26.90	19.17	34.63
116	26.84	19.11	34.56
118	26.70	18.97	34.43
120	26.57	18.84	34.29
122	26.43	18.70	34.16
124	26.30	18.57	34.03
126	26.16	18.43	33.89
128	26.03	18.30	33.76
130	25.89	18.16	33.62
132	25.76	18.03	33.49
134	25.62	17.89	33.35
136	25.49	17.76	33.22
138	25.35	17.62	33.08
140	25.22	17.49	32.95
142	25.08	17.36	32.81
144	24.95	17.22	32.68
146	24.81	17.09	32.54
148	24.68	16.95	32.41
150	25.55	16.82	32.27
152	24.41	16.68	32.14
154	24.28	16.55	32.00
156	24.14	16.41	31.87
158	24.01	16.28	31.73
160	23.87	16.14	31.60
162	23.74	16.01	31.47
164	23.60	15.87	31.33
166	23.47	15.74	31.20
168	23.33	15.60	31.06
170	23.20	15.47	30.93
172	23.06	15.33	30.79
174	22.93	15.20	30.66
176	22.79	15.06	30.52
178	22.66	14.93	30.39
180	22.54	14.80	30.25

Formula: $y = a + b \cdot x$;
$y = \% \frac{RV}{TLC}$ box; x = body height (cm);
$\% \frac{RV}{TLC}$ box = $34.6549 - 0.0673 \cdot$ height (cm);
SD $y \cdot x = \pm 3.91$; $n = 154$; $r = -0.29$.

Table 49. Percentage of residual volume from total lung capacity measured in a body plethysmograph $\left(\% \frac{RV}{TLC} \text{ box}\right)$ in relation to age in boys and girls

Age years	% $\frac{RV}{TLC}$ box		
	mean	lower limits	upper limits
6	26.57	18.70	34.36
7	26.20	18.41	33.99
8	25.83	18.04	33.63
9	25.46	17.67	33.26
10	25.09	17.30	32.89
11	24.73	16.93	32.52
12	24.36	16.56	32.15
13	23.99	16.20	31.78
14	23.62	15.83	31.41
15	23.25	15.46	31.04
16	22.88	15.09	30.67
17	22.51	14.72	30.30

Formula: $y = a + b \cdot x$;
$y = \% \frac{RV}{TLC}$ box; x = age (years);
$\% \frac{RV}{TLC}$ box = $28.7897 - 0.3689 \cdot$ age (years);
SD $y \cdot x = \pm 3.94$; $n = 154$; $r = -0.20$.

Table 50. Percentage of residual volume from total lung capacity measured in a body plethysmograph $\left(\% \frac{RV}{TLC} \text{ box}\right)$ in relation to body surface in boys and girls

Body surface m²	% $\frac{RV}{TLC}$ box		
	mean	lower limits	upper limits
0.60	27.55	19.87	35.23
0.70	27.13	19.46	34.81
0.80	26.71	19.04	34.39
0.90	26.29	18.62	33.97
1.00	25.87	18.20	33.55
1.10	25.45	17.78	33.13
1.20	25.04	17.36	32.71
1.30	24.62	16.94	32.29
1.40	24.20	16.52	31.87
1.50	23.78	16.10	31.45
1.60	23.36	15.68	31.03
1.70	22.94	15.26	30.62
1.80	22.52	14.84	30.20
1.90	22.10	14.42	29.78
2.00	21.68	14.00	29.36

Formula: $y = a + b \cdot x$;
$y = \% \frac{RV}{TLC}$ box; x = body surface (m²);
$\% \frac{RV}{TLC}$ box = $30.0747 - 4.1954 \cdot$ body surface (m²);
SD $y \cdot x = \pm 3.88$; $n = 154$; $r = -0.26$.

Table 51. Ratio of vital capacity to residual volume in a body plethysmograph $\left(\frac{VC}{RV_{box}}\right)$ in relation to body height in boys and girls

Height cm	$\frac{VC}{RV_{box}}$ mean	lower limits	upper limits
115	2.733	1.253	4.212
116	2.746	1.266	4.226
118	2.773	1.293	4.253
120	2.800	1.320	4.280
122	2.827	1.347	4.306
124	2.854	1.374	4.333
126	2.880	1.401	4.360
128	2.907	1.427	4.387
130	2.934	1.454	4.414
132	2.961	1.481	4.441
134	2.988	1.508	4.468
136	3.015	1.535	4.494
138	3.041	1.562	4.521
140	3.068	1.589	4.548
142	3.095	1.615	4.575
144	3.122	1.612	4.602
146	3.149	1.669	4.629
148	3.196	1.696	4.656
150	3.203	1.723	4.682
152	3.229	1.750	4.709
154	3.256	1.776	4.736
156	3.283	1.803	4.763
158	3.310	1.830	4.790
160	3.337	1.857	4.817
162	3.364	1.884	4.844
164	3.391	1.911	4.870
166	3.417	1.938	4.897
168	3.444	1.964	4.924
170	3.471	1.991	4.951
172	3.498	2.018	4.978
174	3.525	2.045	5.005
176	3.552	2.072	5.032
178	3.579	2.099	5.058
180	3.605	2.126	5.085

Formula: $y = a + b \cdot x$;
$y = \frac{VC}{RV_{box}}$; x = body height (cm);
$\frac{VC}{RV_{box}} = 1.1890 + 0.01342 \cdot$ height (cm);
SD $y \cdot x = \pm 0.749$; $n = 154$; $r = +0.25$.

Table 52. Ratio of inspiratory capacity to expiratory reserve volume (IC/ERV) in relation to body height in boys and girls

Height cm	IC/ERV		
	mean	lower limits	upper limits
115	2.26	1.38	3.14
116	2.25	1.37	3.14
118	2.24	1.36	3.12
120	2.23	1.35	3.11
122	2.22	1.34	3.10
124	2.21	1.33	3.09
126	2.20	1.32	3.08
128	2.19	1.30	3.07
130	2.18	1.29	3.06
132	2.16	1.28	3.05
134	2.15	1.27	3.04
136	2.14	1.26	3.02
138	2.13	1.25	3.01
140	2.12	1.24	3.00
142	2.11	1.23	2.99
144	2.10	1.22	2.98
146	2.09	1.20	2.97
148	2.08	1.19	2.96
150	2.07	1.18	2.95
152	2.05	1.17	2.94
154	2.04	1.16	2.93
156	2.03	1.15	2.91
158	2.02	1.14	2.90
160	2.01	1.13	2.89
162	2.00	1.12	2.88
164	1.99	1.11	2.87
166	1.98	1.09	2.86
168	1.97	1.08	2.85
170	1.95	1.07	2.84
172	1.94	1.06	2.83
174	1.93	1.05	2.82
176	1.92	1.04	2.80
178	1.91	1.03	2.79
180	1.90	1.02	2.78

Formula: $y = a + b \cdot x$;
$y = IC/ERV$; x = body height (cm);
$IC/ERV = 2.8981 - 0.00551 \cdot height$ (cm);
$SD = \pm 0.45$; $n = 159$; $r = -0.17$.

Table 53. Ratio of inspiratory capacity to expiratory reserve volume (IC/ERV) in relation to age in boys and girls

Age years	IC/ERV		
	mean	lower limits	upper limits
6	2.26	1.37	3.14
7	2.22	1.34	3.11
8	2.19	1.30	3.07
9	2.15	1.27	3.04
10	2.12	1.24	3.00
11	2.08	1.20	2.97
12	2.05	1.17	2.93
13	2.01	1.13	2.90
14	1.98	1.10	2.86
15	1.95	1.06	2.83
16	1.91	1.03	2.79
17	1.88	0.99	2.76

Formula: $y = a + b \cdot x$;
$y = IC/ERV$; x = age (years);
$IC/ERV = 2.4701 - 0.0346 \cdot age$ (years);
$SD\ y \cdot x = \pm 0.4472$; $n = 159$; $r = -0.16$.

Table 54. Ratio of inspiratory reserve volume to expiratory reserve volume (IRV/ERV) in relation to body height in boys and girls

Height cm	IRV/ERV		
	mean	lower limits	upper limits
115	1.58	0.91	2.26
116	1.58	0.91	2.26
118	1.58	0.90	2.25
120	1.57	0.90	2.25
122	1.57	0.89	2.24
124	1.56	0.89	2.24
126	1.56	0.88	2.23
128	1.55	0.88	2.23
130	1.55	0.87	2.22
132	1.54	0.87	2.22
134	1.54	0.86	2.21
136	1.53	0.86	2.21
138	1.53	0.85	2.20
140	1.52	0.85	2.20
142	1.52	0.84	2.19
144	1,51	0.84	2.19
146	1.51	0.83	2.18
148	1.50	0.83	2.18
150	1.50	0.82	2.17
152	1.49	0.82	2.17
154	1.49	0.81	2.16
156	1.48	0.81	2.16
158	1.48	0.80	2.15
160	1.47	0.80	2.15
162	1.47	0.79	2.14
164	1.46	0.79	2.14
166	1.46	0.78	2.13
168	1.45	0.78	2.13
170	1.45	0.77	2.12
172	1.44	0.77	2.12
174	1.44	0.76	2.11
176	1.43	0.76	2.11
178	1.43	0.75	2.10
180	1.42	0.75	2.10

Formula: $y = a + b \cdot x$;
y = IRV/ERV; x = body height (cm);
IRV/ERV = $1.8770 - 0.00250 \cdot$ height (cm);
SD $y \cdot x = \pm 0.34$; n = 159; r = −0.10.

Table 55. Ratio of inspiratory reserve volume to expiratory reserve volume (IRV/ERV) in relation to age in boys and girls

Age years	IRV/ERV		
	mean	lower limits	upper limits
6	1.61	0.94	2.28
7	1.59	0.92	2.26
8	1.57	0.90	2.24
9	1.55	0.87	2.22
10	1.53	0.85	2.20
11	1.51	0.83	2.18
12	1.49	0.81	2.16
13	1.47	0.79	2.14
14	1.45	0.77	2.12
15	1.43	0.75	2.10
16	1.40	0.73	2.08
17	1.38	0.71	2.06

Formula: $y = a + b \cdot x$;
y = IRV/ERV; x = age (years);
IRV/ERV = $1.7359 - 0.0203 \cdot$ age (years);
SD $y \cdot x = \pm 0.3404$; n = 159; r = −0.12.

Table 56. Total lung capacity measured by a helium-dilution method (TLC$_{He}$) in relation to body height in boys and girls

Height cm	TLC$_{He}$, ml		
	mean	lower limits	upper limits
115	1,844	1,556	2,184
116	1,886	1,592	2,235
118	1,973	1,665	2,337
120	2,062	1,741	2,443
122	2,153	1,818	2,551
124	2,247	1,897	2,662
126	2,344	1,979	2,777
128	2,443	2,062	2,894
130	2,545	2,148	3,014
132	2,649	2,236	3,138
134	2,755	2,326	3,264
136	2,865	2,418	3,394
138	2,977	2,513	3,527
140	3,092	2,610	3,662
142	3,209	2,709	3,801
144	3,329	2,810	3,944
146	3,452	2,914	4,089
148	3,578	3,020	4,238
150	3,706	3,128	4,390
152	3,837	3,239	4,546
154	3,971	3,352	4,704
156	4,108	3,468	4,867
158	4,248	3,586	5,032
160	4,391	3,706	5,201
162	4,536	3,829	5,374
164	4,685	3,955	5,550
166	4,837	4,083	5,730
168	4,991	4,213	5,913
170	5,149	4,346	6,100
172	5,310	4,482	6,290
174	5,473	4,620	6,484
176	5,640	4,761	6,681
178	5,810	4,905	6,883
180	5,983	5,051	7,088

Formula: $\log y = a + b \cdot \log x$;
$y = $ TLC$_{He}$ (ml); $x = $ body height (cm);
$\log$ TLC$_{He}$ (ml) $= -2.1475 + 2.6269 \cdot \log$ height (cm);
SD $\log y \cdot x = \pm 0.0372$; $n = 144$; $r = +0.95$.

Table 57. Total lung capacity measured by a helium-dilution method (TLC$_{He}$) in relation to age in boys and girls

Age years	TLC$_{He}$, ml		
	mean	lower limits	upper limits
6	1,868	1,388	2,513
7	2,197	1,633	2,590
8	2,529	1,880	3,403
9	2,864	2,128	3,853
10	3,200	2,378	4,305
11	3,538	2,630	4,760
12	3,878	2,882	5,217
13	4,219	3,136	5,677
14	4,562	3,391	6,138
15	4,906	3,647	6,601
16	5,251	3,903	7,065
17	5,598	4,161	7,531

Formula: $\log y = a + b \cdot \log x$;
$y = $ TLC$_{He}$ (ml); $x = $ age (years);
$\log$ TLC$_{He}$ (ml) $= 2.4513 + 1.0538 \cdot \log$ age (years);
SD $\log y \cdot x = \pm 0.0651$; $n = 144$; $r = +0.83$.

Table 58. Total lung capacity measured by a helium-dilution method (TLC$_{He}$) in relation to body surface in boys and girls

Body surface m^2	TLC$_{He}$, ml		
	mean	lower limits	upper limits
0.6	1,399	1,120	1,747
0.7	1,696	1,358	2,118
0.8	2,004	1,605	2,502
0.9	2,321	1,859	2,898
1.0	2,648	2,121	3,306
1.1	2,982	2,389	3,724
1.2	3,325	2,663	4,151
1.3	3,674	2,943	4,587
1.4	4,030	3,228	5,032
1.5	4,393	3,519	5,485
1.6	4,762	3,814	5,945
1.7	5,136	4,112	6,413
1.8	5,516	4,418	6,887
1.9	5,901	4,727	7,368
2.0	6,292	5,039	7,855

Formula: $\log y = a + b \cdot \log x$;
$y = $ TLC$_{He}$ (ml); $x = $ body surface (m^2);
$\log$ TLC$_{He}$ (ml) $= 3.4229 + 1.2484 \cdot \log$ body surface (m^2);
SD $\log y \cdot x = \pm 0.0487$; $n = 144$; $r = +0.91$.

Table 59. Total lung capacity measured by a helium-dilution method (TLC$_{He}$) in relation to body height in boys

Height cm	TLC$_{He}$, ml mean	lower limits	upper limits
115	1,869	1,632	2,141
116	1,913	1,670	2,192
118	2,002	1,748	2,294
120	2,094	1,828	2,399
122	2,189	1,910	2,507
124	2,286	1,995	2,619
126	2,385	2,082	2,733
128	2,488	2,172	2,850
130	2,593	2,263	2,971
132	2,701	2,358	3,094
134	2,812	2,454	3,221
136	2,925	2,553	3,351
138	3,041	2,655	3,484
140	3,160	2,759	3,620
142	3,282	2,865	3,760
144	3,407	2,974	3,903
146	3,535	3,086	4,050
148	3,666	3,200	4,199
150	3,799	3,316	4,352
152	3,936	3,436	4,509
154	4,076	3,558	4,669
156	4,219	3,682	4,833
158	4,365	3,810	5,000
160	4,514	3,940	5,171
162	4,666	4,073	5,345
164	4,821	4,208	5,523
166	4,980	4,347	5,705
168	5,141	4,488	5,890
170	5,306	4,632	6,079
172	5,475	4,779	6,272
174	5,646	4,929	6,468
176	5,821	5,081	6,669
178	5,999	5,237	6,873
180	6,181	5,395	7,081

Formula: log y = a + b·log x;
y = TLC$_{He}$ (ml); x = body height (cm);
log TLC$_{He}$ (ml) = −2.2281 + 2.6689·log height (cm);
SD log y·x = ±0.0295; n = 70; r = +0.96.

Table 60. Total lung capacity measured by a helium-dilution method (TLC$_{He}$) in relation to age in boys

Age years	TLC$_{He}$, ml mean	lower limits	upper limits
6	1,929	1,457	2,555
7	2,264	1,710	2,998
8	2,601	1,964	3,443
9	2,939	2,219	3,891
10	3,278	2,476	4,340
11	3,619	2,733	4,791
12	3,960	2,991	5,244
13	4,303	3,250	5,698
14	4,647	3,510	6,153
15	4,992	3,770	6,609
16	5,338	4,032	7,067
17	5,684	4,293	7,526

Formula: log y = a + b·log x;
y = TLC$_{He}$ (ml); x = age (years);
log TLC$_{He}$ (ml) = 2.4783 + 1.0372·log age (years);
SD log y·x = ±0.06107; n = 70; r = +0.83.

Table 61. Total lung capacity measured by a helium-dilution method (TLC$_{He}$) in relation to body surface in boys

Body surface m^2	TLC$_{He}$, ml mean	lower limits	upper limits
0.6	1,417	1,170	1,716
0.7	1,726	1,425	2,089
0.8	2,047	1,691	2,478
0.9	2,379	1,965	2,880
1.0	2,722	2,249	3,295
1.1	3,075	2,540	3,722
1.2	3,436	2,839	4,160
1.3	3,806	3,144	4,608
1.4	4,185	3,457	5,066
1.5	4,570	3,775	5,533
1.6	4,963	4,100	6,008
1.7	5,363	4,430	6,492
1.8	5,769	4,766	6,984
1.9	6,182	5,107	7,484
2.0	6,601	5,453	7,991

Formula: log y = a + b·log x;
y = TLC$_{He}$ (ml); x = body surface (m^2);
log TLC$_{He}$ (ml) = 3.4349 + 1.2777·log body surface (m^2);
SD log y·x = ±0.0415; n = 70; r = +0.93.

Table 62. Total lung capacity measured by a helium-dilution method (TLC$_{He}$) in relation to body height in girls

Height cm	TLC$_{He}$, ml		
	mean	lower limits	upper limits
115	1,828	1,515	2,207
116	1,870	1,549	2,257
118	1,953	1,618	2,358
120	2,040	1,690	2,462
122	2,128	1,763	2,569
124	2,219	1,838	2,678
126	2,312	1,915	2,791
128	2,407	1,994	2,906
130	2,505	2,075	3,024
132	2,605	2,158	3,144
134	2,707	2,243	3,268
136	2,812	2,330	3,395
138	2,920	2,419	3,525
140	3,030	2,510	3,657
142	3,142	2,603	3,793
144	3,257	2,698	3,931
146	3,374	2,795	4,073
148	3,494	2,895	4,218
150	3,617	2,996	4,366
152	3,742	3,100	4,517
154	3,869	3,205	4,671
156	4,000	3,313	4,828
158	4,133	3,424	4,989
160	4,268	3,536	5,152
162	4,407	3,650	5,319
164	4,548	3,767	5,489
166	4,691	3,886	5,663
168	4,838	4,008	5,840
170	4,987	4,131	6,020
172	5,139	4,257	6,203
174	5,294	4,385	6,390
176	5,451	4,516	6,580
178	5,612	4,649	6,774
180	5,775	4,784	6,971

Formula: log y = a + b · log x;
y = TLC$_{He}$ (ml); x = body height (cm);
log TLC$_{He}$ (ml) = −2.0265 + 2.5664 · log height (cm);
SD log y · x = ± 0.0410; n = 74; r = +0.94.

Table 63. Total lung capacity measured by a helium-dilution method (TLC$_{He}$) in relation to age in girls

Age years	TLC$_{He}$, ml		
	mean	lower limits	upper limits
6	1,831	1,337	2,506
7	2,153	1,573	2,948
8	2,478	1,810	3,392
9	2,805	2,049	3,840
10	3,134	2,289	4,291
11	3,465	2,531	4,743
12	3,797	2,774	5,198
13	4,131	3,018	5,655
14	4,465	3,263	6,114
15	4,803	3,508	6,575
16	5,140	3,753	7,037
17	5,479	4,002	7,500

Formula: log y = a + b · log x;
y = TLC$_{He}$ (ml); x = age (years);
log TLC$_{He}$ (ml) = 2.4437 + 1.0524 · log age (years);
SD log y · x = ± 0.0684; n = 74; r = +0.82.

Table 64. Total lung capacity measured by a helium-dilution method (TLC$_{He}$) in relation to body surface in girls

Body surface m^2	TLC$_{He}$, ml		
	mean	lower limits	upper limits
0.6	1,384	1,094	1,750
0.7	1,670	1,321	2,112
0.8	1,965	1,554	2,485
0.9	2,269	1,794	2,869
1.0	2,580	2,040	3,262
1.1	2,898	2,292	3,664
1.2	3,222	2,548	4,074
1.3	3,552	2,810	4,492
1.4	3,888	3,075	4,916
1.5	4,230	3,345	5,348
1.6	4,576	3,619	5,786
1.7	4,927	3,897	6,229
1.8	5,282	4,178	6,679
1.9	5,642	4,462	7,134
2.0	6,006	4,750	7,594

Formula: log y = a + b · log x;
y = TLC$_{He}$ (ml); x = body surface (m^2);
log TLC$_{He}$ (ml) = 3.4116 + 1.2190 · log body surface (m^2);
SD log y · x = ± 0.0511; n = 74; r = +0.90.

Table 65. Functional residual capacity measured by a helium-dilution method (FRC$_{He}$) in relation to body height in boys and girls

Height cm	FRC$_{He}$, ml		
	mean	lower limits	upper limits
115	837	644	1,088
116	858	660	1,115
118	900	693	1,170
120	944	726	1,227
122	989	761	1,286
124	1,036	797	1,346
126	1,084	834	1,408
128	1,133	872	1,472
130	1,183	911	1,538
132	1,236	951	1,606
134	1,289	992	1,675
136	1,344	1,034	1,747
138	1,401	1,078	1,820
140	1,459	1,123	1,896
142	1,518	1,168	1,973
144	1,579	1,215	2,052
146	1,642	1,264	2,134
148	1,706	1,313	2,217
150	1,772	1,364	2,303
152	1,840	1,416	2,391
154	1,909	1,469	2,480
156	1,980	1,523	2,572
158	2,052	1,579	2,666
160	2,126	1,636	2,763
162	2,202	1,695	2,861
164	2,280	1,754	2,962
166	2,359	1,815	3,065
168	2,440	1,878	3,171
170	2,523	1,941	3,278
172	2,607	2,007	3,388
174	2,694	2,073	3,501
176	2,782	2,141	3,615
178	2,872	2,210	3,732
180	2,964	2,281	3,852

Formula: log y = a + b·log x;
y = FRC$_{He}$ (ml); x = body height (cm);
log FRC$_{He}$ (ml) = −2.8899 + 2.8209·log height (cm);
SD log y·x = ±0.0575; n = 144; r = +0.90.

Table 66. Functional residual capacity measured by a helium-dilution method (FRC$_{He}$) in relation to age in boys and girls

Age years	FRC$_{He}$, ml		
	mean	lower limits	upper limits
6	844	586	1,216
7	1,006	698	1,450
8	1,172	813	1,689
9	1,341	931	1,932
10	1,512	1,050	2,179
11	1,686	1,170	2,429
12	1,862	1,292	2,683
13	2,040	1,416	2,939
14	2,220	1,541	3,199
15	2,402	1,667	3,461
16	2,586	1,795	3,726
17	2,771	1,923	3,992

Formula: log y = a + b·log x;
y = FRC$_{He}$ (ml); x = age (years);
log FRC$_{He}$ (ml) = 2.0384 + 1.1412·log age (years);
SD log y·x = ±0.0802; n = 144; r = +0.79.

Table 67. Functional residual capacity measured by a helium-dilution method (FRC$_{He}$) in relation to body surface in boys and girls

Body surface m²	FRC$_{He}$, ml		
	mean	lower limits	upper limits
0.6	649	463	909
0.7	791	565	1,108
0.8	939	671	1,316
0.9	1,093	780	1,531
1.0	1,252	893	1,753
1.1	1,415	1,010	1,982
1.2	1,582	1,130	2,216
1.3	1,754	1,252	2,457
1.4	1,929	1,377	2,702
1.5	2,108	1,505	2,953
1.6	2,290	1,635	3,208
1.7	2,476	1,768	3,468
1.8	2,665	1,902	3,732
1.9	2,856	2,039	4,001
2.0	3,051	2,178	4,274

Formula: log y = a + b·log x;
y = FRC$_{He}$ (ml); x = body surface (m²);
log FRC$_{He}$ (ml) = 3.0976 + 1.2851·log body surface (m²);
SD log y·x = ±0.0740; n = 144; r = +0.82.

Table 68. Functional residual capacity measured by a helium-dilution method (FRC$_{He}$) in relation to body height in boys

Height cm	FRC$_{He}$, ml		
	mean	lower limits	upper limits
115	849	673	1,071
116	870	690	1,098
118	914	724	1,153
120	959	760	1,210
122	1,005	794	1,268
124	1,053	835	1,329
126	1,103	874	1,391
128	1,154	915	1,456
130	1,206	956	1,522
132	1,260	999	1,590
134	1,316	1,043	1,660
136	1,373	1,086	1,732
138	1,431	1,135	1,806
140	1,492	1,182	1,882
142	1,553	1,231	1,960
144	1,617	1,282	2,040
146	1,682	1,333	2,122
148	1,749	1,387	2,206
150	1,818	1,441	2,293
152	1,888	1,497	2,382
154	1,960	1,554	2,473
156	2,034	1,612	2,566
158	2,109	1,672	2,661
160	2,187	1,734	2,759
162	2,266	1,796	2,859
164	2,347	1,861	2,961
166	2,430	1,926	3,066
168	2,515	1,994	3,173
170	2,602	2,062	3,282
172	2,690	2,133	3,394
174	2,781	2,205	3,508
176	2,874	2,278	3,625
178	2,968	2,353	3,744
180	3,065	2,429	3,866

Formula: log y = a + b·log x;
y = FRC$_{He}$ (ml); x = body height (cm);
log FRC$_{He}$ (ml) = −2.9740 + 2.8646·log height (cm);
SD log y·x = ±0.0505; n = 70; r = +0.91.

Table 69. Functional residual capacity measured by a helium-dilution method (FRC$_{He}$) in relation to body height in girls

Height cm	FRC$_{He}$, ml		
	mean	lower limits	upper limits
115	830	624	1,105
116	850	639	1,132
118	892	670	1,187
120	934	701	1,243
122	977	734	1,301
124	1,022	768	1,361
126	1,068	803	1,422
128	1,116	838	1,486
130	1,165	875	1,551
132	1,215	913	1,617
134	1,266	951	1,686
136	1,319	991	1,756
138	1,373	1,032	1,828
140	1,429	1,073	1,902
142	1,486	1,116	1,978
144	1,545	1,160	2,056
146	1,604	1,205	2,136
148	1,666	1,251	2,218
150	1,729	1,299	2,301
152	1,793	1,347	2,387
154	1,859	1,396	2,475
156	1,926	1,447	2,564
158	1,995	1,499	2,656
160	2,066	1,552	2,750
162	2,138	1,606	2,846
164	2,211	1,661	2,944
166	2,287	1,718	3,044
168	2,363	1,775	3,146
170	2,442	1,834	3,251
172	2,522	1,894	3,357
174	2,604	1,956	3,466
176	2,687	2,019	3,577
178	2,772	2,082	3,690
180	2,859	2,148	3,806

Formula: log y = a + b·log x;
y = FRC$_{He}$ (ml); x = body height (cm);
log FRC$_{He}$ (ml) = −2.7651 + 2.7586·log height (cm);
SD log y·x = ±0.0623; n = 74; r = +0.89.

Table 70. Percentage of functional residual capacity from total lung capacity measured by helium-dilution method $\left(\% \frac{FRC}{TLC} He\right)$ in relation to body height in boys and girls

Height cm	$\% \frac{FRC}{TLC} He$		
	mean	lower limits	upper limits
115	45.79	37.84	53.75
116	45.86	37.90	53.81
118	45.98	38.02	53.94
120	46.10	38.15	54.06
122	46.22	38.27	54.18
124	46.35	38.39	54.30
126	46.47	38.51	54.43
128	46.59	38.64	54.55
130	46.72	38.76	54.67
132	46.84	38.88	54.80
134	46.96	39.01	54.92
136	47.09	39.13	55.04
138	47.21	39.26	55.16
140	47.33	39.38	55.29
142	47.45	39.50	55.41
144	47.58	39.62	55.53
146	47.70	39.74	55.66
148	47.82	39.87	55.78
150	47.95	39.99	55.90
152	48.07	40.11	56.03
154	48.19	40.24	56.15
156	48.32	40.36	56.27
158	48.44	40.48	56.39
160	48.56	40.61	56.52
162	48.68	40.73	56.64
164	48.81	40.85	56.76
166	48.93	40.97	56.89
168	49.05	41.10	57.01
170	49.18	41.22	57.13
172	49.30	41.34	57.26
174	49.42	41.47	57.38
176	49.55	41.59	57.50
178	49.67	41.71	57.62
180	49.79	41.84	57.75

Formula: $y = a + b \cdot x$;
$y = \% \frac{FRC}{TLC} He$; x = body height (cm);
$\% \frac{FRC}{TLC} He = 38.7281 + 0.0614 \cdot height (cm)$;
SD $y \cdot x = \pm 4.02$; $n = 144$; $r = +0.21$.

Table 71. Residual volume measured by helium-dilution method (RV_{He}) in relation to body height in boys and girls

Height cm	RV_{He}, ml		
	mean	lower limits	upper limits
115	420	250	707
116	430	255	722
118	448	266	754
120	467	278	785
122	487	289	818
124	506	301	852
126	527	313	886
128	548	326	921
130	569	338	957
132	591	351	994
134	613	365	1,031
136	636	378	1,070
138	660	392	1,109
140	683	406	1,149
142	708	421	1,190
144	733	436	1,232
146	758	451	1,274
148	784	466	1,318
150	810	482	1,362
152	837	498	1,408
154	865	514	1,454
156	893	531	1,501
158	921	548	1,549
160	950	565	1,598
162	980	583	1,647
164	1,010	601	1,698
166	1,041	619	1,749
168	1,072	637	1,802
170	1,103	656	1,855
172	1,136	675	1,910
174	1,169	695	1,965
176	1,202	715	2,021
178	1,236	735	2,078
180	1,271	756	2,136

Formula: $\log y = a + b \cdot \log x$;
$y = RV_{He}$ (ml); x = body height (cm);
$\log RV_{He}$ (ml) $= -2.4585 + 2.4665 \cdot \log$ height (cm);
SD $\log y \cdot x = \pm 0.1141$; $n = 144$; $r = +0.67$.

Table 72. Residual volume measured by helium-dilution method (RV_{He}) in relation to age in boys and girls

Age years	RV_{He}, ml		
	mean	lower limits	upper limits
6	428	242	758
7	498	281	832
8	568	321	1,005
9	637	360	1,128
10	707	399	1,251
11	776	438	1,373
12	845	477	1,495
13	914	516	1,617
14	983	555	1,739
15	1,051	594	1,860
16	1,120	633	1,982
17	1,188	671	2,103

Formula: $\log y = a + b \cdot \log x$;
$y = RV_{He}$ (ml); x = age (years);
$\log RV_{He}$ (ml) $= 1.8704 + 0.9790 \cdot \log$ age (years);
SD $\log y \cdot x = \pm 0.1253$; $n = 144$; $r = +0.58$.

Table 73. Residual volume measured by helium-dilution method (RV_{He}) in relation to body surface in boys and girls

Body surface m^2	RV_{He}, ml		
	mean	lower limits	upper limits
0.6	340	195	594
0.7	404	231	705
0.8	468	268	817
0.9	534	306	931
1.0	600	344	1,046
1.1	667	382	1,163
1.2	734	421	1,281
1.3	803	460	1,400
1.4	871	500	1,580
1.5	941	539	1,640
1.6	1,010	579	1,762
1.7	1,081	620	1,885
1.8	1,151	660	2,008
1.9	1,223	701	2,132
2.0	1,294	742	2,251

Formula: $\log y = a + b \cdot \log x$;
$y = RV_{He}$ (ml); x = body surface (m^2);
$\log RV_{He}$ (ml) $= 2.7784 + 1.1083 \cdot \log$ body surface (m^2);
SD $\log y \cdot x = \pm 0.1221$; $n = 144$; $r = +0.61$.

Table 74. Residual volume measured by a helium-dilution method (RV$_{He}$) in relation to body height in boys

Height cm	RV$_{He}$, ml		
	mean	lower limits	upper limits
115	425	267	678
116	434	272	692
118	452	283	720
120	470	295	748
122	488	306	778
124	507	318	807
126	526	330	838
128	546	342	869
130	566	355	901
132	586	368	934
134	607	381	967
136	628	394	1,001
138	650	408	1,035
140	672	422	1,070
142	694	436	1,106
144	717	450	1,143
146	741	465	1,180
148	765	480	1,218
150	789	495	1,256
152	813	511	1,296
154	838	526	1,336
156	864	542	1,376
158	890	559	1,418
160	916	575	1,460
162	943	592	1,502
164	970	609	1,546
166	998	627	1,590
168	1,026	644	1,635
170	1,055	662	1,680
172	1,084	680	1,726
174	1,113	699	1,773
176	1,143	718	1,821
178	1,174	737	1,869
180	1,205	756	1,919

Formula: log y = a + b·log x;
y = RV$_{He}$ (ml); x = body height (cm);
log RV$_{He}$ (ml) = −2.1543 + 2.3213·log height (cm);
SD log y·x = ±0.1012; n = 70; r = +0.67.

Table 75. Residual volume measured by a helium-dilution method (RV$_{He}$) in relation to body height in girls

Height cm	RV$_{He}$, ml		
	mean	lower limits	upper limits
115	416	234	739
116	425	239	756
118	445	250	791
120	465	261	826
122	485	273	863
124	506	285	900
126	528	297	939
128	550	309	978
130	573	322	1,018
132	596	335	1,060
134	620	349	1,102
136	645	363	1,146
138	670	377	1,190
140	695	391	1,236
142	722	406	1,282
144	748	421	1,330
146	776	436	1,379
148	804	452	1,429
150	833	468	1,480
152	862	485	1,532
154	892	502	1,585
156	922	519	1,639
158	954	536	1,695
160	985	554	1,751
162	1,018	573	1,809
164	1,051	591	1,868
166	1,085	610	1,928
168	1,119	630	1,989
170	1,154	649	2,052
172	1,190	670	2,115
174	1,227	690	2,180
176	1,264	711	2,246
178	1,302	732	2,313
180	1,340	754	2,382

Formula: log y = a + b·log x;
y = RV$_{He}$ (ml); x = body height (cm);
log RV$_{He}$ (ml) = −2.7587 + 2.6099·log height (cm);
SD log y·x = ±0.1252; n = 74; r = +0.67.

Table 76. Difference between FRC_{box} and FRC_{He} as percentage of FRC_{box} $\left(\% \frac{FRC_{box} - FRC_{He}}{FRC_{box}}\right)$ in relation to body height in boys and girls

Height cm	% $\frac{FRC_{box} - FRC_{He}}{FRC_{box}}$		
	mean	lower limits	upper limits
115	8.7	–	24.2
116	8.6	–	24.1
118	8.4	–	23.9
120	8.2	–	23.6
122	7.9	–	23.4
124	7.7	–	23.2
126	7.5	–	23.0
128	7.3	–	22.7
130	7.0	–	22.5
132	6.8	–	22.3
134	6.6	–	22.1
136	6.4	–	21.8
138	6.1	–	21.6
140	5.9	–	21.4
142	5.7	–	21.2
144	5.5	–	20.9
146	5.2	–	20.7
148	5.0	–	20.5
150	4.8	–	20.3
152	4.6	–	20.0
154	4.3	–	19.8
156	4.1	–	19.6
158	3.9	–	19.4
160	3.7	–	19.1
162	3.4	–	18.9
164	3.2	–	18.7
166	3.0	–	18.5
168	2.8	–	18.2
170	2.5	–	18.0
172	2.3	–	17.8
174	2.1	–	17.6
176	1.8	–	17.3
178	1.6	–	17.1
180	1.4	–	16.9

Formula: $y = a + b \cdot x$;
$y = \% \frac{FRC_{box} - FRC_{He}}{FRC_{box}}$; x = body height (cm);
$\% \frac{FRC_{box} - FRC_{He}}{FRC_{box}} = 21.7638 - 0.1128 \cdot height$ (cm);
SD $y \cdot x = \pm 7.81$; $n = 123$; $r = -0.21$.

Table 77. Difference between FRC_{box} and FRC_{He} as percentage of FRC_{box} $\left(\% \frac{FRC_{box} - FRC_{He}}{FRC_{box}}\right)$ in relation to age in boys and girls

Age years	% $\frac{FRC_{box} - FRC_{He}}{FRC_{box}}$		
	mean	lower limits	upper limits
6	9.46	–	24.82
7	8.61	–	23.97
8	7.77	–	23.13
9	6.92	–	22.28
10	6.08	–	21.43
11	5.23	–	20.59
12	4.38	–	19.74
13	3.54	–	18.90
14	2.69	–	18.05
15	1.85	–	17.20
16	1.00	–	16.36
17	0.15	–	15.50

Formula: $y = a + b \cdot x$;
$y = \% \frac{FRC_{box} - FRC_{He}}{FRC_{box}}$; x = age (years);
$\% \frac{FRC_{box} - FRC_{He}}{FRC_{box}} = 14.5408 - 0.8459 \cdot age$ (years);
SD $y \cdot x = \pm 7.75$; $n = 123$; $r = -0.24$.

Table 78. Difference between FRC_{box} and FRC_{He} as percentage of FRC_{box} $\left(\% \frac{FRC_{box} - FRC_{He}}{FRC_{box}}\right)$ in relation to body surface in boys and girls

Body surface m²	% $\frac{FRC_{box} - FRC_{He}}{FRC_{box}}$		
	mean	lower limits	upper limits
0.6	8.47	–	24.07
0.7	7.96	–	23.57
0.8	7.46	–	23.06
0.9	6.95	–	22.56
1.0	6.44	–	22.05
1.1	3.94	–	21.54
1.2	5.43	–	21.04
1.3	4.92	–	20.53
1.4	4.42	–	20.03
1.5	3.91	–	19.52
1.6	3.41	–	19.01
1.7	2.90	–	18.51
1.8	2.39	–	18.00
1.9	1.89	–	17.49
2.0	1.38	–	16.99

Formula: $y = a + b \cdot x$;
$y = \% \frac{FRC_{box} - FRC_{He}}{FRC_{box}}$; x = body surface (m²);
$\% \frac{FRC_{box} - FRC_{He}}{FRC_{box}} = 11.5097 - 5.0615 \cdot body\ surface$ (m²);
SD $y \cdot x = \pm 7.88$; $n = 123$; $r = -0.20$.

Table 79. Tidal volume (V_T) in relation to body height in boys and girls

Height cm	V_T, ml		
	mean	lower limits	upper limits
115	279	185	421
116	283	188	428
118	293	194	442
120	302	200	456
122	311	206	470
124	321	213	484
126	331	219	499
128	341	226	514
130	351	232	529
132	361	239	544
134	371	246	560
136	381	253	575
138	392	260	591
140	403	267	607
142	413	274	624
144	424	281	640
146	435	289	657
148	447	296	674
150	458	303	691
152	469	311	708
154	481	319	726
156	493	327	743
158	505	334	761
160	517	342	779
162	529	350	798
164	541	358	816
166	553	367	835
168	566	375	854
170	578	383	873
172	591	392	892
174	604	400	911
176	617	409	931
178	630	418	951
180	643	426	971

Formula: log y = a + b·log x;
y = V_T (ml); x = body height (cm);
log V_T (ml) = − 1.3956 + 1.8643·log height (cm);
SD log y·x = ± 0.0903; n = 170; r = + 0.65.

Table 80. Tidal volume (V_T) in relation to age in boys and girls

Age years	V_T, ml		
	mean	lower limits	upper limits
6	278	178	432
7	313	201	486
8	347	223	539
9	380	244	590
10	412	265	640
11	443	285	689
12	474	305	737
13	504	324	784
14	534	343	830
15	563	362	875
16	592	381	920
17	620	399	964

Formula: log y = a + b·log x;
y = V_T (ml); x = age (years);
log V_T (ml) = 1.8438 + 0.7713·log age (years);
SD log y·x = ± 0.0969; n = 170; r = + 0.57.

Table 81. Tidal volume (V_T) in relation to body surface in boys and girls

Surface m^2	V_T, ml		
	mean	lower limits	upper limits
0.6	229	150	348
0.7	262	172	400
0.8	295	194	450
0.9	328	215	500
1.0	360	236	549
1.1	392	257	598
1.2	424	278	646
1.3	455	299	694
1.4	486	319	741
1.5	517	339	788
1.6	548	359	835
1.7	578	379	881
1.8	608	399	927
1.9	638	419	973
2.0	668	438	1,018

Formula: log y = a + b·log x;
y = V_T (ml); x = body surface (m^2);
log V_T (ml) = 2.5572 + 0.8897·log body surface (m^2);
SD log y·x = ± 0.0926; n = 170; r = + 0.62.

Table 82. Conversion factors of some lung function parameters from conventional to SI units

Parameter	Conventional unit	SI unit	Conversion factor
Pressure (P)	cm H_2O	kPa	0.0980665; (1 cm $H_2O \cong 0.1$ kPa)
Compliance (C_L)	ml/cm H_2O (ml$\cdot$cm H_2O^{-1})	ml/kPa; (ml$\cdot$kPa^{-1})	10.19716; (1 ml/cm $H_2O \cong 10$ ml/kPa)
Airway, pulmonary resistance (R_{aw}, R_L)	cm H_2O/1/s; (cm $H_2O \cdot l^{-1} \cdot s$)	kPa/l/s; (kPa$\cdot l^{-1} \cdot s$)	0.0980665; (1 cm H_2O/1/s $\cong 0.1$ kPa/l/s)
Airway conductance (G_{aw})	l/s/cm H_2O; (l$\cdot s^{-1} \cdot$cm H_2O^{-1})	l/s/kPa; (l$\cdot s^{-1} \cdot$kPa^{-1})	10.19716; (1 liter/s/cm $H_2O \cong 10$ liters/s/kPa)
'Specific' airway conductance (G_{aw}/TGV)	l/s/cm H_2O/l; (l$\cdot s^{-1} \cdot$cm $H_2O^{-1} \cdot l^{-1}$)	l/s/kPa/l; (l$\cdot s^{-1} \cdot$kPa$^{-1} \cdot l^{-1}$)	10.19716; (l liter/s/cm H_2O/l $\cong 10$ liters/s/kPa/liter)
Work of breathing (W)	kpm/l; kpm/min; (kpm$\cdot l^{-1}$; kpm$\cdot$min^{-1})	J/l; J/min; (J$\cdot l^{-1}$; J$\cdot$min^{-1})	9.8066; (1 kpm/l $\cong 10$ J/l; 1 kpm/min $\cong 10$ J/min)
Lung diffusing capacity (D_L) and membrane component (Dm)	ml/min/Torr (ml$\cdot$min$^{-1} \cdot$Torr^{-1})	mmol/min/kPa; (mmol$\cdot$min$^{-1} \cdot$kPa^{-1})	0.3348; (1 ml/min/Torr $\cong 0.335$ mmol/min/kPa)
Oxygen consumption, CO_2 output	ml/min STPD	mmol/s; (mmol$\cdot s^{-1}$)	$0.7441 \cdot 10^{-3}$ for O_2; $0.7486 \cdot 10^{-3}$ for CO_2

Table 83. Minute ventilation (MV) in relation to body height in boys and girls

Height cm	MV, ml/min		
	mean	lower limits	upper limits
115	5,872	4,454	7,741
116	5,958	4,520	7,855
118	6,132	4,652	8,084
120	6,308	4,785	8,316
122	6,486	4,920	8,550
124	6,666	5,056	8,787
126	6,847	5,194	9,027
128	7,031	5,333	9,269
130	7,217	5,474	9,514
132	7,405	5,617	9,761
134	7,594	5,761	10,011
136	7,786	5,906	10,264
138	7,979	6,053	10,519
140	8,175	6,201	10,777
142	8,372	6,351	11,037
144	8,571	6,502	11,300
146	8,772	6,654	11,565
148	8,976	6,808	11,832
150	9,180	6,964	12,103
152	9,387	7,121	12,375
154	9,596	7,279	12,650
156	9,806	7,439	12,928
158	10,019	7,600	13,208
160	10,233	7,762	13,490
162	10,449	7,926	13,775
164	10,667	8,091	14,062
166	10,886	8,258	14,352
168	11,108	8,426	14,643
170	11,331	8,595	14,938
172	11,556	8,766	15,235
174	11,783	8,938	15,534
176	12,012	9,112	15,835
178	12,242	9,286	16,139
180	12,474	9,463	16,445

Formula: $\log y = a + b \cdot \log x$;
y = MV (ml/min); x = body height (cm);
$\log$ MV (ml/min) = $0.3035 + 1.6815 \cdot \log$ height (cm);
SD $\log y \cdot x = \pm 0.0607$; n = 170; r = +0.75.

Table 84. Minute ventilation (MV) in relation to age in boys and girls

Age years	MV, ml/min		
	mean	lower limits	upper limits
6	5,864	4,287	8,022
7	6,524	4,769	8,924
8	7,154	5,230	9,787
9	7,761	5,674	10,616
10	8,347	6,102	11,418
11	8,916	6,518	12,196
12	9,468	6,922	12,951
13	10,007	7,315	13,688
14	10,532	7,700	14,407
15	11,047	8,076	15,111
16	11,551	8,444	15,800
17	12,045	8,805	16,476

Formula: $\log y = a + b \cdot \log x$;
y = MV (ml/min); x = age (years);
$\log$ MV (ml/min) = $3.2305 + 0.6910 \cdot \log$ age (years);
SD $\log y \cdot x = \pm 0.0689$; n = 170; r = +0.66.

Table 85. Minute ventilation (MV) in relation to body surface in boys and girls

Body surface m²	MV, ml/min		
	mean	lower limits	upper limits
0.6	4,937	3,689	6,607
0.7	5,581	4,170	7,469
0.8	6,206	4,637	8,305
0.9	6,815	5,092	9,121
1.0	7,411	5,537	9,918
1.1	7,994	5,973	10,699
1.2	8,567	6,401	11,465
1.3	9,130	6,822	12,219
1.4	9,684	7,236	12,960
1.5	10,230	7,644	13,691
1.6	10,769	8,046	14,412
1.7	11,301	8,444	15,124
1.8	11,826	8,836	15,827
1.9	12,346	9,225	16,522
2.0	12,859	9,609	17,210

Formula: $\log y = a + b \cdot \log x$;
y = MV (ml/min); x = body surface (m²);
$\log$ MV (ml/min) = $3.8698 + 0.7951 \cdot \log$ body surface (m²);
SD $\log y \cdot x = \pm 0.0641$; n = 170; r = +0.72.

Table 86. Maximal minute ventilation (MMV) in relation to body height in boys and girls

Height cm	MMV, ml/min		
	mean	lower limits	upper limits
115	22,094	13,138	37,154
116	22,683	13,488	38,144
118	23,892	14,207	40,178
120	25,144	14,952	42,284
122	26,439	15,722	44,462
124	27,779	16,518	46,714
126	29,163	17,341	49,041
128	30,592	18,192	51,446
130	32,068	19,069	53,927
132	33,591	19,975	56,488
134	35,162	20,909	59,130
136	36,781	21,872	61,852
138	38,449	22,864	64,658
140	40,168	23,886	67,548
142	41,937	24,938	70,523
144	43,758	26,021	73,585
146	45,631	27,134	76,735
148	47,557	28,280	79,974
150	49,537	29,457	83,304
152	51,572	30,667	86,725
154	53,661	31,910	90,240
156	55,807	33,186	93,849
158	58,010	34,496	97,553
160	60,271	35,840	101,354
162	62,589	37,219	105,253
164	64,967	38,633	109,252
166	67,405	40,082	113,351
168	69,903	41,568	117,552
170	72,463	43,090	121,857
172	75,084	44,649	126,266
174	77,769	46,246	130,781
176	80,518	47,880	135,402
178	83,330	49,553	140,132
180	86,208	51,264	144,972

Formula: log y = a + b·log x;
y = MMV (ml/min); x = body height (cm);
log MMV (ml/min) = − 1.9178 + 3.0388·log height (cm);
SD log y·x = ± 0.1141; n = 140; r = + 0.75.

Table 87. Maximal minute ventilation (MMV) in relation to age in boys and girls

Age years	MMV, ml/min		
	mean	lower limits	upper limits
6	21,749	12,246	38,624
7	26,447	14,892	46,967
8	31,330	17,641	55,639
9	36,380	20,485	64,607
10	41,583	23,415	73,848
11	46,929	26,425	83,341
12	52,406	29,510	93,069
13	58,008	32,664	103,017
14	63,727	35,884	113,174
15	69,558	39,167	123,528
16	75,493	42,510	134,069
17	81,529	45,909	144,788

Formula: log y = a + b·log x;
y = MMV (ml/min); x = age (years);
log MMV (ml/min) = 3.3501 + 1.2687·log age (years);
SD log y·x = ± 0.1261; n = 140; r = + 0.68.

Table 88. Maximal minute ventilation (MMV) in relation to body surface in boys and girls

Body surface m^2	MMV, ml/min		
	mean	lower limits	upper limits
0.6	15,642	9,101	26,884
0.7	19,636	11,425	33,749
0.8	23,912	13,912	41,097
0.9	28,449	16,552	48,896
1.0	33,233	19,336	57,118
1.1	38,250	22,255	65,741
1.2	43,489	25,303	74,745
1.3	48,939	28,474	84,113
1.4	54,593	31,764	93,830
1.5	60,442	35,167	103,882
1.6	66,480	38,680	114,299
1.7	72,699	42,299	124,940
1.8	79,095	46,020	135,941
1.9	83,662	49,841	147,227
2.0	92,395	53,758	158,000

Formula: log y = a + b·log x;
y = MMV (ml/min); x = body surface (m^2);
log MMV (ml/min) = 4.5215 + 1.4751·log body surface (m^2);
SD log y·x = ± 0.1189; n = 140; r = + 0.72.

Table 89. Elastic recoil pressure of the lungs at 25 % of vital capacity (Pst(l)$_{25\%\,VC}$) in relation to body height in boys and girls

Height cm	Pst(l)$_{25\%\,VC}$					
	mean		lower limits		upper limits	
	a	b	a	b	a	b
115	0.093	0.95	−0.246	−2.52	0.432	4.44
116	0.098	1.00	−0.241	−2.47	0.437	4.49
118	0.108	1.11	−0.230	−2.37	0.447	4.59
120	0.118	1.21	−0.220	−2.27	0.457	4.70
122	0.128	1.31	−0.210	−2.16	0.467	4.80
124	0.138	1.42	−0.200	−2.06	0.477	4.90
126	0.148	1.52	−0.190	−1.96	0.487	5.01
128	0.158	1.62	−0.180	−1.85	0.497	5.11
130	0.168	1.73	−0.170	−1.75	0.508	5.21
132	0.179	1.83	−0.160	−1.65	0.518	5.32
134	0.189	1.93	−0.150	−1.54	0.528	5.42
136	0.199	2.04	−0.139	−1.44	0.538	5.52
138	0.209	2.14	−0.129	−1.34	0.548	5.63
140	0.219	2.24	−0.119	−1.23	0.558	5.73
142	0.229	2.35	−0.109	−1.13	0.568	5.83
144	0.239	2.45	−0.099	−1.03	0.578	5.94
146	0.249	2.55	−0.089	−0.92	0.589	6.04
148	0.260	2.66	−0.079	−0.82	0.599	6.14
150	0.270	2.76	−0.069	−0.72	0.609	6.25
152	0.280	2.86	−0.058	−0.61	0.619	6.35
154	0.290	2.97	−0.048	−0.51	0.629	6.45
156	0.300	3.07	−0.038	−0.41	0.639	6.56
158	0.310	3.17	−0.028	−0.30	0.649	6.66
160	0.320	3.28	−0.018	−0.20	0.659	6.76
162	0.330	3.38	−0.008	−0.10	0.669	6.87
164	0.340	3.48	0.001	0.06	0.680	6.97
166	0.351	3.59	0.011	0.10	0.690	7.07
168	0.361	3.69	0.022	0.20	0.700	7.18
170	0.371	3.79	0.032	0.31	0.710	7.28
172	0.381	3.90	0.042	0.41	0.720	7.38
174	0.391	4.00	0.052	0.51	0.730	7.49
176	0.401	4.10	0.062	0.62	0.740	7.59
178	0.411	4.21	0.072	0.72	0.750	7.69
180	0.422	4.31	0.082	0.82	0.761	7.80

Formula: $y = a + b \cdot x$;
$y = Pst(l)_{25\%\,VC}$ (kPa or cm H$_2$O); x = body height (cm);
$Pst(l)_{25\%\,VC}$ (kPa) $= -0.48894 + 5.06023 \cdot 10^{-3} \cdot$ height;
SD y·x = ±0.171; n = 106; r = +0.40.
$Pst(l)_{25\%\,VC}$ (cm H$_2$O) $= -4.9859 + 0.0516 \cdot x$;
SD y·x = ±1.75.
a = kPa; b = cm H$_2$O.

Table 90. Elastic recoil pressure of the lungs at 25 % vital capacity (Pst(l)$_{25\%\,VC}$) in relation to age in boys and girls

Age years	Pst(l)$_{25\%\,VC}$					
	mean		lower limits		upper limits	
	a	b	a	b	a	b
6	0.118	1.20	−0.230	−2.37	0.467	4.78
7	0.146	1.49	−0.202	−2.08	0.495	5.07
8	0.175	1.78	−0.174	−1.79	0.524	5.36
9	0.203	2.07	−0.145	−1.50	0.552	5.65
10	0.231	2.36	−0.117	−1.21	0.580	5.94
11	0.259	2.64	−0.089	−0.96	0.608	6.22
12	0.287	2.93	−0.061	−0.67	0.636	6.51
13	0.316	3.22	−0.033	−0.35	0.665	6.80
14	0.344	3.51	−0.004	−0.06	0.693	7.09
15	0.372	3.79	0.023	0.21	0.721	7.37
16	0.400	4.08	0.051	0.50	0.749	7.66
17	0.428	4.37	0.079	0.79	0.777	7.95

Formula: $y = a + b \cdot x$;
$y = Pst(l)_{25\%\,VC}$ (kPa or cm H$_2$O); x = age (years);
$Pst(l)_{25\%\,VC}$ (kPa) $= -0.05070 + 0.02821 \cdot$ age (years);
SD y·x = ±0.176; n = 106; r = +0.34.
$Pst(l)_{25\%\,VC}$ (cm H$_2$O) $= -0.5170 + 0.2877 \cdot x$;
SD y·x = ±1.80.
a = kPa; b = cm H$_2$O.

Table 91. Elastic recoil pressure of the lungs at 25 % of vital capacity (Pst(l)$_{25\%\,VC}$) in relation body surface in boys and girls

Body surface m^2	Pst(l)$_{25\%\,VC}$					
	mean		lower limits		upper limits	
	a	b	a	b	a	b
0.60	0.090	0.92	−0.258	−2.64	0.440	4.50
0.70	0.115	1.18	−0.233	−2.39	0.464	4.75
0.80	0.140	1.43	−0.208	−2.14	0.489	5.00
0.90	0.165	1.68	−0.183	−1.88	0.514	5.26
1.00	0.190	1.94	−0.158	−1.63	0.539	5.51
1.10	0.215	2.19	−0.133	−1.38	0.564	5.76
1.20	0.240	2.44	−0.109	−1.12	0.589	6.02
1.30	0.264	2.70	−0.084	−0.87	0.613	6.27
1.40	0.289	2.95	−0.059	−0.61	0.638	6.52
1.50	0.314	3.20	−0.034	−0.36	0.663	6.78
1.60	0.339	3.46	−0.009	−0.11	0.688	7.03
1.70	0.364	3.71	0.015	0.14	0.713	7.28
1.80	0.389	3.96	0.040	0.39	0.738	7.54
1.90	0.414	4.22	0.065	0.64	0.763	7.79
2.00	0.438	4.47	0.086	0.90	0.791	8.04

Formula: $y = a + b \cdot x$;
$y = Pst(l)_{25\%\,VC}$ (kPa or cm H$_2$O); x = body surface (m^2);
$Pst(l)_{25\%\,VC}$ (kPa) $= -0.05817 + 0.24852 \cdot$ body surface (m^2);
SD y·x = ±0.176; n = 106; r = +0.35.
$Pst(l)_{25\%\,VC}$ (cm H$_2$O) $= -0.5932 + 2.5342 \cdot x$;
SD y·x = ±1.80.
a = kPa; b = cm H$_2$O.

Table 92. Elastic recoil pressure of the lungs measured at 30% of vital capacity (Pst(l)$_{30\%\,VC}$) in relation to body height in boys and girls

Height cm	Pst(l)$_{30\%\,VC}$					
	mean		lower limits		upper limits	
	a	b	a	b	a	b
115	0.164	1.68	−1.191	−1.96	0.521	5.34
116	0.171	1.75	−0.185	−1.90	0.527	5.40
118	0.183	1.87	−0.173	−1.77	0.539	5.52
120	0.195	2.00	−0.160	−1.65	0.551	5.65
122	0.207	2.12	−0.148	−1.52	0.563	5.77
124	0.219	2.24	−0.136	−1.40	0.576	5.90
126	0.232	2.37	−0.124	−1.27	0.588	6.02
128	0.244	2.49	−0.112	−1.15	0.600	6.15
130	0.256	2.62	−0.099	−1.02	0.612	6.27
132	0.268	2.74	−0.087	−0.90	0.624	6.40
134	0.280	2.87	−0.075	−0.78	0.637	6.52
136	0.293	2.99	−0.063	−0.65	0.649	6.64
138	0.305	3.12	−0.051	−0.53	0.661	6.77
140	0.317	3.24	−0.038	−0.40	0.673	6.89
142	0.329	3.37	−0.026	−0.28	0.685	7.02
144	0.341	3.49	−0.014	−0.15	0.698	7.14
146	0.354	3.61	−0.002	−0.03	0.710	7.27
148	0.366	3.74	0.010	0.01	0.722	7.39
150	0.378	3.86	0.022	0.21	0.734	7.52
152	0.390	3.99	0.034	0.34	0.746	7.64
154	0.402	4.11	0.046	0.46	0.759	7.77
156	0.415	4.24	0.058	0.58	0.771	7.89
158	0.427	4.36	0.071	0.71	0.783	8.01
160	0.439	4.49	0.083	0.83	0.795	8.14
162	0.451	4.61	0.095	0.96	0.807	8.26
164	0.463	4.74	0.107	1.08	0.819	8.39
166	0.476	4.86	0.119	1.21	0.832	8.51
168	0.488	4.98	0.132	1.33	0.844	8.64
170	0.500	5.11	0.144	1.46	0.856	8.76
172	0.512	5.23	0.156	1.58	0.868	8.89
174	0.524	5.36	0.168	1.71	0.880	9.01
176	0.537	5.48	0.180	1.83	0.893	9.14
178	0.549	5.61	0.193	1.95	0.905	9.26
180	0.561	5.73	0.205	2.08	0.917	9.38

Formula: y = a + b·x;
y = Pst(l)$_{30\%\,VC}$ (kPa or cm H$_2$O); x = body height (cm);
Pst(l)$_{30\%\,VC}$ (kPa) = −0.53658 + 6.09967·10^{-3}· height;
SD y·x = ±0.180; n = 130; r = +0.46.
Pst(l)$_{30\%\,VC}$ (cm H$_2$O) = −5.4716 + 0.0622·x;
SD y·x = ±1.84.
a = kPa; b = cm H$_2$O.

Table 93. Elastic recoil pressure of the lungs at 30% of vital capacity (Pst(l)$_{30\%\,VC}$ in relation to age in boys and girls

Age years	Pst(l)$_{30\%\,VC}$					
	mean		lower limits		upper limits	
	a	b	a	b	a	b
6	0.185	2.02	−0.184	−1.76	0.555	5.81
7	0.218	2.36	−0.151	−1.42	0.588	6.15
8	0.251	2.70	−0.118	−1.08	0.621	6.49
9	0.285	3.04	−0.085	−0.74	0.655	6.83
10	0.318	3.38	−0.051	−0.40	0.688	7.17
11	0.351	3.72	−0.018	−0.06	0.721	7.51
12	0.385	4.06	0.015	0.27	0.755	7.85
13	0.418	4.40	0.048	0.61	0.788	8.19
14	0.451	4.74	0.081	0.95	0.821	8.53
15	0.485	5.08	0.114	1.29	0.855	8.87
16	0.518	5.42	0.148	1.63	0.888	9.21
17	0.551	5.76	0.181	1.97	0.921	9.55

Formula: y = a + b·x;
y = Pst(l)$_{30\%\,VC}$ (kPa or cm H$_2$O); x = age (years);
Pst(l)$_{30\%\,VC}$ (kPa) = −0.01483 + 0.03332·age (years);
SD y·x = ±0.187; n = 130; r = +0.38.
Pst(l)$_{30\%\,VC}$ (cm H$_2$O) = −0.01513 + 0.3398·x;
SD y·x = ±1.91.
a = kPa; b = cm H$_2$O.

Table 94. Elastic recoil pressure of the lungs measured at 30% vital capacity (Pst(l)$_{30\%\,VC}$) in relation to body surface in boys and girls

Body surface m^2	Pst(l)$_{30\%\,VC}$					
	mean		lower limits		upper limits	
	a	b	a	b	a	b
0.60	0.145	1.51	−0.218	−2.21	0.513	5.24
0.70	0.177	1.83	−0.186	−1.89	0.541	5.56
0.80	0.209	2.16	−0.154	−1.56	0.573	5.89
0.90	0.241	2.49	−0.122	−1.24	0.605	6.22
1.00	0.273	2.81	−0.090	−0.91	0.637	6.54
1.10	0.305	3.14	−0.058	−0.58	0.669	6.87
1.20	0.337	3.47	−0.026	−0.26	0.701	7.20
1.30	0.369	3.79	0.005	0.06	0.733	7.52
1.40	0.401	4.12	0.037	0.39	0.765	7.85
1.50	0.433	4.44	0.069	0.71	0.797	8.18
1.60	0.465	4.77	0.101	1.04	0.829	8.50
1.70	0.497	5.10	0.133	1.37	0.861	8.83
1.80	0.529	5.42	0.165	1.69	0.893	9.15
1.90	0.561	5.75	0.197	2.02	0.925	9.48
2.00	0.593	6.08	0.229	2.34	0.961	9.81

Formula: y = a + b·x;
y = Pst(l)$_{30\%\,VC}$ (kPa or cm H$_2$O); x = body surface (m^2);
Pst(l)$_{30\%\,VC}$ (kPa) = −0.04666 + 0.32001·body surface (m^2);
SD y·x = ±0.184; n = 130; r = +0.42.
Pst(l)$_{30\%\,VC}$ (cm H$_2$O) = −0.4758 + 3.2632·x;
SD y·x = ±1.88.
a = kPa; b = cm H$_2$O.

Table 95. Elastic recoil pressure of the lungs measured at 40% of vital capacity ($Pst(l)_{40\% VC}$) in relation to body height in boys and girls

Height cm	$Pst(l)_{40\% VC}$ mean		lower limits		upper limits	
	a	b	a	b	a	b
115	0.350	3.56	0.000	0.00	0.694	7.10
116	0.356	3.64	0.009	0.10	0.701	7.17
118	0.370	3.78	0.023	0.24	0.715	7.31
120	0.384	3.92	0.037	0.38	0.728	7.45
122	0.398	4.06	0.051	0.52	0.742	7.59
124	0.412	4.20	0.064	0.66	0.756	7.74
126	0.426	4.34	0.078	0.80	0.770	7.88
128	0.439	4.48	0.093	0.95	0.784	8.02
130	0.453	4.62	0.106	1.09	0.798	8.16
132	0.467	4.76	0.120	1.23	0.811	8.30
134	0.481	4.90	0.134	1.37	0.825	8.44
136	0.495	5.05	0.148	1.51	0.839	8.58
138	0.509	5.19	0.162	1.65	0.853	8.72
140	0.522	5.33	0.175	1.79	0.867	8.86
142	0.536	5.47	0.189	1.93	0.880	9.00
144	0.550	5.61	0.203	2.07	0.894	9.15
146	0.564	5.75	0.216	2.21	0.908	9.29
148	0.578	5.89	0.231	2.36	0.922	9.43
150	0.592	6.03	0.245	2.50	0.936	9.57
152	0.605	6.17	0.259	2.64	0.950	9.71
154	0.619	6.31	0.272	2.78	0.963	9.85
156	0.633	6.46	0.286	2.92	0.977	9.99
158	0.647	6.60	0.300	3.06	0.991	10.13
160	0.661	6.74	0.313	3.20	1.005	10.27
162	0.674	6.88	0.327	3.34	1.019	10.41
164	0.688	7.02	0.341	3.48	1.033	10.56
166	0.702	7.16	0.355	3.63	1.046	10.70
168	0.716	7.30	0.369	3.77	1.060	10.84
170	0.730	7.44	0.383	3.91	1.074	10.98
172	0.744	7.58	0.396	4.05	1.088	11.12
174	0.757	7.73	0.410	4.19	1.102	11.26
176	0.771	7.87	0.424	4.33	1.116	11.40
178	0.785	8.01	0.438	4.47	1.129	11.54
180	0.799	8.15	0.451	4.61	1.143	11.68

Formula: $y = a + b \cdot x$;
$y = Pst(l)_{40\% VC}$ (kPa or cm H_2O); x = body height (cm);
$Pst(l)_{40\% VC}$ (kPa) = $-0.44509 + 6.91361 \cdot 10^{-3} \cdot$ height (cm);
SD $y \cdot x = \pm 0.174$; n = 130; r = +0.51.
$Pst(l)_{40\% VC}$ (cm H_2O) = $-4.5388 + 0.0705 \cdot x$;
SD $y \cdot x = \pm 1.78$.
a = kPa; b = cm H_2O.

Table 96. Elastic recoil pressure of the lungs measured at 40% of vital capacity ($Pst(l)_{40\% VC}$) in relation to age in boys and girls

Age years	$Pst(l)_{40\% VC}$ mean		lower limits		upper limits	
	a	b	a	b	a	b
6	0.378	3.86	0.017	0.18	0.739	7.54
7	0.418	4.26	0.057	0.58	0.776	7.94
8	0.457	4.66	0.096	0.98	0.815	8.34
9	0.496	5.06	0.135	1.38	0.854	8.74
10	0.536	5.46	0.174	1.78	0.894	9.14
11	0.575	5.86	0.214	2.18	0.933	9.54
12	0.614	6.27	0.254	2.59	0.972	9.95
13	0.654	6.67	0.293	2.99	1.012	10.35
14	0.693	7.07	0.332	3.39	1.051	10.75
15	0.732	7.47	0.371	3.79	1.090	11.15
16	0.772	7.87	0.410	4.19	1.130	11.55
17	0.811	8.27	0.450	4.59	1.169	11.95

Formula: $y = a + b \cdot x$;
$y = Pst(l)_{40\% VC}$ (kPa or cm H_2O); x = age (years);
$Pst(l)_{40\% VC}$ (kPa) = $0.14253 + 0.03935 \cdot$ age (years);
SD $y \cdot x = \pm 0.181$; n = 130; r = +0.44.
$Pst(l)_{40\% VC}$ (cm H_2O) = $1.4535 + 0.4013 \cdot x$;
SD $y \cdot x = \pm 1.85$.
a = kPa; b = cm H_2O.

Table 97. Elastic recoil pressure of the lungs measured at 40% of vital capacity ($Pst(l)_{40\% VC}$) in relation to body surface in boys and girls

Body surface m^2	$Pst(l)_{40\% VC}$ mean		lower limits		upper limits	
	a	b	a	b	a	b
0.60	0.327	3.34	-0.027	-0.28	0.683	6.96
0.70	0.364	3.71	0.007	0.08	0.720	7.34
0.80	0.400	4.08	0.044	0.46	0.756	7.71
0.90	0.437	4.46	0.081	0.83	0.793	8.08
1.00	0.474	4.83	0.117	1.20	0.830	8.46
1.10	0.510	5.20	0.154	1.58	0.866	8.83
1.20	0.547	5.58	0.191	1.95	0.903	9.20
1.30	0.584	5.95	0.227	2.32	0.940	9.58
1.40	0.620	6.32	0.264	2.70	0.976	9.95
1.50	0.657	6.70	0.301	3.07	1.013	10.32
1.60	0.693	7.07	0.337	3.45	1.050	10.70
1.70	0.730	7.45	0.374	3.82	1.086	11.07
1.80	0.767	7.82	0.411	4.19	1.123	11.45
1.90	0.803	8.19	0.447	4.57	1.160	11.82
2.00	0.841	8.57	0.481	4.94	1.201	12.19

Formula: $y = a + b \cdot x$;
$y = Pst(l)_{40\% VC}$ (kPa or cm H_2O); x = body surface (m^2);
$Pst(l)_{40\% VC}$ (kPa) = $0.10757 + 0.36647 \cdot$ body surface (m^2);
SD $y \cdot x = \pm 0.180$; n = 130; r = +0.47.
$Pst(l)_{40\% VC}$ (cm H_2O) = $1.0970 + 3.7370 \cdot x$;
SD $y \cdot x = \pm 1.832$.
a = kPa; b = cm H_2O.

Table 98. Elastic recoil pressure of the lungs measured at 50% of vital capacity (Pst(l)$_{50\% \text{VC}}$) in relation to body height in boys and girls

Height cm	Pst(l)$_{50\% \text{VC}}$					
	mean		lower limits		upper limits	
	a	b	a	b	a	b
115	0.536	5.47	0.186	1.87	0.886	9.06
116	0.544	5.54	0.194	1.95	0.984	9.14
118	0.559	5.70	0.209	2.11	0.909	9.29
120	0.574	5.85	0.224	2.26	0.924	9.45
122	0.589	6.01	0.239	2.41	0.939	9.60
124	0.604	6.16	0.254	2.57	0.954	9.76
126	0.619	6.32	0.269	2.72	0.970	9.91
128	0.634	6.47	0.284	2.88	0.985	10.06
130	0.650	6.62	0.299	3.03	1.000	10.22
132	0.665	6.78	0.314	3.18	1.015	10.37
134	0.680	6.93	0.330	3.34	1.030	10.53
136	0.695	7.09	0.345	3.49	1.045	10.68
138	0.710	7.24	0.360	3.65	1.060	10.83
140	0.725	7.39	0.375	3.80	1.075	10.99
142	0.740	7.55	0.390	3.95	1.090	11.14
144	0.755	7.70	0.405	4.11	1.106	11.30
146	0.770	7.86	0.420	4.26	1.121	11.45
148	0.786	8.01	0.435	4.42	1.136	11.60
150	0.801	8.16	0.450	4.57	1.151	11.76
152	0.816	8.32	0.466	4.72	1.166	11.91
154	0.831	8.47	0.481	4.88	1.181	12.07
156	0.846	8.63	0.496	5.03	1.196	12.22
158	0.861	8.78	0.511	5.19	1.211	12.37
160	0.876	8.93	0.526	5.34	1.226	12.53
162	0.891	9.09	0.541	5.50	1.242	12.68
164	0.906	9.24	0.556	5.65	1.257	12.84
166	0.922	9.40	0.571	5.80	1.272	12.99
168	0.937	9.55	0.586	5.96	1.287	13.15
170	0.952	9.71	0.602	6.11	1.302	13.30
172	0.967	9.86	0.617	6.27	1.317	13.45
174	0.982	10.01	0.632	6.42	1.332	13.61
176	0.997	10.17	0.647	6.57	1.347	13.76
178	1.012	10.32	0.662	6.73	1.362	13.92
180	1.027	10.48	0.677	6.88	1.378	14.07

Formula: $y = a + b \cdot x$;
$y = $ Pst(l)$_{50\% \text{VC}}$ (kPa or cm H_2O); $x = $ body height (cm);
Pst(l)$_{50\% \text{VC}}$ (kPa) $= -0.33216 + 7.55504 \cdot 10^{-3} \cdot$ height (cm);
SD $y \cdot x = \pm 0.177$; $n = 130$; $r = +0.54$.
Pst(l)$_{50\% \text{VC}}$ (cm H_2O) $= -3.3871 + 0.07704 \cdot x$;
SD $y \cdot x = \pm 1.81$.
$a = $ kPa; $b = $ cm H_2O.

Table 99. Elastic recoil pressure of the lungs measured at 50% of vital capacity (Pst(l)$_{50\% \text{VC}}$) in relation to age in boys and girls

Age years	Pst(l)$_{50\% \text{VC}}$					
	mean		lower limits		upper limits	
	a	b	a	b	a	b
6	0.566	5.77	0.200	2.02	0.932	9.53
7	0.609	6.21	0.243	2.46	0.975	9.97
8	0.653	6.66	0.287	2.90	1.019	10.41
9	0.696	7.10	0.330	3.34	1.062	10.85
10	0.739	7.54	0.373	3.78	1.105	11.29
11	0.782	7.98	0.416	4.22	1.148	11.74
12	0.826	8.42	0.460	4.66	1.192	12.18
13	0.869	8.86	0.503	5.11	1.235	12.62
14	0.912	9.30	0.546	5.55	1.278	13.06
15	0.955	9.74	0.589	5.99	1.322	13.50
16	0.999	10.19	0.633	6.43	1.365	13.94
17	1.042	10.63	0.676	6.87	1.408	14.38

Formula: $y = a + b \cdot x$;
$y = $ Pst(l)$_{50\% \text{VC}}$ (kPa or cm H_2O); $x = $ age (years);
Pst(l)$_{50\% \text{VC}}$ (kPa) $= 0.30685 + 0.04327 \cdot$ age (years);
SD $y \cdot x = \pm 0.185$; $n = 130$; $r = +0.48$.
Pst(l)$_{50\% \text{VC}}$ (cm H_2O) $= 3.1290 + 0.4413 \cdot x$;
SD $y \cdot x = \pm 1.89$.
$a = $ kPa; $b = $ cm H_2O.

Table 100. Elastic recoil pressure of the lungs measured at 50% of vital capacity (Pst(l)$_{50\% \text{VC}}$) in relation to body surface in boys and girls

Body surface m^2	Pst(l)$_{50\% \text{VC}}$					
	mean		lower limits		upper limits	
	a	b	a	b	a	b
0.60	0.508	5.18	0.148	1.50	0.868	8.87
0.70	0.549	5.60	0.189	1.91	0.909	9.28
0.80	0.589	6.01	0.229	2.32	0.949	9.69
0.90	0.630	6.42	0.270	2.74	0.990	10.11
1.00	0.670	6.84	0.310	3.15	1.031	10.52
1.10	0.711	7.25	0.351	3.56	1.071	10.93
1.20	0.751	7.66	0.391	3.98	1.112	11.35
1.30	0.792	8.08	0.432	4.39	1.152	11.76
1.40	0.832	8.49	0.472	4.80	1.193	12.17
1.50	0.873	8.90	0.513	5.22	1.233	12.59
1.60	0.913	9.31	0.553	5.63	1.274	13.00
1.70	0.954	9.73	0.594	6.04	1.314	13.41
1.80	0.994	10.14	0.634	6.46	1.355	13.83
1.90	1.035	10.55	0.675	6.87	1.395	14.24
2.00	1.076	10.97	0.715	7.28	1.436	14.65

Formula: $y = a + b \cdot x$;
$y = $ Pst(l)$_{50\% \text{VC}}$ (kPa or cm H_2O); $x = $ body surface (m^2);
Pst(l)$_{50\% \text{VC}}$ (kPa) $= 0.26570 + 0.40513 \cdot$ body surface (m^2);
SD $y \cdot x = \pm 0.182$; $n = 130$; $r = +0.51$.
Pst(l)$_{50\% \text{VC}}$ (cm H_2O) $= 2.7094 + 4.1312 \cdot x$;
SD $y \cdot x = \pm 1.8625$.
$a = $ kPa; $b = $ cm H_2O.

Table 101. Elastic recoil pressure of the lung measured at 60% of vital capacity ($Pst(l)_{60\% VC}$) in relation to body height in boys and girls

Height cm	Pst(l)$_{60\% VC}$ mean		lower limits		upper limits	
	a	b	a	b	a	b
115	0.694	7.08	0.332	3.37	1.056	10.80
116	0.703	7.17	0.341	3.46	1.065	10.89
118	0.720	7.35	0.358	3.63	1.082	11.07
120	0.738	7.53	0.376	3.81	1.100	11.25
122	0.755	7.71	0.393	3.99	1.117	11.43
124	0.773	7.89	0.411	4.17	1.135	11.61
126	0.790	8.07	0.428	4.35	1.152	11.79
128	0.808	8.25	0.446	4.53	1.170	11.97
130	0.825	8.43	0.463	4.71	1.187	12.14
132	0.843	8.60	0.481	4.89	1.205	12.32
134	0.860	8.78	0.498	5.06	1.222	12.50
136	0.878	8.96	0.516	5.24	1.240	12.68
138	0.895	9.14	0.533	5.42	1.258	12.86
140	0.913	9.32	0.551	5.60	1.275	13.04
142	0.930	9.50	0.568	5.78	1.293	13.22
144	0.948	9.68	0.586	5.96	1.310	13.40
146	0.965	9.86	0.603	6.14	1.328	13.57
148	0.983	10.03	0.621	6.32	1.345	13.75
150	1.000	10.21	0.638	6.49	1.363	13.93
152	1.018	10.39	0.656	6.67	1.380	14.11
154	1.036	10.57	0.673	6.85	1.398	14.29
156	1.053	10.75	0.691	7.03	1.415	14.47
158	1.071	10.93	0.708	7.21	1.433	14.65
160	1.088	11.11	0.726	7.39	1.450	14.83
162	1.106	11.29	0.743	7.57	1.468	15.00
164	1.123	11.46	0.761	7.75	1.485	15.18
166	1.141	11.64	0.779	7.92	1.503	15.36
168	1.158	11.82	0.796	8.10	1.520	15.54
170	1.176	12.00	0.814	8.28	1.538	15.72
172	1.193	12.18	0.831	8.46	1.555	15.90
174	1.211	12.36	0.849	8.64	1.573	16.08
176	1.228	12.54	0.866	8.82	1.590	16.26
178	1.246	12.72	0.884	9.00	1.608	16.43
180	1.263	12.89	0.901	9.18	1.625	16.61

Formula: $y = a + b \cdot x$;
$y = Pst(l)_{60\% VC}$ (kPa or cm H_2O); x = body height (cm);
$Pst(l)_{60\% VC}$ (kPa) $= -0.31265 + 8.75733 \cdot 10^{-3} \cdot$ height (cm);
SD $y \cdot x = \pm 0.183$; n = 130; r = +0.58.
$Pst(l)_{60\% VC}$ (cm H_2O) $= -3.1882 + 0.0893 \cdot x$;
SD $y \cdot x = \pm 1.87$.
a = kPa; b = cm H_2O.

Table 102. Elastic recoil pressure of the lungs measured at 60% of vital capacity ($Pst(l)_{60\% VC}$) in relation to age in boys and girls

Age years	Pst(l)$_{60\% VC}$ mean		lower limits		upper limits	
	a	b	a	b	a	b
6	0.727	7.41	0.345	3.50	1.109	11.33
7	0.778	7.93	0.396	4.02	1.160	11.85
8	0.828	8.45	0.447	4.53	1.210	12.36
9	0.879	8.96	0.497	5.05	1.261	12.88
10	0.930	9.48	0.548	5.57	1.312	13.40
11	0.980	10.00	0.598	6.08	1.362	13.91
12	1.031	10.51	0.649	6.60	1.413	14.43
13	1.082	11.03	0.700	7.12	1.464	14.95
14	1.132	11.55	0.750	7.63	1.514	15.46
15	1.183	12.06	0.801	8.15	1.565	15.98
16	1.234	12.58	0.852	8.66	1.615	16.50
17	1.284	13.10	0.902	9.18	1.666	17.01

Formula: $y = a + b \cdot x$;
$y = Pst(l)_{60\% VC}$ (kPa or cm H_2O); x = age (years);
$Pst(l)_{60\% VC}$ (kPa) $= 0.42366 + 0.05065 \cdot$ age (years);
SD $y \cdot x = \pm 0.193$; n = 130; r = +0.52.
$Pst(l)_{60\% VC}$ (cm H_2O) $= 4.3202 + 0.5165 \cdot x$;
SD $y \cdot x = \pm 1.97$.
a = kPa; b = cm H_2O.

Table 103. Elastic recoil pressure of the lungs measured at 60% of vital capacity ($Pst(l)_{60\% VC}$) in relation to body surface in boys and girls

Body surface m^2	Pst(l)$_{60\% VC}$ mean		lower limits		upper limits	
	a	b	a	b	a	b
0.60	0.662	6.75	0.286	2.91	1.038	10.58
0.70	0.709	7.23	0.333	3.39	1.085	11.06
0.80	0.756	7.71	0.380	3.87	1.132	11.54
0.90	0.803	8.19	0.427	4.35	1.179	12.02
1.00	0.850	8.67	0.474	4.84	1.226	12.50
1.10	0.897	9.15	0.521	5.32	1.273	12.98
1.20	0.944	9.63	0.568	5.80	1.320	13.46
1.30	0.991	10.11	0.615	6.28	1.367	13.94
1.40	1.039	10.59	0.663	6.76	1.415	14.42
1.50	1.086	11.07	0.710	7.24	1.462	14.90
1.60	1.133	11.55	0.757	7.72	1.509	15.38
1.70	1.180	12.03	0.804	8.20	1.556	15.86
1.80	1.227	12.51	0.851	8.68	1.603	16.34
1.90	1.274	12.99	0.898	9.16	1.650	16.83
2.00	1.321	13.47	0.945	9.64	1.697	17.31

Formula: $y = a + b \cdot x$;
$y = Pst(l)_{60\% VC}$ (kPa or cm H_2O); x = body surface (m^2);
$Pst(l)_{60\% VC}$ (kPa) $= 0.37936 + 0.47117 \cdot$ body surface (m^2);
SD $y \cdot x = \pm 0.190$; n = 130; r = +0.54.
$Pst(l)_{60\% VC}$ (cm H_2O) $= 3.8684 + 4.8046 \cdot x$;
SD $y \cdot x = \pm 1.937$.
a = kPa; b = cm H_2O.

Table 104. Elastic recoil pressure of the lungs measured at 70% of vital capacity (Pst(l)$_{70\%\,VC}$) in relation to body height in boys and girls

Height cm	Pst(l)$_{70\%\,VC}$					
	mean		lower limits		upper limits	
	a	b	a	b	a	b
115	0.877	8.95	0.472	4.80	1.283	13.10
116	0.887	9.04	0.481	4.89	1.292	13.20
118	0.905	9.23	0.500	5.08	1.311	13.39
120	0.924	9.42	0.518	5.27	1.330	13.58
122	0.943	9.62	0.537	5.46	1.348	13.77
124	0.961	9.81	0.556	5.65	1.367	13.96
126	0.980	10.00	0.574	5.84	1.386	14.15
128	0.999	10.19	0.593	6.04	1.404	14.34
130	1.018	10.38	0.612	6.23	1.423	14.53
132	1.036	10.57	0.631	6.42	1.442	14.72
134	1.055	10.76	0.649	6.61	1.461	14.91
136	1.074	10.95	0.668	6.80	1.479	15.10
138	1.092	11.14	0.687	6.99	1.498	15.29
140	1.111	11.33	0.705	7.18	1.517	15.49
142	1.130	11.52	0.724	7.37	1.535	15.68
144	1.148	11.71	0.743	7.56	1.554	15.87
146	1.167	11.91	0.762	7.75	1.573	16.06
148	1.186	12.10	0.780	7.94	1.592	16.25
150	1.205	12.29	0.799	8.13	1.610	16.44
152	1.223	12.48	0.818	8.33	1.629	16.63
154	1.242	12.67	0.836	8.52	1.648	16.82
156	1.261	12.86	0.855	8.71	1.666	17.01
158	1.279	13.05	0.874	8.90	1.685	17.20
160	1.298	13.24	0.893	9.09	1.704	17.39
162	1.317	13.43	0.911	9.28	1.723	17.58
164	1.336	13.62	0.930	9.47	1.741	17.78
166	1.354	13.81	0.949	9.66	1.760	17.97
168	1.373	14.01	0.967	9.85	1.779	18.16
170	1.392	14.20	0.986	10.04	1.797	18.35
172	1.410	14.39	1.005	10.23	1.816	18.54
174	1.429	14.58	1.024	10.43	1.835	18.73
176	1.448	14.77	1.042	10.62	1.853	18.92
178	1.467	14.96	1.061	10.81	1.872	19.11
180	1.485	15.15	1.080	11.00	1.891	19.30

Formula: y = a + b·x;
y = Pst(l)$_{70\%\,VC}$ (kPa or cm H$_2$O); x = body height (cm);
Pst(l)$_{70\%\,VC}$ (kPa) = −0.19826 + 9.35554·10^{-3}·height (cm);
SD y·x = ± 0.205; n = 130; r = +0.58.
Pst(l)$_{70\%\,VC}$ (cm H$_2$O) = −2.0217 + 0.0954·x;
SD y·x = ± 2.09.
a = kPa; b = cm H$_2$O.

Table 105. Elastic recoil pressure of the lungs measured at 70% of vital capacity Pst(l)$_{70\%\,VC}$ in relation to age in boys and girls

Age years	Pst(l)$_{70\%\,VC}$					
	mean		lower limits		upper limits	
	a	b	a	b	a	b
6	0.904	9.22	0.485	4.91	1.324	13.54
7	0.960	9.79	0.540	5.48	1.379	14.10
8	1.015	10.35	0.596	6.04	1.435	14.67
9	1.071	10.92	0.651	6.61	1.490	15.23
10	1.126	11.49	0.707	7.17	1.546	15.80
11	1.182	12.05	0.763	7.74	1.601	16.37
12	1.238	12.62	0.818	8.31	1.657	16.93
13	1.293	13.19	0.874	8.87	1.713	17.50
14	1.349	13.75	0.929	9.44	1.768	18.07
15	1.404	14.32	0.985	10.01	1.824	18.63
16	1.460	14.89	1.040	10.57	1.879	19.20
17	1.515	15.45	1.096	11.14	1.935	19.76

Formula: y = a + b·x;
y = Pst(l)$_{70\%\,VC}$ (kPa or cm H$_2$O); x = age (years);
Pst(l)$_{70\%\,VC}$ (kPa) = 0.57162 + 0.05553·age (years);
SD y·x = ± 0.212; n = 130; r = +0.52.
Pst(l)$_{70\%\,VC}$ (cm H$_2$O) = 5.8289 + 0.5663·x;
SD y·x = ± 2.17.
a = kPa; b = cm H$_2$O.

Table 106. Elastic recoil pressure of the lungs measured at 70% of vital capacity (Pst(l)$_{70\%\,VC}$) in relation to body surface in boys and girls

Body surface m^2	Pst(l)$_{70\%\,VC}$					
	mean		lower limits		upper limits	
	a	b	a	b	a	b
0.60	0.844	8.61	0.425	4.33	1.264	12.89
0.70	0.894	9.12	0.475	4.84	1.314	13.40
0.80	0.944	9.63	0.525	5.35	1.364	13.91
0.90	0.994	10.14	0.575	5.86	1.414	14.42
1.00	1.044	10.65	0.625	6.37	1.464	14.93
1.10	1.094	11.16	0.675	6.88	1.514	15.44
1.20	1.144	11.67	0.725	7.39	1.564	15.95
1.30	1.194	12.18	0.775	7.90	1.614	16.46
1.40	1.244	12.69	0.825	8.41	1.664	16.97
1.50	1.294	13.20	0.875	8.92	1.714	17.48
1.60	1.344	13.71	0.925	9.43	1.764	17.99
1.70	1.394	14.22	0.975	9.94	1.814	18.50
1.80	1.444	14.73	1.025	10.45	1.864	19.01
1.90	1.494	15.24	1.075	10.96	1.914	19.52
2.00	1.544	15.75	1.125	11.47	1.964	20.03

Formula: y = a + b·x;
y = Pst(l)$_{70\%\,VC}$ (kPa or cm H$_2$O); x = body surface (m^2);
Pst(l)$_{70\%\,VC}$ (kPa) = 0.54450 + 0.50008·body surface (m^2);
SD y·x = ± 0.212; n = 130; r = +0.53.
Pst(l)$_{70\%\,VC}$ (cm H$_2$O) = 5.5524 + 5.0994·x;
SD y·x = ± 2.16.
a = kPa; b = cm H$_2$O.

Table 107. Elastic recoil pressure of the lungs measured at 75 % of vital capacity ($Pst(l)_{75\% VC}$) in relation to body height in boys and girls

Height cm	Pst(l)$_{75\% VC}$					
	mean		lower limits		upper limits	
	a	b	a	b	a	b
115	1.027	10.47	0.607	6.18	1.446	14.77
116	1.034	10.55	0.614	6.25	1.453	14.84
118	1.049	10.70	0.629	6.40	1.468	14.99
120	1.064	10.85	0.644	6.55	1.483	15.15
122	1.079	11.01	0.660	6.71	1.499	15.31
124	1.095	11.17	0.675	6.87	1.514	15.47
126	1.111	11.34	0.692	7.04	1.531	15.63
128	1.128	11.50	0.708	7.21	1.547	15.80
130	1.145	11.68	0.725	7.38	1.564	15.98
132	1.162	11.86	0.743	7.56	1.582	16.15
134	1.180	12.04	0.760	7.74	1.599	16.33
136	1.198	12.22	0.779	7.93	1.618	16.52
138	1.217	12.41	0.797	8.12	1.636	16.71
140	1.236	12.61	0.816	8.31	1.655	16.90
142	1.255	12.80	0.835	8.51	1.674	17.10
144	1.275	13.00	0.855	8.71	1.694	17.30
146	1.295	13.21	0.875	8.91	1.714	17.51
148	1.315	13.42	0.896	9.12	1.735	17.72
150	1.336	13.63	0.917	9.33	1.756	17.93
152	1.357	13.85	0.938	9.55	1.777	18.15
154	1.379	14.07	0.960	9.77	1.799	18.37
156	1.401	14.29	0.982	10.00	1.821	18.59
158	1.424	14.52	1.004	10.23	1.843	18.82
160	1.446	14.76	1.027	10.46	1.866	19.05
162	1.470	14.99	1.050	10.70	1.889	19.29
164	1.493	15.24	1.074	10.94	1.913	19.53
166	1.517	15.48	1.098	11.18	1.937	19.78
168	1.542	15.73	1.122	11.43	1.961	20.03
170	1.567	15.98	1.147	11.69	1.986	20.28
172	1.592	16.24	1.172	11.94	2.011	20.54
174	1.617	16.50	1.198	12.20	2.037	20.80
176	1.643	16.76	1.224	12.47	2.063	21.06
178	1.670	17.03	1.250	12.74	2.089	21.33
180	1.696	17.31	1.277	13.01	2.116	21.60

Formula: $y = a + b \cdot x + c \cdot x^2$;
$y = Pst(l)_{75\% VC}$ (kPa or cm H$_2$O); x = body height (cm);
$Pst(l)_{75\% VC}$ (kPa) =
   $0.85085 - 4.06975 \cdot 10^{-3} \cdot \text{height} + 4.87194 \cdot 10^{-5} \cdot \text{height}^2$;
SD y·x = ± 0.212; n = 130; r = +0.60.
$Pst(l)_{75\% VC}$ (cm H$_2$O) =
   $8.6763 - 0.0415 \cdot x + 0.4968 \cdot 10^{-3} \cdot x^2$;
SD y·x = ± 2.17.
a = kPa; b = cm H$_2$O.

Table 108. Elastic recoil pressure of the lungs measured at 75 % of vital capacity ($Pst(l)_{75\% VC}$) in relation to age in boys and girls

Age years	Pst(l)$_{75\% VC}$					
	mean		lower limits		upper limits	
	a	b	a	b	a	b
6	1.000	10.19	0.560	5.69	1.439	14.69
7	1.067	10.88	0.628	6.38	1.506	15.38
8	1.133	11.56	0.694	7.05	1.573	16.06
9	1.198	12.22	0.759	7.72	1.638	16.72
10	1.262	12.87	0.823	8.37	1.702	17.37
11	1.325	13.51	0.886	9.01	1.765	18.02
12	1.387	14.14	0.948	9.64	1.826	18.64
13	1.447	14.76	1.008	10.26	1.887	19.26
14	1.507	15.37	1.068	10.86	1.946	19.87
15	1.565	15.96	1.126	11.46	2.004	20.46
16	1.622	16.54	1.183	12.04	2.062	21.04
17	1.678	17.11	1.239	12.61	2.118	21.61

Formula: $y = a + b \cdot x + c \cdot x^2$;
$y = Pst(l)_{75\% VC}$ (kPa or cm H$_2$O); x = age (years);
$Pst(l)_{75\% VC}$ (kPa) =
   $0.57152 + 0.07485 \cdot \text{age} - 5.71727 \cdot 10^{-4} \cdot \text{age}^2$ (years);
SD y·x = ± 0.222; n = 130; r = +0.55.
$Pst(l)_{75\% VC}$ (cm H$_2$O) = $5.8279 + 0.7633 \cdot x - 0.00583 \cdot x^2$;
SD y·x = ± 2.27.
a = kPa; b = cm H$_2$O.

Table 109. Elastic recoil pressure of the lungs measured at 75 % of vital capacity ($Pst(l)_{75\% VC}$) in relation to body surface in boys and girls

Body surface m^2	Pst(l)$_{75\% VC}$					
	mean		lower limits		upper limits	
	a	b	a	b	a	b
0.60	0.943	9.62	0.510	5.18	1.377	14.05
0.70	0.999	10.19	0.566	5.75	1.433	14.63
0.80	1.055	10.76	0.622	6.32	1.489	15.20
0.90	1.111	11.37	0.678	6.90	1.545	15.77
1.00	1.167	11.90	0.734	7.47	1.601	16.34
1.10	1.224	12.48	0.790	8.04	1.657	16.91
1.20	1.280	13.05	0.846	8.61	1.713	17.48
1.30	1.336	13.62	0.902	9.18	1.769	18.06
1.40	1.392	14.19	0.958	9.75	1.825	18.63
1.50	1.448	14.76	1.014	10.33	1.881	19.20
1.60	1.504	15.33	1.071	10.90	1.937	19.77
1.70	1.560	15.91	1.127	11.47	1.993	20.34
1.80	1.616	16.48	1.183	12.04	2.049	20.92
1.90	1.672	17.05	1.239	12.61	2.105	21.49
2.00	1.728	17.62	1.295	13.18	2.161	22.06

Formula: $y = a + b \cdot x$;
$y = Pst(l)_{75\% VC}$ (kPa or cm H$_2$O); x = body surface (m^2);
$Pst(l)_{75\% VC}$ (kPa) = $0.60726 + 0.56065 \cdot$ body surface (m^2);
SD y·x = ± 0.219; n = 130; r = +0.56.
$Pst(l)_{75\% VC}$ (cm H$_2$O) = $6.1924 + 5.7171 \cdot x$;
SD y·x = ± 2.24.
a = kPa; b = cm H$_2$O.

Table 110. Elastic recoil pressure of the lung measured at 80% of vital capacity (Pst(l)$_{80\% VC}$) in relation to body height in boys and girls

Height cm	Pst(l)$_{80\% VC}$					
	mean		lower limits		upper limits	
	a	b	a	b	a	b
115	1.169	11.91	0.743	7.54	1.594	16.28
116	1.177	11.99	0.751	7.62	1.602	16.36
118	1.192	12.15	0.767	7.78	1.618	16.52
120	1.208	12.31	0.783	7.94	1.634	16.68
122	1.225	12.48	0.799	8.11	1.650	16.85
124	1.242	12.65	0.816	8.28	1.667	17.02
126	1.259	12.83	0.833	8.46	1.684	17.20
128	1.276	13.01	0.851	8.64	1.702	17.38
130	1.295	13.19	0.869	8.82	1.720	17.56
132	1.313	13.38	0.888	9.01	1.738	17.75
134	1.332	13.57	0.906	9.20	1.757	17.94
136	1.351	13.77	0.926	9.40	1.777	18.14
138	1.371	13.97	0.945	9.60	1.796	18.34
140	1.391	14.17	0.965	9.80	1.816	18.54
142	1.411	14.38	0.986	10.01	1.837	18.75
144	1.432	14.59	1.007	10.22	1.858	18.96
146	1.453	14.81	1.028	10.44	1.879	19.18
148	1.475	15.03	1.050	10.66	1.901	19.40
150	1.497	15.26	1.072	10.88	1.923	19.63
152	1.520	15.48	1.094	11.11	1.945	19.86
154	1.542	15.72	1.117	11.35	1.968	20.09
156	1.566	15.95	1.140	11.58	1.991	20.33
158	1.589	16.20	1.164	11.82	2.015	20.57
160	1.613	16.44	1.188	12.07	2.039	20.81
162	1.638	16.69	1.212	12.32	2.063	21.06
164	1.663	16.94	1.237	12.57	2.088	21.32
166	1.688	17.20	1.263	12.83	2.113	21.57
168	1.714	17.46	1.288	13.09	2.139	21.83
170	1.740	17.73	1.314	13.36	2.165	22.10
172	1.766	18.00	1.341	13.63	2.192	22.37
174	1.793	18.27	1.368	13.90	2.219	22.64
176	1.820	18.55	1.395	14.18	2.246	22.92
178	1.848	18.83	1.423	14.46	2.273	23.20
180	1.876	19.12	1.451	14.75	2.302	23.49

Formula: $y = a + b \cdot x + c \cdot x^2$;
$y = $ Pst(l)$_{80\% VC}$ (kPa or cm H_2O); x = body height (cm);
Pst(l)$_{80\% VC}$ (kPa) =
$\quad 0.95333 - 3.87362 \cdot 10^{-3} \cdot$ height $+ 5.00139 \cdot 10^{-5} \cdot$ height^2;
SD $y \cdot x = \pm 0.215$; n = 130; r = +0.61.
Pst(l)$_{80\% VC}$ (cm H_2O) =
$\quad 9.7213 - 0.0395 \cdot x + 0.5100 \cdot 10^{-3} \cdot x^2$;
SD $y \cdot x = \pm 2.20$.
a = kPa; b = cm H_2O.

Table 111. Elastic recoil pressure of the lungs measured at 80% of vital capacity (Pst(l)$_{80\% VC}$) in relation to age in boys and girls

Age years	Pst(l)$_{80\% VC}$					
	mean		lower limits		upper limits	
	a	b	a	b	a	b
6	1.136	11.58	0.689	7.01	1.583	16.15
7	1.208	12.32	0.761	7.75	1.655	16.89
8	1.279	13.04	0.831	8.47	1.726	17.61
9	1.348	13.75	0.901	9.18	1.795	18.32
10	1.417	14.44	0.969	9.87	1.864	19.01
11	1.484	15.13	1.036	10.56	1.931	19.70
12	1.550	15.80	1.102	11.23	1.997	20.37
13	1.614	16.46	1.167	11.88	2.061	21.03
14	1.678	17.10	1.230	12.53	2.125	21.67
15	1.740	17.73	1.293	13.16	2.187	22.31
16	1.801	18.35	1.353	13.78	2.248	22.93
17	1.860	18.96	1.413	14.39	2.308	23.53

Formula: $y = a + b \cdot x + c \cdot x^2$;
$y = $ Pst(l)$_{80\% VC}$ (kPa or cm H_2O); x = age (years);
Pst(l)$_{80\% VC}$ (kPa) =
$\quad 0.67812 + 0.08007 \cdot$ age $- 6.17818 \cdot 10^{-4} \cdot$ age^2 (years);
SD $y \cdot x = \pm 0.226$; n = 130; r = +0.56.
Pst(l)$_{80\% VC}$ (cm H_2O) = $6.9149 + 0.8168 \cdot x - 0.0063 \cdot x^2$;
SD $y \cdot x = \pm 2.31$.
a = kPa; b = cm H_2O.

Table 112. Elastic recoil pressure of the lungs measured at 80% of vital capacity (Pst(l)$_{80\% VC}$) in relation to body surface in boys and girls

Body surface m^2	Pst(l)$_{80\% VC}$					
	mean		lower limits		upper limits	
	a	b	a	b	a	b
0.60	1.099	11.21	0.660	6.71	1.539	15.72
0.70	1.152	11.75	0.713	7.24	1.591	16.25
0.80	1.206	12.30	0.766	7.79	1.645	16.80
0.90	1.260	12.85	0.821	8.35	1.700	17.36
1.00	1.316	13.43	0.877	8.92	1.755	17.93
1.10	1.373	14.00	0.934	9.50	1.812	18.51
1.20	1.431	14.60	0.992	10.09	1.870	19.10
1.30	1.490	15.20	1.051	10.70	1.929	19.71
1.40	1.550	15.82	1.111	11.31	1.990	20.32
1.50	1.612	16.44	1.173	11.94	2.051	20.95
1.60	1.674	17.08	1.235	12.57	2.114	21.59
1.70	1.738	17.73	1.299	13.22	2.177	22.23
1.80	1.803	18.39	1.363	13.88	2.242	22.90
1.90	1.869	19.06	1.429	14.56	2.308	23.57
2.00	1.936	19.74	1.496	15.24	2.375	24.25

Formula: $y = a + b \cdot x + c \cdot x^2$;
$y = $ Pst(l)$_{80\% VC}$ (kPa or cm H_2O); x = body surface (m^2);
Pst(l)$_{80\% VC}$ (kPa) =
$\quad 0.80851 + 0.45266 \cdot$ body surface $+ 0.05573 \cdot$ body surface^2 (m^2);
SD $y \cdot x = \pm 0.222$; n = 130; r = +0.58.
Pst(l)$_{80\% VC}$ (cm H_2O) = $8.2445 + 4.6159 \cdot x + 0.5683 \cdot x^2$;
SD $y \cdot x = \pm 2.27$.
a = kPa; b = cm H_2O.

Table 113. Elastic recoil pressure of the lungs measured at 90 % of vital capacity (Pst(l)$_{90\% \text{VC}}$) in relation to body height in boys and girls

Height cm	Pst(l)$_{90\% \text{VC}}$					
	mean		lower limits		upper limits	
	a	b	a	b	a	b
115	1.474	15.04	0.934	9.52	2.015	20.56
116	1.488	15.18	0.948	9.65	2.028	20.70
118	1.515	15.45	0.975	9.93	2.055	20.98
120	1.542	15.73	1.002	10.21	2.082	21.25
122	1.570	16.01	1.029	10.49	2.110	21.53
124	1.597	16.29	1.057	10.77	2.137	21.81
126	1.625	16.57	1.085	11.05	2.165	22.10
128	1.653	16.86	1.112	11.34	2.193	22.38
130	1.681	17.14	1.140	11.62	2.221	22.67
132	1.709	17.43	1.169	11.91	2.249	22.95
134	1.737	17.72	1.197	12.20	2.277	23.24
136	1.766	18.01	1.225	12.49	2.306	23.53
138	1.794	18.30	1.254	12.78	2.335	23.83
140	1.823	18.60	1.283	13.07	2.363	24.12
142	1.852	18.89	1.312	13.37	2.392	24.42
144	1.881	19.19	1.341	13.67	2.421	24.71
146	1.911	19.49	1.370	13.97	2.451	25.01
148	1.940	19.79	1.400	14.27	2.480	25.31
150	1.970	20.09	1.429	14.57	2.510	25.61
152	1.999	20.39	1.459	14.87	2.540	25.92
154	2.029	20.70	1.489	15.18	2.569	26.22
156	2.059	21.01	1.519	15.48	2.600	26.53
158	2.090	21.32	1.549	15.79	2.630	26.84
160	2.120	21.63	1.580	16.10	2.660	27.15
162	2.150	21.94	1.610	16.41	2.691	27.46
164	2.181	22.25	1.641	16.73	2.721	27.77
166	2.212	22.56	1.672	17.04	2.752	28.09
168	2.243	22.88	1.703	17.36	2.783	28.40
170	2.274	23.20	1.734	17.68	2.814	28.72
172	2.306	23.52	1.765	18.00	2.846	29.04
174	2.337	23.84	1.797	18.32	2.877	29.36
176	2.369	24.16	1.828	18.64	2.909	29.69
178	2.400	24.19	1.860	18.96	2.941	30.01
180	2.432	24.81	1.892	19.29	2.973	30.34

Formula: y = a + b·x + c·x^2;
y = Pst(l)$_{90\% \text{VC}}$ (kPa or cm H$_2$O); x = body height (cm);
Pst(l)$_{90\% \text{VC}}$ (kPa) =
    $0.18712 + 8.93385 \cdot 10^{-3} \cdot$ height $+ 1.96819 \cdot 10^{-5} \cdot$ height^2;
SD y·x = ± 0.273; n = 130; r = + 0.65.
Pst(l)$_{90\% \text{VC}}$ (cm H$_2$O) =
    $1.9081 + 0.0911 \cdot x + 0.2007 \cdot 10^{-3} \cdot x^2$;
SD y·x = ± 2.79.
a = kPa; b = cm H$_2$O.

Table 114. Elastic recoil pressure of the lungs measured at 90 % of vital capacity (Pst(l)$_{90\% \text{VC}}$) in relation to age in boys and girls

Age years	Pst(l)$_{90\% \text{VC}}$					
	mean		lower limits		upper limits	
	a	b	a	b	a	b
6	1.413	14.41	0.851	8.66	1.975	20.16
7	1.536	15.66	0.974	9.91	2.098	21.41
8	1.652	16.84	1.090	11.10	2.214	22.59
9	1.761	17.95	1.199	12.21	2.323	23.70
10	1.863	18.99	1.301	13.24	2.425	24.74
11	1.958	19.96	1.396	14.21	2.520	25.70
12	2.045	20.85	1.483	15.10	2.607	26.60
13	2.126	21.67	1.564	15.92	2.688	27.42
14	2.199	22.41	1.637	16.66	2.761	28.16
15	2.265	23.09	1.703	17.34	2.827	28.84
16	2.324	23.69	1.763	17.94	2.886	29.44
17	2.377	24.22	1.815	18.47	2.939	29.97

Formula: y = a + b·x + c·x^2;
y = Pst(l)$_{90\% \text{VC}}$ (kPa or cm H$_2$O); x = age (years);
Pst(l)$_{90\% \text{VC}}$ (kPa) =
    $0.52589 + 0.16924 \cdot$ age $- 3.55000 \cdot 10^{-3} \cdot$ age^2;
SD y·x = ± 0.284; n = 130; r = + 0.59.
Pst(l)$_{90\% \text{VC}}$ (cm H$_2$O) = $5.3626 + 1.7258 \cdot x - 0.0362 \cdot x^2$;
SD y·x = ± 2.90.
a = kPa; b = cm H$_2$O.

Table 115. Elastic recoil pressure of the lungs measured at 90 % of vital capacity (Pst(l)$_{90\% \text{VC}}$) in relation to body surface in boys and girls

Body surface m^2	Pst(l)$_{90\% \text{VC}}$					
	mean		lower limits		upper limits	
	a	b	a	b	a	b
0.60	1.338	13.64	0.784	7.97	1.892	19.23
0.70	1.434	14.62	0.880	8.95	1.988	20.30
0.80	1.528	15.58	0.974	9.91	2.082	21.26
0.90	1.620	16.52	1.066	10.84	2.174	22.19
1.00	1.709	17.43	1.155	11.76	2.263	23.11
1.10	1.797	18.32	1.243	12.65	2.351	24.00
1.20	1.882	19.19	1.328	13.52	2.436	24.87
1.30	1.965	20.04	1.411	14.36	2.519	25.71
1.40	2.046	20.86	1.492	15.19	2.600	26.54
1.50	2.125	21.66	1.571	15.99	2.679	27.34
1.60	2.201	22.45	1.647	16.77	2.755	28.12
1.70	2.275	23.20	1.721	17.53	2.830	28.88
1.80	2.348	23.94	1.794	18.26	2.902	29.61
1.90	2.418	24.65	1.864	18.98	2.972	30.33
2.00	2.486	25.34	1.931	19.67	3.040	31.02

Formula: y = a + b·x + c·x^2;
y = Pst(l)$_{90\% \text{VC}}$ (kPa or cm H$_2$O); x = body surface (m^2);
Pst(l)$_{90\% \text{VC}}$ (kPa) =
    $0.71615 + 1.10242 \cdot$ body surface $- 0.10876 \cdot$ body surface^2 (m^2);
SD y·x = ± 0.280; n = 130; r = + 0.61.
Pst(l)$_{90\% \text{VC}}$ (cm H$_2$O) = $7.3027 + 11.2416 \cdot x - 1.1091 \cdot x^2$;
SD y·x = ± 2.86.
a = kPa; b = cm H$_2$O.

Table 116. Elastic recoil pressure of the lungs at 40 % of total lung capacity (Pst(l)$_{40\% \text{ TLC}}$) in relation to body height in boys and girls

Height cm	Pst(l)$_{40\% \text{ TLC}}$					
	mean		lower limits		upper limits	
	a	b	a	b	a	b
115	0.008	0.09	−0.311	−3.18	0.329	3.38
116	0.013	0.14	−0.307	−3.14	0.334	3.43
118	0.022	0.23	−0.298	−3.04	0.343	3.52
120	0.031	0.33	−0.288	−2.95	0.352	3.61
122	0.041	0.42	−0.279	−2.85	0.361	3.71
124	0.050	0.52	−0.270	−2.76	0.371	3.80
126	0.059	0.61	−0.261	−2.67	0.388	3.90
128	0.068	0.71	−0.251	−2.57	0.389	3.99
130	0.078	0.80	−0.242	−2.48	0.398	4.09
132	0.087	0.89	−0.233	−2.38	0.408	4.18
134	0.096	0.99	−0.224	−2.29	0.417	4.27
136	0.105	1.08	−0.215	−2.19	0.426	4.37
138	0.114	1.18	−0.205	−2.10	0.435	4.46
140	0.124	1.27	−0.196	−2.01	0.444	4.56
142	0.133	1.36	−0.187	−1.91	0.454	4.65
144	0.142	1.46	−0.178	−1.82	0.463	4.74
146	0.151	1.55	−0.169	−1.72	0.472	4.84
148	0.161	1.65	−0.159	−1.63	0.481	4.93
150	0.170	1.74	−0.150	−1.54	0.490	5.03
152	0.179	1.83	−0.141	−1.44	0.500	5.12
154	0.188	1.93	−0.132	−1.35	0.509	5.22
156	0.197	2.02	−0.122	−1.25	0.518	5.31
158	0.207	2.12	−0.113	−1.16	0.527	5.40
160	0.216	2.21	−0.104	−1.07	0.537	5.50
162	0.225	2.31	−0.095	−0.97	0.546	5.59
164	0.234	2.40	−0.086	−0.88	0.555	5.69
166	0.243	2.49	−0.076	−0.78	0.564	5.78
168	0.253	2.59	−0.067	−0.69	0.573	5.87
170	0.262	2.68	−0.058	−0.59	0.583	5.97
172	0.271	2.78	−0.049	−0.50	0.592	6.06
174	0.280	2.87	−0.039	−0.41	0.601	6.16
176	0.290	2.96	−0.030	−0.31	0.610	6.25
178	0.299	3.06	−0.021	−0.22	0.620	6.34
180	0.308	3.15	−0.012	−0.12	0.629	6.44

Formula: $y = a + b \cdot x$;
$y = $ Pst(l)$_{40\% \text{ TLC}}$ (kPa or cm H$_2$O); x = body height (cm);
Pst(l)$_{40\% \text{ TLC}}$ (kPa) = $-0.52117 + 4.60912 \cdot 10^{-3} \cdot$ height;
SD y·x = ±0.162; n = 122; r = +0.39.
Pst(l)$_{40\% \text{ TLC}}$ (cm H$_2$O) = $-5.3145 + 0.0470 \cdot$ x;
SD y·x = ±1.65.
a = kPa; b = cm H$_2$O.

Table 117. Elastic recoil pressure of the lungs at 40 % of total lung capacity (Pst(l)$_{40\% \text{ TLC}}$) in relation to age in boys and girls

Age years	Pst(l)$_{40\% \text{ TLC}}$					
	mean		lower limits		upper limits	
	a	b	a	b	a	b
6	0.038	0.39	−0.292	−2.99	0.369	3.78
7	0.063	0.64	−0.267	−2.74	0.393	4.03
8	0.087	0.89	−0.243	−2.49	0.418	4.27
9	0.111	1.14	−0.218	−2.24	0.442	4.52
10	0.136	1.38	−0.194	−1.19	0.466	4.77
11	0.160	1.63	−0.170	−1.74	0.491	5.02
12	0.185	1.88	−0.145	−1.50	0.515	5.27
13	0.209	2.13	−0.121	−1.25	0.540	5.52
14	0.233	2.38	−0.098	−1.00	0.564	5.77
15	0.258	2.63	−0.072	−0.75	0.588	6.02
16	0.282	2.88	−0.048	−0.50	0.613	6.26
17	0.306	3.13	−0.023	−0.25	0.637	6.51

Formula: $y = a + b \cdot x$;
$y = $ Pst(l)$_{40\% \text{ TLC}}$ (kPa or cm H$_2$O); x = age (years);
Pst(l)$_{40\% \text{ TLC}}$ (kPa) = $-0.10761 + 0.02438 \cdot$ age (years);
SD y·x = ±0.167; n = 122; r = +0.32.
Pst(l)$_{40\% \text{ TLC}}$ (cm H$_2$O) = $-1.0973 + 0.2486 \cdot$ x;
SD y·x = ±1.71.
a = kPa; b = cm H$_2$O.

Table 118. Elastic recoil pressure of the lungs at 40 % of total lung capacity (Pst(l)$_{40\% \text{ TLC}}$) in relation to body surface in boys and girls

Body surface m^2	Pst(l)$_{40\% \text{ TLC}}$					
	mean		lower limits		upper limits	
	a	b	a	b	a	b
0.60	0.003	0.03	−0.325	−3.321	0.331	3.38
0.70	0.026	0.26	−0.302	−3.084	0.355	3.62
0.80	0.049	0.50	−0.279	−2.848	0.378	3.85
0.90	0.072	0.74	−0.255	−2.611	0.401	4.09
1.00	0.096	0.97	−0.232	−2.374	0.424	4.33
1.10	0.119	1.21	−0.209	−2.137	0.447	4.56
1.20	0.142	1.45	−0.186	−1.901	0.471	4.80
1.30	0.165	1.68	−0.163	−1.664	0.494	5.04
1.40	0.188	1.92	−0.139	−1.427	0.517	5.27
1.50	0.212	2.16	−0.116	−1.191	0.540	5.51
1.60	0.235	2.39	−0.093	−1.095	0.563	5.75
1.70	0.258	2.63	−0.070	−0.071	0.587	5.98
1.80	0.281	2.87	−0.047	−0.048	0.610	6.22
1.90	0.304	3.10	−0.023	−0.024	0.633	6.46
2.00	0.328	3.34	−0.000	−0.006	0.656	6.69

Formula: $y = a + b \cdot x$;
$y = $ Pst(l)$_{40\% \text{ TLC}}$ (kPa or cm H$_2$O); x = body surface (m^2);
Pst(l)$_{40\% \text{ TLC}}$ (kPa) =
    $-0.13613 + 0.23212 \cdot$ body surface (m^2);
SD y·x = ±0.166; n = 122; r = +0.34.
Pst(l)$_{40\% \text{ TLC}}$ (cm H$_2$O) = $-1.3881 + 2.3670 \cdot$ x;
SD y·x = ±1.69.
a = kPa; b = cm H$_2$O.

Table 119. Elastic recoil pressure of the lungs at 50% of total lung capacity (Pst(l)$_{50\% \text{ TLC}}$) in relation to body height in boys and girls

Height cm	Pst(l)$_{50\% \text{ TLC}}$					
	mean		lower limits		upper limits	
	a	b	a	b	a	b
115	0.203	2.08	−0.166	−1.71	0.573	5.88
116	0.210	2.15	−0.159	−1.63	0.580	5.95
118	0.225	2.31	−0.144	−1.48	0.595	6.10
120	0.240	2.46	−0.129	−1.33	0.610	6.25
122	0.255	2.61	−0.114	−1.18	0.625	6.41
124	0.270	2.76	−0.099	−1.03	0.640	6.56
126	0.285	2.91	−0.085	−0.88	0.655	6.71
128	0.299	3.06	−0.070	−0.72	0.669	6.86
130	0.314	3.22	−0.055	−0.57	0.684	7.01
132	0.329	3.37	−0.040	−0.42	0.699	7.17
134	0.344	3.52	−0.025	−0.27	0.714	7.32
136	0.359	3.67	−0.010	−0.12	0.729	7.47
138	0.374	3.82	0.004	0.03	0.744	7.62
140	0.389	3.97	0.019	0.18	0.759	7.77
142	0.403	4.13	0.033	0.33	0.773	7.92
144	0.418	4.28	0.048	0.48	0.788	8.08
146	0.433	4.43	0.063	0.63	0.803	8.23
148	0.448	4.58	0.078	0.78	0.818	8.38
150	0.463	4.73	0.093	0.94	0.833	8.53
152	0.478	4.89	0.108	1.09	0.848	8.68
154	0.493	5.04	0.123	1.24	0.863	8.83
156	0.508	5.19	0.137	1.39	0.878	8.99
158	0.522	5.34	0.152	1.54	0.892	9.14
160	0.537	5.49	0.167	1.70	0.907	9.29
162	0.552	5.64	0.182	1.85	0.922	9.44
164	0.567	5.80	0.197	2.00	0.937	9.59
166	0.582	5.95	0.212	2.15	0.952	9.75
168	0.597	6.10	0.227	2.30	0.967	9.90
170	0.612	6.25	0.242	2.45	0.982	10.05
172	0.626	6.40	0.256	2.61	0.996	10.20
174	0.641	6.56	0.271	2.76	1.011	10.35
176	0.656	6.71	0.286	2.91	1.026	10.50
178	0.671	6.86	0.301	3.06	1.041	10.66
180	0.686	7.01	0.316	3.21	1.056	10.81

Formula: $y = a + b \cdot x$;
$y = $ Pst(l)$_{50\% \text{ TLC}}$ (kPa or cm H_2O); x = body height (cm);
Pst(l)$_{50\% \text{ TLC}}$ (kPa) =
   $-0.65164 + 7.43344 \cdot 10^{-3} \cdot$ body height (cm);
SD $y \cdot x = \pm 0.187$; n = 130; r = +0.51.
Pst(l)$_{50\% \text{ TLC}}$ (cm H_2O) $= -6.6449 + 0.0758 \cdot x$;
SD $y \cdot x = \pm 1.91$.
a = kPa; b = cm H_2O.

Table 120. Elastic recoil pressure of the lungs at 50% of total lung capacity (Pst(l)$_{50\% \text{ TLC}}$) in relation to age in boys and girls

Age years	Pst(l)$_{50\% \text{ TLC}}$					
	mean		lower limits		upper limits	
	a	b	a	b	a	b
6	0.248	2.43	−0.139	−1.53	0.636	6.41
7	0.290	2.86	−0.097	−1.10	0.678	6.83
8	0.331	3.28	−0.056	−0.68	0.719	7.25
9	0.373	3.71	−0.014	−0.16	0.761	7.68
10	0.414	4.13	0.027	0.26	0.802	8.10
11	0.456	4.55	0.068	0.58	0.844	8.53
12	0.498	4.98	0.110	1.01	0.886	8.95
13	0.539	5.40	0.151	1.43	0.927	9.37
14	0.581	5.83	0.193	1.85	0.969	9.80
15	0.622	6.25	0.235	2.28	1.010	10.22
16	0.664	6.68	0.276	2.70	1.052	10.65
17	0.706	7.10	0.318	3.13	1.094	11.07

Formula: $y = a + b \cdot x$;
$y = $ Pst(l)$_{50\% \text{ TLC}}$ (kPa or cm H_2O); x = age (years);
Pst(l)$_{50\% \text{ TLC}}$ (kPa) $= -1.05029 \cdot 10^{-3} + 0.04160 \cdot$ age (years);
SD $y \cdot x = \pm 0.196$; n = 130; r = +0.44.
Pst(l)$_{50\% \text{ TLC}}$ (cm H_2O) $= -0.1071 + 0.4242 \cdot x$;
SD $y \cdot x = \pm 2.00$.
a = kPa; b = cm H_2O.

Table 121. Elastic recoil pressure of the lungs at 50% of total lung capacity (Pst(l)$_{50\% \text{ TLC}}$) in relation to body surface in boys and girls

Body surface m^2	Pst(l)$_{50\% \text{ TLC}}$					
	mean		lower limits		upper limits	
	a	b	a	b	a	b
0.60	0.175	1.79	−0.204	−2.08	0.555	5.67
0.70	0.215	2.20	−0.164	−1.67	0.595	6.08
0.80	0.255	2.60	−0.124	−1.27	0.635	6.48
0.90	0.295	3.01	−0.084	−0.86	0.675	6.89
1.00	0.335	3.42	−0.044	−0.45	0.715	7.30
1.10	0.376	3.83	−0.004	−0.04	0.755	7.71
1.20	0.416	4.24	0.036	0.36	0.795	8.12
1.30	0.456	4.65	0.076	0.77	0.836	8.52
1.40	0.496	5.05	0.116	1.17	0.876	8.93
1.50	0.536	5.46	0.156	1.58	0.916	9.34
1.60	0.576	5.87	0.196	1.99	0.956	9.75
1.70	0.616	6.28	0.236	2.40	0.996	10.16
1.80	0.656	6.69	0.276	2.81	1.036	10.57
1.90	0.696	7.09	0.316	3.21	1.176	10.97
2.00	0.736	7.50	0.356	3.62	1.116	11.38

Formula: $y = a + b \cdot x$;
$y = $ Pst(l)$_{50\% \text{ TLC}}$ (kPa or cm H_2O); x = body surface (m^2);
Pst(l)$_{50\% \text{ TLC}}$ (kPa) $= -0.06433 + 0.40027 \cdot$ body surface (m^2);
SD $y \cdot x = \pm 0.192$; n = 130; r = +0.48.
Pst(l)$_{50\% \text{ TLC}}$ (cm H_2O) $= -0.6560 + 4.0816 \cdot x$;
SD $y \cdot x = \pm 1.96$.
a = kPa; b = cm H_2O.

Table 122. Elastic recoil pressure of the lungs at 60% of total lung capacity (Pst(l)$_{60\% \text{ TLC}}$) in relation to body height in boys and girls

Height cm	Pst(l)$_{60\% \text{ TLC}}$					
	mean		lower limits		upper limits	
	a	b	a	b	a	b
115	0.453	4.62	0.111	1.11	0.796	8.13
116	0.462	4.71	0.119	1.20	0.804	8.22
118	0.478	4.87	0.136	1.36	0.820	8.38
120	0.494	5.04	0.152	1.53	0.837	8.55
122	0.511	5.21	0.168	1.70	0.853	8.72
124	0.527	5.37	0.185	1.86	0.869	8.88
126	0.543	5.54	0.201	2.03	0.886	9.05
128	0.560	5.71	0.217	2.20	0.902	9.22
130	0.576	5.87	0.234	2.36	0.918	9.38
132	0.592	6.04	0.250	2.53	0.934	9.55
134	0.609	6.21	0.266	2.70	0.951	9.71
136	0.625	6.37	0.283	2.86	0.967	9.88
138	0.641	6.54	0.299	3.03	0.983	10.05
140	0.657	6.70	0.315	3.20	1.000	10.21
142	0.674	6.87	0.332	3.36	1.016	10.38
144	0.690	7.04	0.348	3.53	1.032	10.55
146	0.706	7.20	0.364	3.69	1.049	10.71
148	0.723	7.37	0.380	3.86	1.065	10.88
150	0.739	7.54	0.397	4.03	1.081	11.05
152	0.755	7.70	0.413	4.19	1.098	11.21
154	0.772	7.87	0.429	4.36	1.114	11.38
156	0.788	8.04	0.446	4.53	1.130	11.55
158	0.804	8.20	0.462	4.69	1.147	11.71
160	0.821	8.37	0.478	4.86	1.163	11.88
162	0.837	8.54	0.495	5.03	1.179	12.05
164	0.853	8.70	0.511	5.19	1.196	12.21
166	0.870	8.87	0.527	5.36	1.212	12.38
168	0.886	9.04	0.544	5.53	1.228	12.55
170	0.902	9.20	0.560	5.69	1.245	12.71
172	0.919	9.37	0.576	5.86	1.261	12.88
174	0.935	9.54	0.593	6.03	1.277	13.04
176	0.951	9.70	0.609	6.19	1.294	13.21
178	0.968	9.87	0.625	6.36	1.310	13.38
180	0.984	10.03	0.642	6.53	1.326	13.54

Formula: y = a + b·x;
y = Pst(l)$_{60\% \text{ TLC}}$ (kPa or cm H$_2$O); x = body height (cm);
Pst(l)$_{60\% \text{ TLC}}$ (kPa) =
  $-0.48502 + 8.16403 \cdot 10^{-3} \cdot$ body height (cm);
SD y·x = ±0.173; n = 130; r = +0.58.
Pst(l)$_{60\% \text{ TLC}}$ (cm H$_2$O) = −4.9458 + 0.08325·x;
SD y·x = ±1.78.
a = kPa; b = cm H$_2$O.

Table 123. Elastic recoil pressure of the lungs at 60% of total lung capacity (Pst(l)$_{60\% \text{ TLC}}$) in relation to age in boys and girls

Age years	Pst(l)$_{60\% \text{ TLC}}$					
	mean		lower limits		upper limits	
	a	b	a	b	a	b
6	0.484	4.94	0.124	1.24	0.845	8.63
7	0.531	5.42	0.171	1.72	0.892	9.11
8	0.578	5.90	0.218	2.20	0.939	9.59
9	0.625	6.38	0.265	2.68	0.986	10.07
10	0.672	6.86	0.312	3.16	1.033	10.55
11	0.719	7.34	0.359	3.64	1.080	11.03
12	0.766	7.82	0.406	4.12	1.127	11.51
13	0.813	8.30	0.453	4.60	1.174	11.99
14	0.860	8.77	0.500	5.08	1.221	12.47
15	0.907	9.25	0.547	5.56	1.268	12.95
16	0.955	9.73	0.594	6.04	1.315	13.43
17	1.002	10.21	0.641	6.52	1.362	13.91

Formula: y = a + b·x;
y = Pst(l)$_{60\% \text{ TLC}}$ (kPa or cm H$_2$O); x = age (years);
Pst(l)$_{60\% \text{ TLC}}$ (kPa) = 0.20279 + 0.04701·age (years);
SD y·x = ±0.182; n = 130; r = +0.51.
Pst(l)$_{60\% \text{ TLC}}$ (cm H$_2$O) = 2.0679 + 0.4794·x;
SD y·x = ±1.86.
a = kPa; b = cm H$_2$O.

Table 124. Elastic recoil pressure of the lungs at 60% of total lung capacity Pst(l)$_{60\% \text{ TLC}}$ in relation to body surface in boys and girls

Body surface m^2	Pst(l)$_{60\% \text{ TLC}}$					
	mean		lower limits		upper limits	
	a	b	a	b	a	b
0.60	0.420	4.28	0.068	0.68	0.772	7.89
0.70	0.464	4.84	0.112	1.13	0.817	8.34
0.80	0.509	5.19	0.156	1.58	0.861	8.79
0.90	0.553	5.64	0.201	2.03	0.905	9.24
1.00	0.597	6.09	0.245	2.48	0.949	9.69
1.10	0.641	6.54	0.289	2.94	0.994	10.14
1.20	0.686	6.99	0.333	3.39	1.038	10.59
1.30	0.730	7.44	0.378	3.84	1.082	11.04
1.40	0.774	7.89	0.422	4.29	1.126	11.50
1.50	0.818	8.34	0.466	4.74	1.170	11.95
1.60	0.862	8.79	0.510	5.19	1.215	12.40
1.70	0.907	9.24	0.554	5.64	1.259	12.65
1.80	0.951	9.69	0.599	6.09	1.303	13.30
1.90	0.995	10.15	0.643	6.54	1.347	13.75
2.00	1.039	10.60	0.687	6.99	1.391	14.20

Formula: y = a + b·x;
y = Pst(l)$_{60\% \text{ TLC}}$ (kPa or cm H$_2$O); x = body surface (m^2);
Pst(l)$_{60\% \text{ TLC}}$ (kPa) = 0.15541 + 0.44212·body surface (m^2);
SD y·x = ±0.178; n = 130; r = +0.55.
Pst(l)$_{60\% \text{ TLC}}$ (cm H$_2$O) = 1.5847 + 4.5084·x;
SD y·x = ±1.82.
a = kPa; b = cm H$_2$O.

Table 125. Elastic recoil pressure of the lungs at 70% of total lung capacity (Pst(l)$_{70\% TLC}$) in relation to body height in boys and girls

Height cm	Pst(l)$_{70\% TLC}$ mean		lower limits		upper limits	
	a	b	a	b	a	b
115	0.704	7.19	0.332	3.37	1.076	11.01
116	0.712	7.27	0.340	3.45	1.084	11.09
118	0.727	7.43	0.355	3.61	1.099	11.24
120	0.743	7.59	0.371	3.77	1.115	11.40
122	0.759	7.75	0.387	3.93	1.131	11.57
124	0.775	7.91	0.403	4.09	1.147	11.73
126	0.791	8.08	0.419	4.26	1.163	11.90
128	0.807	8.24	0.435	4.43	1.179	12.06
130	0.824	8.41	0.452	6.60	1.196	12.23
132	0.841	8.59	0.469	4.77	1.213	12.40
134	0.858	8.76	0.486	4.94	1.230	12.58
136	0.875	8.94	0.503	5.12	1.247	12.75
138	0.892	9.11	0.520	5.29	1.264	12.93
140	0.910	9.29	0.538	5.47	1.282	13.11
142	0.928	9.47	0.556	5.65	1.300	13.29
144	0.946	9.66	0.574	5.84	1.318	13.48
146	0.964	9.84	0.592	6.02	1.336	13.66
148	0.982	10.03	0.610	6.21	1.354	13.85
150	1.001	10.22	0.629	6.40	1.373	14.04
152	1.019	10.41	0.647	6.59	1.391	14.23
154	1.038	10.60	0.666	6.78	1.410	14.42
156	1.057	10.80	0.685	6.98	1.429	14.62
158	1.077	10.99	0.705	7.17	1.449	14.81
160	1.096	11.19	0.724	7.37	1.468	15.01
162	1.116	11.39	0.744	7.57	1.488	15.21
164	1.136	11.60	0.764	7.78	1.508	15.41
166	1.156	11.80	0.784	7.98	1.528	15.62
168	1.176	12.01	0.804	8.19	1.548	15.83
170	1.196	12.22	0.824	8.40	1.568	16.03
172	1.217	12.43	0.845	8.61	1.589	16.24
174	1.238	12.64	0.866	8.82	1.610	16.46
176	1.259	12.85	0.887	9.03	1.631	16.67
178	1.280	13.07	0.908	9.25	1.652	16.89
180	1.301	13.29	0.929	9.47	1.673	17.11

Formula: $y = a + b \cdot x + c \cdot x^2$;
$y = $ Pst(l)$_{70\% TLC}$ (kPa or cm H$_2$O); x = body height (cm);
Pst(l)$_{70\% TLC}$ (kPa) = $0.13906 + 2.18688 \cdot 10^{-3} \cdot$ body height $+ 2.3732 \cdot 10^{-5} \cdot$ height^2;
SD y·x = ±0.188; n = 130; r = +0.60.
Pst(l)$_{70\% TLC}$ (cm H$_2$O) = $1.4180 + 0.0223 \cdot x + 0.242 \cdot 10^{-3} \cdot x^2$;
SD y·x = ±1.92.
a = kPa; b = cm H$_2$O.

Table 126. Elastic recoil pressure of the lungs at 70% of total lung capacity (Pst(l)$_{70\% TLC}$) in relation to age in boys and girls

Age years	Pst(l)$_{70\% TLC}$ mean		lower limits		upper limits	
	a	b	a	b	a	b
6	0.716	7.30	0.323	3.28	1.110	11.32
7	0.770	7.84	0.376	3.82	1.164	11.86
8	0.824	8.39	0.430	4.37	1.217	12.41
9	0.878	8.94	0.484	4.92	1.271	12.95
10	0.932	9.49	0.538	5.47	1.326	13.50
11	0.986	10.04	0.593	6.02	1.380	14.06
12	1.041	10.59	0.647	6.57	1.435	14.61
13	1.096	11.15	0.702	7.13	1.490	15.17
14	1.151	11.71	0.757	7.69	1.545	15.72
15	1.207	12.27	0.813	8.25	1.600	16.28
16	1.262	12.83	0.868	8.81	1.656	16.85
17	1.318	13.39	0.924	9.37	1.712	17.41

Formula: $y = a + b \cdot x + c \cdot x^2$;
$y = $ Pst(l)$_{70\% TLC}$ (kPa or cm H$_2$O); x = age (years);
Pst(l)$_{70\% TLC}$ (kPa) = $0.40061 + 0.05199 \cdot$ age $+ 1.17875 \cdot 10^{-4} \cdot$ age^2 (years);
SD y·x = ±0.199; n = 130; r = +0.54.
Pst(l)$_{70\% TLC}$ (cm H$_2$O) = $4.0851 + 0.5302 \cdot x + 0.001202 \cdot x^2$;
SD y·x = ±2.03.
a = kPa; b = cm H$_2$O.

Table 127. Elastic recoil pressure of the lungs at 70% of total lung capacity (Pst(l)$_{70\% TLC}$) in relation to body surface in boys and girls

Body surface m^2	Pst(l)$_{70\% TLC}$ mean		lower limits		upper limits	
	a	b	a	b	a	b
0.60	0.627	6.39	0.249	2.51	1.005	10.27
0.70	0.681	6.94	0.303	3.06	1.059	10.82
0.80	0.734	7.49	0.356	3.61	1.112	11.37
0.90	0.788	8.03	0.410	4.15	1.166	11.91
1.00	0.841	8.57	0.463	4.70	1.219	12.45
1.10	0.893	9.11	0.516	5.23	1.271	12.99
1.20	0.946	9.64	0.568	5.77	1.324	13.52
1.30	0.998	10.17	0.620	6.30	1.376	14.05
1.40	1.049	10.70	0.672	6.82	1.427	14.58
1.50	1.101	11.22	0.723	7.35	1.479	15.10
1.60	1.152	11.74	0.774	7.87	1.530	15.62
1.70	1.202	12.26	0.824	8.38	1.580	16.14
1.80	1.253	12.77	0.875	8.90	1.631	16.65
1.90	1.303	13.28	0.925	9.41	1.681	17.16
2.00	1.352	13.79	0.974	9.91	1.730	17.67

Formula: $y = a + b \cdot x + c \cdot x^2$;
$y = $ Pst(l)$_{70\% TLC}$ (kPa or cm H$_2$O); x = body surface (m^2);
Pst(l)$_{70\% TLC}$ (kPa) = $0.29567 + 0.56261 \cdot$ body surface $- 0.01703 \cdot$ body surface^2 (m^2);
SD y·x = ±0.191; n = 130; r = +0.58.
Pst(l)$_{70\% TLC}$ (cm H$_2$O) = $3.0150 + 5.7370 \cdot x - 0.1737 \cdot x^2$;
SD y·x = ±1.95.
a = kPa; b = cm H$_2$O.

Table 128. Elastic recoil pressure of the lungs at 80% of total lung capacity (Pst(l)$_{80\% TLC}$) in relation to body height in boys and girls

Height cm	Pst(l)$_{80\% TLC}$					
	mean		lower limits		upper limits	
	a	b	a	b	a	b
115	0.944	9.63	0.534	5.44	1.354	13.82
116	0.954	9.73	0.544	5.54	1.363	13.92
118	0.974	9.93	0.564	5.74	1.383	14.12
120	0.993	10.13	0.584	5.94	1.403	14.32
122	1.013	10.33	0.604	6.15	1.423	14.52
124	1.033	10.54	0.624	6.35	1.443	14.73
126	1.054	10.75	0.644	6.56	1.463	14.93
128	1.074	10.95	0.665	6.77	1.484	15.14
130	1.095	11.16	0.685	6.98	1.504	15.35
132	1.115	11.38	0.706	7.19	1.525	15.56
134	1.136	11.59	0.727	7.40	1.546	15.78
136	1.157	11.80	0.748	7.61	1.567	15.99
138	1.178	12.02	0.769	7.83	1.588	16.21
140	1.200	12.24	0.790	8.05	1.609	16.42
142	1.221	12.45	0.812	8.27	1.631	16.64
144	1.243	12.67	0.833	8.49	1.652	16.86
146	1.265	12.90	0.855	8.71	1.674	17.08
148	1.286	13.12	0.877	8.93	1.696	17.31
150	1.308	13.34	0.899	9.16	1.718	17.53
152	1.331	13.57	0.921	9.38	1.740	17.76
154	1.353	13.80	0.943	9.61	1.763	17.99
156	1.375	14.03	0.966	9.84	1.785	18.22
158	1.398	14.26	0.989	10.07	1.808	18.45
160	1.421	14.49	1.011	10.30	1.831	18.68
162	1.444	14.73	1.034	10.54	1.853	18.91
164	1.467	14.96	1.057	10.77	1.877	19.15
166	1.490	15.20	1.081	11.01	1.900	19.39
168	1.513	15.44	1.104	11.25	1.923	19.62
170	1.537	15.68	1.127	11.49	1.947	19.86
172	1.561	15.92	1.151	11.73	1.970	20.11
174	1.584	16.16	1.175	11.97	1.994	20.35
176	1.608	16.40	1.199	12.22	2.018	20.59
178	1.633	16.65	1.223	12.46	2.042	20.84
180	1.657	16.90	1.247	12.71	2.066	21.09

Formula: $y = a + b \cdot x + c \cdot x^2$;
$y = $ Pst(l)$_{80\% TLC}$ (kPa or cm H$_2$O); x = body height (cm);
Pst(l)$_{80\% TLC}$ (kPa) $= 0.06549 + 5.52114 \cdot 10^{-3} \cdot$
   body height $+ 1.84561 \cdot 10^{-5} \cdot$ height^2;
SD $x \cdot y = \pm 0.207$; n = 130; r = +0.63.
Pst(l)$_{80\% TLC}$ (cm H$_2$O) $= 0.6678 + 0.0563 \cdot x + 0.1882 \cdot 10^{-3} \cdot x^2$;
SD $y \cdot x = \pm 2.116$.
a = kPa; b = cm H$_2$O.

Table 129. Elastic recoil pressure of the lungs at 80% of total lung capacity (Pst(l)$_{80\% TLC}$) in relation to age in boys and girls

Age years	Pst(l)$_{80\% TLC}$					
	mean		lower limits		upper limits	
	a	b	a	b	a	b
6	0.939	9.57	0.442	5.11	1.436	14.04
7	1.015	10.35	0.519	5.89	1.512	14.81
8	1.089	11.10	0.592	6.64	1.586	15.56
9	1.160	11.82	0.663	7.36	1.657	16.29
10	1.228	12.52	0.732	8.06	1.725	16.98
11	1.294	13.19	0.797	8.72	1.791	17.65
12	1.357	13.83	0.860	9.37	1.854	18.29
13	1.417	14.44	0.921	9.98	1.914	18.91
14	1.475	15.03	0.979	10.57	1.972	19.50
15	1.530	15.59	1.034	11.13	2.027	20.06
16	1.583	16.13	1.086	11.66	2.080	20.59
17	1.633	16.63	1.136	12.17	2.130	21.70

Formula: $y = a + b \cdot x + c \cdot x^2$;
$y = $ Pst(l)$_{80\% TLC}$ (kPa or cm H$_2$O); x = age (years);
Pst(l)$_{80\% TLC}$ (kPa) $=$
   $0.42712 + 0.09330 \cdot$ age $- 1.31409 \cdot 10^{-3} \cdot$ age^2 (years);
SD $y \cdot x = \pm 0.251$; n = 130; r = +0.56.
Pst(l)$_{80\% TLC}$ (cm H$_2$O) $= 4.3554 + 0.9514 \cdot x - 0.0134 \cdot x^2$;
SD $y \cdot x = \pm 2.56$.
a = kPa; b = cm H$_2$O.

Table 130. Elastic recoil pressure of the lungs at 80% of total lung capacity (Pst(l)$_{80\% TLC}$) in relation to body surface in boys and girls

Body surface m^2	Pst(l)$_{80\% TLC}$					
	mean		lower limits		upper limits	
	a	b	a	b	a	b
0.60	0.853	8.70	0.429	4.35	1.276	13.04
0.70	0.921	9.39	0.498	5.05	1.345	13.74
0.80	0.989	10.08	0.565	5.74	1.412	14.42
0.90	1.054	10.75	0.631	6.41	1.478	15.09
1.00	1.119	11.41	0.695	7.07	1.542	15.75
1.10	1.182	12.05	0.759	7.71	1.606	16.40
1.20	1.244	12.69	0.821	8.34	1.668	17.03
1.30	1.305	13.30	0.881	8.96	1.728	17.64
1.40	1.364	13.91	0.940	9.57	1.787	18.25
1.50	1.422	14.50	0.998	10.16	1.845	18.84
1.60	1.478	15.08	1.055	10.73	1.902	19.42
1.70	1.534	15.64	1.110	11.30	1.957	19.98
1.80	1.588	16.19	1.164	11.85	2.011	20.53
1.90	1.640	16.73	1.217	12.30	2.064	21.07
2.00	1.692	17.25	1.268	12.91	2.115	21.59

Formula: $y = a + b \cdot x + c \cdot x^2$;
$y = $ Pst(l)$_{80\% TLC}$ (kPa or cm H$_2$O); x = body surface (m^2);
Pst(l)$_{80\% TLC}$ (kPa) $= 0.41449 + 0.77105 \cdot$ body surface $-$
   $0.06614 \cdot$ body surface^2 (m^2);
SD $y \cdot x = \pm 0.214$; n = 130; r = +0.59.
Pst(l)$_{80\% TLC}$ (cm H$_2$O) $= 4.2266 + 7.8625 \cdot x - 0.6744 \cdot x^2$;
SD $y \cdot x = \pm 2.19$.
a = kPa; b = cm H$_2$O.

Table 131. Elastic recoil pressure of the lungs at 90 % of total lung capacity (Pst(l)$_{90\% \text{ TLC}}$) in relation to body height in boys and girls

Height cm	Pst(l)$_{90\% \text{ TLC}}$					
	mean		lower limits		upper limits	
	a	b	a	b	a	b
115	1.262	12.87	0.793	8.07	1.730	17.66
116	1.277	13.02	0.808	8.23	1.746	17.82
118	1.308	13.34	0.839	8.54	1.777	18.13
120	1.338	13.65	0.869	8.85	1.807	18.44
122	1.369	13.96	0.900	9.16	1.838	18.75
124	1.399	14.27	0.930	9.47	1.868	19.06
126	1.429	14.58	0.960	9.78	1.898	19.37
128	1.459	14.88	0.990	10.09	1.928	19.68
130	1.489	15.19	1.020	10.39	1.958	19.98
132	1.519	15.49	1.050	10.70	1.988	20.28
134	1.549	15.79	1.080	11.00	2.018	20.59
136	1.578	16.09	1.109	11.30	2.047	20.89
138	1.607	16.39	1.138	11.60	2.076	21.19
140	1.636	16.69	1.167	11.89	2.105	21.48
142	1.665	16.98	1.197	12.19	2.134	21.78
144	1.694	17.28	1.225	12.48	2.163	22.07
146	1.723	17.57	1.254	12.78	2.192	22.37
148	1.752	17.86	1.283	13.07	2.221	22.66
150	1.780	18.15	1.311	13.36	2.249	22.95
152	1.808	18.44	1.339	13.65	2.277	23.24
154	1.836	18.73	1.368	13.93	2.305	23.52
156	1.864	19.01	1.396	14.22	2.333	23.81
158	1.892	19.30	1.423	14.50	2.361	24.09
160	1.920	19.58	1.451	14.78	2.389	24.37
162	1.948	19.86	1.479	15.06	2.417	24.65
164	1.975	20.14	1.506	15.34	2.444	24.93
166	2.002	20.42	1.533	15.62	2.471	25.21
168	2.029	20.69	1.560	15.90	2.498	25.49
170	2.056	20.97	1.587	16.17	2.525	25.76
172	2.083	21.24	1.614	16.45	2.552	26.04
174	2.110	21.51	1.641	16.72	2.579	26.31
176	2.136	21.78	1.667	16.99	2.605	26.58
178	2.163	22.05	1.694	17.26	2.632	26.85
180	2.189	22.32	1.720	17.53	2.658	27.12

Formula: $y = a + b \cdot x + c \cdot x^2$;
$y = $ Pst(l)$_{90\% \text{ TLC}}$ (kPa or cm H_2O); $x = $ body height (cm);
Pst(l)$_{90\% \text{ TLC}}$ (kPa) $= -0.7565 + 0.01965 \cdot$ body height $- 1.82403 \cdot 10^{-5} \cdot$ height^2 (cm);
SD $y \cdot x = \pm 0.237$; n = 130; r = +0.67.
Pst(l)$_{90\% \text{ TLC}}$ (cm H_2O) $= -7.7149 + 0.2004 \cdot x - 0.000186 \cdot x^2$;
SD $y \cdot x = \pm 2.42$.
a = kPa; b = cm H_2O.

Table 132. Elastic recoil pressure of the lungs at 90 % of total lung capacity (Pst(l)$_{90\% \text{ TLC}}$) in relation to age in boys and girls

Age years	Pst(l)$_{90\% \text{ TLC}}$					
	mean		lower limits		upper limits	
	a	b	a	b	a	b
6	1.227	12.51	0.730	7.43	1.724	17.59
7	1.351	13.78	0.855	8.70	1.848	18.86
8	1.467	14.96	0.971	9.88	1.964	20.04
9	1.575	16.06	1.078	10.98	2.072	21.14
10	1.674	17.06	1.177	11.99	2.171	22.14
11	1.764	17.99	1.268	12.91	2.261	23.07
12	1.846	18.82	1.350	13.74	2.343	23.90
13	1.920	19.57	1.423	14.49	2.416	24.65
14	1.984	20.23	1.488	15.15	2.481	25.31
15	2.041	20.80	1.544	15.72	2.537	25.88
16	2.089	21.29	1.592	16.21	2.585	26.37
17	2.128	21.68	1.631	16.61	2.624	26.76

Formula: $y = a + b \cdot x + c \cdot x^2$;
$y = $ Pst(l)$_{90\% \text{ TLC}}$ (kPa or cm H_2O); $x = $ age (years);
Pst(l)$_{90\% \text{ TLC}}$ (kPa) $= 0.30076 + 0.18002 \cdot$ age $- 4.26589 \cdot 10^{-3} \cdot$ age^2 (years);
SD $y \cdot x = \pm 0.251$; n = 130; r = +0.61.
Pst(l)$_{90\% \text{ TLC}}$ (cm H_2O) $= 3.0669 + 1.8357 \cdot x - 0.0435 \cdot x^2$;
SD $y \cdot x = \pm 2.56$.
a = kPa; b = cm H_2O.

Table 133. Elastic recoil pressure of the lungs at 90 % of total lung capacity (Pst(l)$_{90\% \text{ TLC}}$) in relation to body surface in boys and girls

Body surface m²	Pst(l)$_{90\% \text{ TLC}}$					
	mean		lower limits		upper limits	
	a	b	a	b	a	b
0.60	1.111	11.33	0.626	6.38	1.596	16.27
0.70	1.219	12.43	0.734	7.48	1.704	17.38
0.80	1.323	13.49	0.838	8.54	1.808	18.44
0.90	1.422	14.50	0.937	9.55	1.907	19.45
1.00	1.517	15.47	1.032	10.52	2.002	20.42
1.10	1.607	16.39	1.122	11.44	2.092	21.34
1.20	1.693	17.27	1.208	12.32	2.178	22.21
1.30	1.775	18.10	1.290	13.15	2.260	23.05
1.40	1.852	18.88	1.367	13.94	2.337	23.83
1.50	1.925	19.62	1.440	14.68	2.409	24.57
1.60	1.993	20.32	1.508	15.37	2.477	25.27
1.70	2.056	20.97	1.572	16.02	2.541	25.92
1.80	2.116	21.57	1.631	16.63	2.601	26.52
1.90	2.171	22.13	1.686	17.19	2.655	27.08
2.00	2.221	22.65	1.736	17.70	2.706	27.59

Formula: $y = a + b \cdot x + c \cdot x^2$;
$y = $ Pst(l)$_{90\% \text{ TLC}}$ (kPa or cm H_2O); $x = $ body surface (m²);
Pst(l)$_{90\% \text{ TLC}}$ (kPa) $= 0.36857 + 1.37110 \cdot$ body surface $- 0.22234 \cdot$ body surface^2 (m²);
SD $y \cdot x = \pm 0.245$; n = 130; r = +0.64.
Pst(l)$_{90\% \text{ TLC}}$ (cm H_2O) $= 3.7584 + 13.9813 \cdot x - 2.2672 \cdot x^2$;
SD $y \cdot x = \pm 2.50$.
a = kPa; b = cm H_2O.

Table 134. Elastic recoil pressure of the lungs at 100% of total lung capacity (Pst(l)$_{100\% \text{ TLC}}$) in relation to body height in boys and girls

Height cm	Pst(l)$_{100\% \text{ TLC}}$					
	mean		lower limits		upper limits	
	a	b	a	b	a	b
115	2.381	24.27	1.225	12.36	3.536	36.18
116	2.414	24.62	1.259	12.71	3.570	36.53
118	2.481	25.30	1.326	13.39	3.637	37.21
120	2.548	25.98	1.392	14.07	3.703	37.89
122	2.613	26.65	1.458	14.74	3.769	38.56
124	2.678	27.31	1.523	15.40	3.834	39.22
126	2.742	27.96	1.587	16.05	3.898	39.87
128	2.806	28.61	1.650	16.70	3.961	40.52
130	2.868	29.24	1.713	17.34	4.024	41.15
132	2.930	29.87	1.774	17.97	4.086	41.78
134	2.991	30.50	1.836	18.59	4.147	42.41
136	3.052	31.11	1.896	19.20	4.207	43.02
138	3.111	31.72	1.956	19.81	4.267	43.63
140	3.170	32.32	2.014	20.41	4.326	44.23
142	3.228	32.91	2.072	21.00	4.384	44.82
144	3.285	33.50	2.130	21.59	4.441	45.41
146	3.342	34.08	2.186	22.17	4.498	45.98
148	3.398	34.64	2.242	22.74	4.554	46.55
150	3.453	35.21	2.298	23.30	4.609	47.12
152	3.508	35.76	2.352	23.85	4.663	47.67
154	3.561	36.31	2.406	24.40	4.717	48.22
156	3.614	36.85	2.458	24.94	4.770	48.76
158	3.666	37.38	2.511	25.47	4.822	49.29
160	3.718	37.90	2.562	25.99	4.873	49.81
162	3.768	38.42	2.613	26.51	4.924	50.33
164	3.818	38.93	2.663	27.02	4.974	50.84
166	3.867	39.43	2.712	27.52	5.023	51.34
168	3.916	39.92	2.760	28.01	5.071	51.83
170	3.963	40.41	2.808	28.50	5.119	52.32
172	4.010	40.89	2.855	28.98	5.166	52.79
174	4.057	41.36	2.901	29.45	5.212	53.27
176	4.102	41.82	2.946	29.91	5.258	53.73
178	4.147	42.28	2.991	30.37	5.302	54.18
180	4.191	42.72	3.035	30.81	5.346	54.63

Formula: $y = a + b \cdot x + c \cdot x^2$;
$y = $ Pst(l)$_{100\% \text{ TLC}}$ (kPa or cm H$_2$O); x = body height (cm);
Pst(l)$_{100\% \text{ TLC}}$ (kPa) = $-2.75204 + 0.05536 \cdot$ height $-$
9.32612 $\cdot 10^{-5} \cdot$ height^2 (cm);
SD y·x = ±0.584; n = 130; r = +0.59.
Pst(l)$_{100\% \text{ TLC}}$ (cm H$_2$O) = $-28.0630 + 0.5645 \cdot x - 0.000951 \cdot x^2$;
SD y·x = ±6.02.
a = kPa; b = cm H$_2$O.

Table 135. Elastic recoil pressure of the lungs at 100% of total lung capacity (Pst(l)$_{100\% \text{ TLC}}$) in relation to age in boys and girls

Age years	Pst(l)$_{100\% \text{ TLC}}$					
	mean		lower limits		upper limits	
	a	b	a	b	a	b
6	2.149	21.91	0.977	9.84	3.320	33.98
7	2.481	25.29	1.309	13.22	3.652	37.36
8	2.777	28.31	1.606	16.25	3.949	40.38
9	3.039	30.98	1.868	18.91	4.210	43.05
10	3.266	33.29	2.094	21.22	4.437	45.36
11	3.457	35.24	2.286	23.18	4.629	47.31
12	3.614	36.84	2.443	24.77	4.786	48.91
13	3.736	38.08	2.565	26.01	4.907	50.15
14	3.823	38.96	2.651	26.89	4.994	51.03
15	3.874	39.49	2.703	27.42	5.046	51.55
16	3.891	39.65	2.720	27.59	5.063	51.72
17	3.873	39.46	2.701	27.40	5.044	51.53

Formula: $y = a + b \cdot x + c \cdot x^2$;
$y = $ Pst(l)$_{100\% \text{ TLC}}$ (kPa or cm H$_2$O); x = age (years);
Pst(l)$_{100\% \text{ TLC}}$ (kPa) =
$-0.57619 + 0.55924 \cdot$ age $- 0.01750 \cdot$ age^2 (years);
SD y·x = ±0.592; n = 130; r = +0.54.
Pst(l)$_{100\% \text{ TLC}}$ (cm H$_2$O) = $-5.8755 + 5.7027 \cdot x - 0.1785 \cdot x^2$;
SD y·x = ±6.09.
a = kPa; b = cm H$_2$O.

Table 136. Elastic recoil pressure of the lungs at 100% of total lung capacity (Pst(l)$_{100\% \text{ TLC}}$) in relation to body surface in boys and girls

Body surface m^2	Pst(l)$_{100\% \text{ TLC}}$					
	mean		lower limits		upper limits	
	a	b	a	b	a	b
0.60	2.060	21.01	0.875	8.79	3.245	33.22
0.70	2.296	23.42	1.111	11.20	3.482	35.63
0.80	2.520	25.69	1.335	13.48	3.705	37.91
0.90	2.730	27.84	1.545	15.63	3.916	40.05
1.00	2.928	29.86	1.743	17.65	4.113	42.07
1.10	3.113	31.74	1.928	19.53	4.298	43.95
1.20	3.285	33.50	2.100	21.28	4.470	45.71
1.30	3.444	35.12	2.259	22.91	4.629	47.33
1.40	3.590	36.61	2.405	24.40	4.775	48.82
1.50	3.723	37.97	2.538	25.76	4.909	50.18
1.60	3.844	39.20	2.659	26.98	5.029	51.41
1.70	3.951	40.29	2.766	28.08	5.137	52.50
1.80	4.046	41.26	2.861	29.05	5.231	53.47
1.90	4.128	42.09	2.943	29.88	5.313	54.30
2.00	4.197	42.79	3.011	30.58	5.382	55.01

Formula: $y = a + b \cdot x + c \cdot x^2$;
$y = $ Pst(l)$_{100\% \text{ TLC}}$ (kPa or cm H$_2$O); x = body surface (m^2);
Pst(l)$_{100\% \text{ TLC}}$ (kPa) = $0.37204 + 3.20043 \cdot$ body surface $-$
0.64393 · body surface^2 (m^2);
SD y·x = ±0.599; n = 130; r = +0.54.
Pst(l)$_{100\% \text{ TLC}}$ (cm H$_2$O) = $3.7938 + 32.6354 \cdot x - 6.5663 \cdot x^2$;
SD y·x = ±6.17.
a = kPa; b = cm H$_2$O.

Table 137. Static lung compliance (Cst) in relation to body height in boys and girls

Height cm	Cst					
	mean		lower limits		upper limits	
	a	b	a	b	a	b
115	847.91	83.15	601.69	59.00	1,194.91	117.18
116	863.34	84.66	612.63	60.08	1,216.64	119.31
118	894.61	87.73	634.82	62.25	1,260.71	123.63
120	926.47	90.85	657.43	64.47	1,305.60	128.04
122	958.90	94.03	680.44	66.73	1,351.31	132.52
124	991.91	97.27	703.87	69.02	1,397.84	137.08
126	1,025.51	100.57	727.71	71.36	1,445.18	141.72
128	1,059.69	103.92	751.96	73.74	1,493.34	146.45
130	1,094.45	107.33	776.63	76.16	1,542.33	151.25
132	1,129.79	110.79	801.71	78.62	1,592.13	156.14
134	1,165.72	114.32	827.20	81.12	1,642.76	161.10
136	1,202.23	117.90	853.11	83.66	1,694.21	166.15
138	1,239.33	121.54	879.43	86.24	1,746.49	171.28
140	1,277.01	125.23	906.17	88.86	1,799.59	176.48
142	1,315.28	128.99	933.33	91.53	1,853.53	181.77
144	1,354.13	132.80	960.90	94.23	1,908.29	187.14
146	1,393.58	136.66	988.90	96.98	1,963.88	192.59
148	1,433.62	140.59	1,017.31	99.76	2,020.29	198.13
150	1,474.24	144.58	1,046.13	102.59	2,077.54	203.74
152	1,515.45	148.62	1,075.38	105.46	2,135.62	209.44
154	1,557.26	152.72	1,105.04	108.37	2,194.53	215.22
156	1,599.66	156.87	1,135.13	111.32	2,254.28	221.07
158	1,642.64	161.09	1,165.63	114.31	2,314.86	227.02
160	1,686.23	165.36	1,196.56	117.34	2,376.28	233.04
162	1,730.40	169.70	1,227.91	120.42	2,438.53	239.14
164	1,775.17	174.09	1,259.67	123.53	2,501.62	245.33
166	1,820.53	178.54	1,291.36	126.69	2,565.54	251.60
168	1,866.49	183.04	1,324.48	129.89	2,630.31	257.95
170	1,913.04	187.61	1,357.51	133.13	2,695.92	264.39
172	1,960.19	192.23	1,390.97	136.41	2,762.36	270.90
174	2,007.94	196.92	1,424.85	139.73	2,829.65	277.50
176	2,056.25	201.66	1,459.16	143.10	2,897.78	284.18
178	2,105.23	206.46	1,493.88	146.50	2,966.74	290.95
180	2,154.77	211.32	1,529.04	149.95	3,036.56	297.79

Formula: log y = a + b·log x;
y = Cst (ml/kPa or ml/cm H$_2$O); x = body height (cm);
log Cst (ml/kPa) = –1.3614 + 2.0817·log height (cm);
SD log y·x = ±0.0753; n = 131; r = +0.78.
log Cst (ml/cm H$_2$O) = –2.3699 + 2.0817·log x;
SD log y·x = ±0.0753.
a = ml/kPa; b = ml/cm H$_2$O.

Table 138. Static lung compliance (Cst) in relation to age in boys and girls

Age years	Cst					
	mean		lower limits		upper limits	
	a	b	a	b	a	b
6	846.88	83.07	571.58	56.05	1,254.78	123.11
7	968.61	95.01	653.73	64.11	1,435.13	140.81
8	1,088.10	106.75	734.39	72.01	1,612.19	158.18
9	1,205.69	118.27	813.75	79.80	1,786.40	175.27
10	1,321.60	129.64	891.98	87.47	1,958.14	192.13
11	1,436.02	140.86	969.20	95.04	2,127.67	208.76
12	1,549.11	151.95	1,045.53	102.53	2,295.23	225.20
13	1,660.99	162.93	1,121.04	109.93	2,461.00	241.47
14	1,771.76	173.80	1,195.81	117.27	2,625.13	257.57
15	1,881.52	184.56	1,269.89	124.53	2,787.76	273.53
16	1,990.35	195.24	1,343.33	131.73	2,948.99	289.35
17	2,098.29	205.83	1,416.19	138.85	3,108.93	305.04

Formula: log y = a + b·log x;
y = Cst (ml/kPa or ml/cm H$_2$O); x = age (years);
log Cst (ml/kPa) = 2.2499 + 0.8712·log age (years);
SD log y·x = ±0.0863; n = 131; r = +0.69.
log Cst (ml/cm H$_2$O) = 1.2415 + 0.8712·log x;
SD log y·x = ±0.0863.
a = ml/kPa; b = ml/cm H$_2$O.

Table 139. Static lung compliance (Cst) in relation to body surface in boys and girls

Body surface m^2	Cst					
	mean		lower limits		upper limits	
	a	b	a	b	a	b
0.60	691.41	67.82	475.88	46.68	1,004.56	98.55
0.70	802.96	78.77	552.66	54.21	1,166.63	114.45
0.80	914.04	89.66	629.11	61.71	1,328.02	130.28
0.90	1,024.71	100.52	705.28	69.18	1,488.80	146.06
1.00	1,135.01	111.34	781.20	76.63	1,649.06	161.78
1.10	1,244.98	122.13	856.87	84.05	1,808.84	177.46
1.20	1,354.65	132.89	932.38	91.46	1,968.18	193.09
1.30	1,464.06	143.62	1,007.67	98.84	2,127.14	208.68
1.40	1,573.21	154.33	1,082.80	106.21	2,285.73	224.24
1.50	1,682.13	165.02	1,157.77	113.57	2,443.98	239.77
1.60	1,790.84	175.68	1,232.59	120.91	2,601.92	255.27
1.70	1,899.34	186.33	1,307.27	128.23	2,759.57	270.07
1.80	2,007.66	196.95	1,381.82	135.55	2,916.94	286.17
1.90	2,115.80	207.56	1,456.25	142.85	3,074.05	301.59
2.00	2,223.76	218.15	1,524.36	150.14	3,244.06	316.98

Formula: log y = a + b·log x;
y = Cst (ml/kPa or ml/cm H$_2$O); x = body surface (m^2);
log Cst (ml/kPa) = 3.0550 + 0.9703·log body surface (m^2);
SD log y·x = ±0.0820; n = 131; r = +0.73.
log Cst (ml/cm H$_2$O) = 2.0466 + 0.9703·log x;
SD log y·x = ±0.0820.
a = ml/kPa; b = ml/cm H$_2$O.

Table 140. Static lung compliance (Cst) in relation to vital capacity (VC) in boys and girls

VC ml	Cst					
	mean		lower limits		upper limits	
	a	b	a	b	a	b
1,250	795.4	78.09	356.0	35.00	1,234.8	121.19
1,500	900.2	88.38	460.8	45.29	1,339.6	131.48
2,000	1,109.8	108.97	670.4	65.87	1,549.2	152.06
2,500	1,319.3	129.55	879.9	86.46	1,758.7	172.65
3,000	1,528.9	150.14	1,089.5	107.04	1,968.3	193.23
3,500	1,738.4	170.72	1,299.0	127.62	2,177.8	213.82
4,000	1,948.0	191.31	1,508.6	148.21	2,387.4	234.40
4,500	2,157.5	211.89	1,718.1	168.79	2,596.9	254.99
5,000	2,367.1	232.47	1,927.7	189.38	2,806.5	275.57
5,250	2,471.8	242.77	2,027.7	199.67	2,916.1	285.86

Formula: $y = a + b \cdot x$;
y = Cst (ml/kPa or ml/cm H_2O); x = VC (ml);
Cst (ml/kPa) = $271.6074 + 0.4191 \cdot$ VC (ml);
SD $y \cdot x = \pm 222.09$; n = 131; r = +0.85.
Cst (ml/cm H_2O) = $26.6356 + 0.0411 \cdot x$;
SD $y \cdot x = \pm 21.78$.
a = ml/kPa; b = ml/cm H_2O.

Table 142. Static lung compliance (Cst) in relation to functional residual capacity measured in a body plethysmograph (FRC$_{box}$) in boys and girls

FRC$_{box}$ ml	Cst					
	mean		lower limits		upper limits	
	a	b	a	b	a	b
900	900.38	88.34	372.94	36.60	1,427.81	140.08
1,000	959.93	94.18	432.49	42.44	1,487.36	145.93
1,500	1,257.68	123.41	730.24	71.67	1,785.11	175.15
2,000	1,555.43	152.64	1,027.99	100.90	2,082.86	204.38
2,500	1,853.18	181.86	1,325.74	130.12	2,380.61	233.60
3,000	2,150.93	211.09	1,623.49	159.35	2,678.36	262.83
3,500	2,448.68	240.31	1,921.24	188.57	2,976.11	292.05

Formula: $y = a + b \cdot x$;
y = Cst (ml/kPa or ml/cm H_2O); x = FRC$_{box}$ (ml);
Cst (ml/kPa) = $364.4322 + 0.5955 \cdot$ FRC$_{box}$ (ml);
SD $y \cdot x = \pm 266.34$; n = 120; r = +0.79.
Cst (ml/cm H_2O) = $35.7386 + 0.0584 \cdot x$;
SD $y \cdot x = \pm 26.12$.
a = ml/kPa; b = ml/cm H_2O.

Table 141. Static lung compliance (Cst) in relation to total lung capacity TLC measured in a body plethysmograph (TLC$_{box}$) in boys and girls

TLC$_{box}$ ml	Cst					
	mean		lower limits		upper limits	
	a	b	a	b	a	b
1,750	785.03	77.11	321.76	31.68	1,248.31	122.54
2,000	868.88	85.35	405.61	39.92	1,332.16	130.78
2,500	1,036.58	101.83	573.31	56.40	1,499.86	147.26
3,000	1,204.28	118.31	741.01	72.88	1,667.56	163.74
3,500	1,371.98	134.79	908.71	89.36	1,835.26	180.22
4,000	1,539.68	151.27	1,076.41	105.84	2,002.96	196.70
4,500	1,707.38	167.76	1,244.11	122.33	2,170.66	213.19
5,000	1,875.08	184.24	1,411.81	138.81	2,338.36	229.67
5,500	2,042.78	200.72	1,579.51	155.29	2,506.06	246.15
6,000	2,210.48	217.20	1,747.21	171.77	2,673.76	262.63
6,500	2,378.18	233.68	1,914.91	188.25	2,841.46	279.11
6,620	2,418.44	237.64	1,950.59	192.21	2,886.28	283.07

Formula: $y = a + b \cdot x$;
y = Cst (ml/kPa or ml/cm H_2O); x = TLC$_{box}$ (ml);
Cst (ml/kPa) = $198.0890 + 0.3354 \cdot$ TLC$_{box}$ (ml);
SD $y \cdot x = \pm 233.92$; n = 120; r = +0.84.
Cst (ml/cm H_2O) = $19.4259 + 0.0329 \cdot x$;
SD $y \cdot x = \pm 22.94$.
a = ml/kPa; b = ml/cm H_2O.

Table 143. Static lung compliance (Cst) in relation to residual volume measured in a body plethysmograph (RV$_{box}$) in boys and girls

RV$_{box}$ ml	Cst					
	mean		lower limits		upper limits	
	a	b	a	b	a	b
417	1,014.87	99.55	320.02	31.41	1,709.72	167.69
500	1,092.82	107.20	397.97	39.06	1,787.66	175.34
750	1,327.59	130.24	632.74	62.10	2,022.44	198.39
1,000	1,562.37	153.29	867.52	85.15	2,257.21	221.43
1,250	1,797.14	176.33	1,102.29	108.19	2,491.99	244.47
1,500	2,031.92	199.37	1,337.07	131.23	2,726.76	267.51
1,750	2,266.69	222.42	1,571.84	154.27	2,961.54	290.56
1,870	2,379.39	233.48	1,677.62	165.33	3,081.14	301.62

Formula: $y = a + b \cdot x$;
y = Cst (ml/kPa or ml/cm H_2O); x = RV$_{box}$ (ml);
Cst (ml/kPa) = $623.2718 + 0.9391 \cdot$ RV$_{box}$ (ml);
SD $y \cdot x = \pm 350.88$; n = 120; r = +0.59.
Cst (ml/cm H_2O) = $61.1221 + 0.0921 \cdot x$;
SD $y \cdot x = \pm 34.41$.
a = ml/kPa; b = ml/cm H_2O.

Table 144. Static lung compliance (Cst) in relation to total lung capacity measured by helium-dilution method (TLC$_{He}$) in boys and girls

TLC$_{He}$ ml	Cst					
	mean		lower limits		upper limits	
	a	b	a	b	a	b
1,930	914.47	89.75	457.58	44.94	1,371.36	134.56
2,000	937.38	92.00	480.49	47.19	1,394.27	136.81
2,500	1,101.03	108.07	644.14	63.25	1,557.92	152.88
3,000	1,264.68	124.14	807.79	79.38	1,721.57	168.95
3,500	1,428.33	140.21	971.44	95.39	1,885.22	185.02
4,000	1,591.98	156.27	1,135.09	111.64	2,048.87	201.09
4,500	1,755.63	172.34	1,298.74	127.53	2,212.52	217.16
5,000	1,919.28	188.41	1,462.39	143.60	2,376.17	233.22
5,500	2,082.93	204.48	1,626.04	159.67	2,539.82	249.29
6,000	2,246.58	220.55	1,789.69	175.73	2,703.47	265.36
6,500	2,410.23	236.62	1,953.34	191.80	2,867.12	281.43
6,640	2,456.05	241.12	1,995.15	196.30	2,916.95	285.93

Formula: $y = a + b \cdot x$;
$y = Cst$ (ml/kPa or ml/cm H$_2$O); $x = TLC_{He}$ (ml);
Cst (ml/kPa) = $282.7815 + 0.3273 \cdot TLC_{He}$ (ml);
SD $y \cdot x = \pm 230.45$; $n = 108$; $r = +0.84$.
Cst (ml/cm H$_2$O) = $27.7314 + 0.0321 \cdot x$;
SD $y \cdot x = \pm 22.6$.
a = ml/kPa; b = ml/cm H$_2$O.

Table 146. Static lung compliance (Cst) in relation to residual volume measured by helium-dilution method (RV$_{He}$) in boys and girls

RV$_{He}$ ml	Cst					
	mean		lower limits		upper limits	
	a	b	a	b	a	b
500	1,246.91	122.28	553.47	54.26	1,940.34	190.29
750	1,447.53	141.95	754.10	73.94	2,140.97	209.97
1,000	1,648.16	161.63	954.72	93.61	2,341.59	229.65
1,250	1,848.78	181.31	1,155.35	113.29	2,542.22	249.32
1,500	2,049.41	200.98	1,355.97	132.97	2,742.84	269.00
1,645	2,250.03	212.39	1,556.60	144.38	2,943.47	280.41

Formula: $y = a + b \cdot x$;
$y = Cst$ (ml/kPa or ml/cm H$_2$O); $x = RV_{He}$ (ml);
Cst (ml/kPa) = $845.6627 + 0.8025 \cdot RV_{He}$ (ml);
SD $y \cdot x = \pm 349.76$; $n = 108$; $r = +0.57$.
Cst (ml/cm H$_2$O) = $82.9312 + 0.0787 \cdot x$;
SD $y \cdot x = \pm 34.30$.
a = ml/kPa; b = ml/cm H$_2$O.

Table 145. Static lung compliance (Cst) in relation to functional residual capacity measured by a helium-dilution method (FRC$_{He}$) in boys and girls

FRC$_{He}$ ml	Cst					
	mean		lower limits		upper limits	
	a	b	a	b	a	b
930	1,030.92	101.11	490.13	48.07	1,571.72	154.15
1,000	1,069.54	104.89	528.74	51.85	1,610.33	157.93
1,500	1,345.34	131.95	804.54	78.91	1,886.13	184.99
2,000	1,621.14	159.00	1,080.34	105.96	2,161.93	212.04
2,500	1,896.94	186.05	1,356.14	133.01	2,437.73	239.09
3,000	2,172.74	213.11	1,631.94	160.07	2,713.53	266.15
3,500	2,448.54	240.16	1,907.74	187.12	2,989.33	293.20

Formula: $y = a + b \cdot x$;
$y = Cst$ (ml/kPa or ml/cm H$_2$O); $x = FRC_{He}$ (ml);
Cst (ml/kPa) = $517,9402 + 0.5516 \cdot FRC_{He}$ (ml);
SD $y \cdot x = \pm 272,77$; $n = 108$; $r = +0.77$.
Cst (ml/cm H$_2$O) = $50.7926 + 0.0541 \cdot x$;
SD $y \cdot x = \pm 26.75$.
a = ml/kPa; b = ml/cm H$_2$O.

Table 147. Static lung complicance per milliliter of TLC_{box} $\left(\frac{Cst}{TLC_{box}}\right)$ in relation to body height in boys and girls

Height cm	$\frac{Cst}{TLC_{box}}$ mean		lower limits		upper limits	
	a	b	a	b	a	b
115	0.437	0.0428	0.317	0.0311	0.556	0.0545
116	0.435	0.0427	0.316	0.0310	0.555	0.0544
118	0.433	0.0424	0.313	0.0307	0.552	0.0542
120	0.430	0.0422	0.311	0.0304	0.549	0.0539
122	0.427	0.0419	0.308	0.0302	0.547	0.0536
124	0.425	0.0416	0.305	0.0299	0.544	0.0534
126	0.422	0.0414	0.303	0.0296	0.541	0.0531
128	0.419	0.0411	0.300	0.0294	0.539	0.0528
130	0.417	0.0408	0.297	0.0291	0.536	0.0526
132	0.414	0.0406	0.294	0.0288	0.533	0.0523
134	0.411	0.0403	0.292	0.0286	0.530	0.0520
136	0.408	0.0401	0.289	0.0283	0.528	0.0518
138	0.406	0.0398	0.286	0.0281	0.525	0.0515
140	0.403	0.0395	0.284	0.0278	0.522	0.0513
142	0.400	0.0393	0.281	0.0275	0.520	0.0510
144	0.398	0.0390	0.278	0.0273	0.517	0.0507
146	0.395	0.0387	0.276	0.0270	0.514	0.0505
148	0.392	0.0385	0.273	0.0267	0.512	0.0502
150	0.390	0.0382	0.270	0.0265	0.509	0.0499
152	0.387	0.0379	0.268	0.0262	0.506	0.0497
154	0.384	0.0377	0.265	0.0259	0.504	0.0494
156	0.382	0.0374	0.262	0.0257	0.501	0.0492
158	0.379	0.0372	0.260	0.0254	0.498	0.0489
160	0.376	0.0369	0.257	0.0252	0.496	0.0486
162	0.374	0.0366	0.254	0.0249	0.493	0.0484
164	0.371	0.0364	0.252	0.0246	0.490	0.0481
166	0.368	0.0361	0.249	0.0244	0.488	0.0478
168	0.366	0.0358	0.246	0.0241	0.485	0.0476
170	0.363	0.0356	0.244	0.0238	0.482	0.0473
172	0.360	0.0353	0.241	0.0236	0.479	0.0470
174	0.357	0.0350	0.238	0.0233	0.477	0.0468
176	0.355	0.0348	0.235	0.0231	0.474	0.0465
178	0.352	0.0345	0.233	0.0228	0.471	0.0463
180	0.349	0.0343	0.230	0.0225	0.469	0.0460

$a = \frac{ml/kPa}{ml}$; $b = \frac{ml/cm\ H_2O}{ml}$.

$\frac{Cst}{TLC_{box}} \left(\frac{ml/cm\ H_2O}{ml}\right) = 0.0580 - 0.1316 \cdot 10^{-3} \cdot x$;

SD $y \cdot x = \pm 0.00592$.

Formula: $y = a + b \cdot x$;

$y = \frac{Cst}{TLC_{box}} \left(\frac{ml/kPa}{ml} \text{ or } \frac{ml/cm\ H_2O}{ml}\right)$; x = body height (cm);

$\frac{Cst}{TLC_{box}} \left(\frac{ml/kPa}{ml}\right) = 0.5914 - 1.3419 \cdot 10^{-3} \cdot$ body height (cm);

SD $y \cdot x = \pm 0.0603$; n = 130; r = -0.32.

Table 148. Static lung compliance per milliliter of TLC_{box} $\left(\frac{Cst}{TLC_{box}}\right)$ in relation to age in boys and girls

Age years	$\frac{Cst}{TLC_{box}}$ mean		lower limits		upper limits	
	a	b	a	b	a	b
6	0.43	0.042	0.31	0.030	0.55	0.054
7	0.42	0.041	0.30	0.030	0.54	0.053
8	0.41	0.041	0.29	0.029	0.53	0.052
9	0.40	0.040	0.29	0.028	0.52	0.052
10	0.40	0.039	0.28	0.027	0.52	0.051
11	0.39	0.038	0.27	0.026	0.51	0.050
12	0.38	0.037	0.26	0.025	0.50	0.049
13	0.37	0.036	0.25	0.025	0.49	0.048
14	0.36	0.036	0.24	0.024	0.48	0.047
15	0.36	0.035	0.24	0.023	0.47	0.047
16	0.35	0.034	0.23	0.022	0.47	0.046
17	0.34	0.033	0.22	0.021	0.46	0.045

$a = \frac{ml/kPa}{ml}$; $b = \frac{ml/cm\ H_2O}{ml}$.

$\frac{Cst}{TLC_{box}} \left(\frac{ml/cm\ H_2O}{ml}\right) = 0.0474 - 0.8047 \cdot 10^{-3} \cdot x$;

SD $y \cdot x = \pm 0.0059$.

Formula: $y = a + b \cdot x$;

$y = \frac{Cst}{TLC_{box}} \left(\frac{ml/kPa}{ml} \text{ or } \frac{ml/cm\ H_2O}{ml}\right)$; x = age (years);

$\frac{Cst}{TLC_{box}} \left(\frac{ml/kPa}{ml}\right) = 0.4833 + 8.2056 \cdot 10^{-3} \cdot$ age (years);

SD $y \cdot x = \pm 0.0601$; n = 130; r = -0.30.

Table 149. Static lung compliance per milliliter of TLC_{box} $\left(\frac{Cst}{TLC_{box}}\right)$ in relation to body surface in boys and girls

Body surface m²	$\frac{Cst}{TLC_{box}}$ mean		lower limits		upper limits	
	a	b	a	b	a	b
0.60	0.448	0.0439	0.329	0.0323	0.567	0.0556
0.70	0.440	0.0431	0.321	0.0315	0.558	0.0548
0.80	0.431	0.0423	0.313	0.0307	0.550	0.0540
0.90	0.423	0.0415	0.304	0.0299	0.542	0.0532
1.00	0.415	0.0407	0.296	0.0291	0.534	0.0524
1.10	0.407	0.0400	0.288	0.0283	0.526	0.0516
1.20	0.399	0.0392	0.280	0.0275	0.518	0.0508
1.30	0.391	0.0384	0.272	0.0267	0.510	0.0500
1.40	0.383	0.0376	0.264	0.0259	0.502	0.0492
1.50	0.375	0.0368	0.256	0.0251	0.494	0.0484
1.60	0.367	0.0360	0.248	0.0243	0.486	0.0476
1.70	0.359	0.0352	0.240	0.0235	0.478	0.0468
1.80	0.351	0.0344	0.232	0.0227	0.469	0.0461
1.90	0.342	0.0336	0.224	0.0219	0.461	0.0453
2.00	0.335	0.0328	0.215	0.0211	0.455	0.0445

$a = \frac{ml/kPa}{ml}$; $b = \frac{ml/cm\ H_2O}{ml}$.

$\frac{Cst}{TLC_{box}} \left(\frac{ml/cm\ H_2O}{ml}\right) = 0.0487 - 0.00794 \cdot x$;

SD $y \cdot x = \pm 0.00589$.

Formula: $y = a + b \cdot x$;

$y = \frac{Cst}{TLC_{box}} \left(\frac{ml/kPa}{ml} \text{ or } \frac{ml/cm\ H_2O}{ml}\right)$; x = body surface (m²);

$\frac{Cst}{TLC_{box}} \left(\frac{ml/kPa}{ml}\right) = 0.4966 - 0.0809 \cdot$ body surface (m²);

SD $y \cdot x = \pm 0.0601$; n = 130; r = -0.34.

Table 150. Static lung compliance per milliliter of VC $\left(\frac{Cst}{VC}\right)$ in relation to body height in boys and girls

Height cm	$\frac{Cst}{VC}$ mean		lower limits		upper limits	
	a	b	a	b	a	b
115	0.593	0.0582	0.440	0.0431	0.747	0.0733
116	0.591	0.0580	0.438	0.0429	0.744	0.0731
118	0.587	0.0576	0.434	0.0425	0.740	0.0727
120	0.583	0.0572	0.429	0.0421	0.736	0.0723
122	0.578	0.0568	0.425	0.0417	0.731	0.0719
124	0.574	0.0563	0.421	0.0412	0.727	0.0714
126	0.570	0.0559	0.416	0.0408	0.723	0.0710
128	0.565	0.0555	0.412	0.0404	0.718	0.0706
130	0.561	0.0551	0.408	0.0400	0.714	0.0702
132	0.557	0.0546	0.403	0.0395	0.710	0.0697
134	0.552	0.0542	0.399	0.0391	0.705	0.6935
136	0.548	0.0538	0.395	0.0387	0.701	0.0689
138	0.544	0.0534	0.390	0.0383	0.697	0.0685
140	0.539	0.0529	0.386	0.0378	0.692	0.0680
142	0.535	0.0525	0.382	0.0374	0.688	0.0676
144	0.531	0.0521	0.377	0.0370	0.684	0.0672
146	0.526	0.0517	0.373	0.0659	0.679	0.0668
148	0.522	0.0512	0.369	0.3617	0.675	0.0663
150	0.518	0.0508	0.364	0.0357	0.671	0.0659
152	0.513	0.0504	0.360	0.0353	0.666	0.0655
154	0.507	0.0499	0.356	0.0348	0.662	0.0651
156	0.505	0.0495	0.351	0.0344	0.658	0.0646
158	0.500	0.0491	0.347	0.0340	0.653	0.0642
160	0.496	0.0487	0.343	0.0336	0.649	0.0638
162	0.491	0.0482	0.338	0.0331	0.645	0.0634
164	0.487	0.0478	0.334	0.0327	0.640	0.0629
166	0.483	0.0474	0.330	0.0323	0.636	0.0625
168	0.478	0.0470	0.325	0.0319	0.632	0.0621
170	0.474	0.0465	0.321	0.0314	0.627	0.0616
172	0.470	0.0461	0.317	0.0310	0.623	0.0612
174	0.465	0.0457	0.312	0.0306	0.619	0.0608
176	0.461	0.0453	0.308	0.0302	0.614	0.0604
178	0.457	0.0448	0.304	0.0297	0.610	0.0599
180	0.452	0.0444	0.299	0.0293	0.606	0.0595

$a = \frac{ml/kPa}{ml}$; $b = \frac{ml/cm\ H_2O}{ml}$.

$\frac{Cst}{VC}\left(\frac{ml/cm\ H_2O}{ml}\right) = 0.0827 - 0.2127 \cdot 10^{-3} \cdot x$;

SD $y \cdot x = \pm 0.0076$.

Formula: $y = a + b \cdot x$;

$y = \frac{Cst}{VC}\left(\frac{ml/kPa}{ml}\ or\ \frac{ml/cm\ H_2O}{ml}\right)$; $x = $ height (cm);

$\frac{Cst}{VC}\left(\frac{ml/kPa}{ml}\right) = 0.8433 - 2.1689 \cdot 10^{-3} \cdot $ height (cm);

SD $y \cdot x = \pm 0.0774$; $n = 130$; $r = -0.39$.

Table 151. Static lung compliance per milliliter of VC $\left(\frac{Cst}{VC}\right)$ in relation to age in boys and girls

Age years	$\frac{Cst}{VC}$ mean		lower limits		upper limits	
	a	b	a	b	a	b
6	0.586	0.057	0.431	0.042	0.741	0.072
7	0.573	0.056	0.418	0.040	0.729	0.071
8	0.561	0.055	0.406	0.039	0.716	0.070
9	0.549	0.053	0.393	0.038	0.704	0.069
10	0.536	0.052	0.381	0.037	0.692	0.067
11	0.524	0.051	0.369	0.035	0.679	0.066
12	0.511	0.050	0.356	0.034	0.667	0.065
13	0.499	0.048	0.344	0.033	0.654	0.064
14	0.487	0.047	0.331	0.032	0.642	0.063
15	0.474	0.046	0.319	0.031	0.630	0.061
16	0.462	0.045	0.307	0.029	0.617	0.060
17	0.449	0.044	0.294	0.028	0.605	0.059

$a = \frac{ml/kPa}{ml}$; $b = \frac{ml/cm\ H_2O}{ml}$.

$\frac{Cst}{VC}\left(\frac{ml/cm\ H_2O}{ml}\right) = 0.0648 - 0.00122 \cdot x$;

SD $y \cdot x = \pm 0.0077$.

Formula: $y = a + b \cdot x$;

$y = \frac{Cst}{VC}\left(\frac{ml/kPa}{ml}\ or\ \frac{ml/cm\ H_2O}{ml}\right)$; $x = $ age (years);

$\frac{Cst}{VC}\left(\frac{ml/kPa}{ml}\right) = 0.6607 - 0.0124 \cdot $ age (years);

SD $y \cdot x = \pm 0.0785$; $n = 130$; $r = -0.34$.

Table 152. Static lung compliance per milliliter of VC $\left(\frac{Cst}{VC}\right)$ in relation to body surface in boys and girls

Body surface m²	$\frac{Cst}{VC}$ mean		lower limits		upper limits	
	a	b	a	b	a	b
0.60	0.611	0.0599	0.458	0.0449	0.763	0.0749
0.70	0.598	0.0587	0.445	0.0437	0.751	0.0736
0.80	0.585	0.0574	0.433	0.0424	0.738	0.0724
0.90	0.572	0.0561	0.420	0.0411	0.725	0.0711
1.00	0.559	0.0549	0.407	0.0399	0.712	0.0698
1.10	0.547	0.0536	0.394	0.0386	0.699	0.0686
1.20	0.534	0.0523	0.381	0.0373	0.686	0.0673
1.30	0.521	0.0511	0.368	0.0361	0.673	0.0660
1.40	0.508	0.0498	0.356	0.0348	0.661	0.0648
1.50	0.495	0.0485	0.343	0.0335	0.648	0.0635
1.60	0.482	0.0473	0.330	0.0323	0.635	0.0622
1.70	0.470	0.0460	0.317	0.0310	0.622	0.0610
1.80	0.457	0.0447	0.304	0.0297	0.609	0.0597
1.90	0.444	0.0434	0.291	0.0285	0.596	0.0584
2.00	0.432	0.0422	0.277	0.0272	0.586	0.0572

$a = \frac{ml/kPa}{ml}$; $b = \frac{ml/cm\ H_2O}{ml}$.

$\frac{Cst}{VC}\left(\frac{ml/cm\ H_2O}{ml}\right) = 0.0675 - 0.0126 \cdot x$;

SD $y \cdot x = \pm 0.00757$.

Formula: $y = a + b \cdot x$;

$y = \frac{Cst}{VC}\left(\frac{ml/kPa}{ml}\ or\ \frac{ml/cm\ H_2O}{ml}\right)$; $x = $ body surface (m²);

$\frac{Cst}{VC}\left(\frac{ml/kPa}{ml}\right) = 0.6883 - 0.1284 \cdot $ body surface (m²);

SD $y \cdot x = \pm 0.0771$; $n = 130$; $r = -0.40$.

Table 153. Static lung compliance per milliliter of FRC_{box} $\left(\frac{Cst}{FRC_{box}}\right)$ in relation to body height in boys and girls

Body height cm	$\frac{Cst}{FRC_{box}}$ mean		lower limits		upper limits	
	a	b	a	b	a	b
115	0.911	0.0893	0.614	0.0600	1.208	0.1187
116	0.908	0.0891	0.611	0.0597	1.205	0.1184
118	0.902	0.0885	0.605	0.0591	1.199	0.1178
120	0.896	0.0879	0.599	0.0585	1.193	0.1173
122	0.890	0.0873	0.593	0.0579	1.187	0.1167
124	0.884	0.0867	0.587	0.0573	1.181	0.1161
126	0.878	0.0961	0.584	0.0568	1.175	0.1155
128	0.872	0.0855	0.575	0.0562	1.169	0.1149
130	0.866	0.0850	0.565	0.0556	1.163	0.1143
132	0.860	0.0844	0.563	0.0550	1.157	0.1138
134	0.854	0.0838	0.558	0.0544	1.151	0.1132
136	0.848	0.0832	0.552	0.0538	1.145	0.1126
138	0.842	0.0826	0.546	0.0532	1.139	0.1120
140	0.836	0.0820	0.540	0.0527	1.133	0.1114
142	0.831	0.0815	0.534	0.0521	1.127	0.1108
144	0.825	0.0809	0.528	0.0515	1.121	0.1102
146	0.819	0.0803	0.522	0.0509	1.115	0.1097
148	0.813	0.0797	0.516	0.0503	1.109	0.1091
150	0.807	0.0791	0.510	0.0497	1.103	0.1085
152	0.801	0.0785	0.504	0.0492	1.098	0.1079
154	0.795	0.0779	0.498	0.0486	1.092	0.1073
156	0.789	0.0774	0.492	0.0480	1.086	0.1067
158	0.783	0.0768	0.486	0.0474	1.080	0.1062
160	0.777	0.0762	0.480	0.0468	1.074	0.1056
162	0.771	0.0756	0.474	0.0462	1.068	0.1050
164	0.765	0.0750	0.468	0.0456	1.062	0.1044
166	0.759	0.0774	0.462	0.0451	1.056	0.1038
168	0.753	0.0739	0.456	0.0445	1.050	0.1032
170	0.747	0.0733	0.450	0.0439	1.044	0.1026
172	0.741	0.0727	0.444	0.0433	1.038	0.1021
174	0.735	0.0721	0.438	0.0427	1.032	0.1015
176	0.729	0.0715	0.432	0.0421	1.026	0.1009
178	0.723	0.0709	0.426	0.0416	1.020	0.1003
180	0.717	0.0703	0.420	0.0410	1.014	0.0997

$a = \frac{ml/kPa}{ml}$; $b = \frac{ml/cm\ H_2O}{ml}$.

$\frac{Cst}{FRC_{box}}\left(\frac{ml/cm\ H_2O}{ml}\right) = 0.1230 - 0.2923 \cdot 10^{-3} \cdot x$;

SD $y \cdot x = \pm 0.0148$.

Formula: $y = a + b \cdot x$;

$y = \frac{Cst}{FRC_{box}}\left(\frac{ml/kPa}{ml}\ or\ \frac{ml/cm\ H_2O}{ml}\right)$; x = body height (cm);

$\frac{Cst}{FRC_{box}}\left(\frac{ml/kPa}{ml}\right) = 1.2542 - 2.9806 \cdot 10^{-3} \cdot height\ (cm)$;

SD $y \cdot x = \pm 0.150$; n = 130; r = −0.28.

Table 154. Static lung compliance per milliliter of FRC_{box} $\left(\frac{Cst}{FRC_{box}}\right)$ in relation to age in boys and girls

Age years	$\frac{Cst}{FRC_{box}}$ mean		lower limits		upper limits	
	a	b	a	b	a	b
6	0.902	0.088	0.601	0.058	1.203	0.118
7	0.884	0.086	0.584	0.057	1.185	0.116
8	0.867	0.085	0.566	0.055	1.168	0.114
9	0.849	0.083	0.549	0.053	1.150	0.112
10	0.832	0.081	0.531	0.052	1.133	0.111
11	0.814	0.079	0.514	0.050	1.115	0.109
12	0.797	0.078	0.496	0.048	1.098	0.107
13	0.779	0.076	0.479	0.046	1.080	0.106
14	0.762	0.074	0.461	0.045	1.063	0.104
15	0.744	0.072	0.444	0.043	1.045	0.102
16	0.727	0.071	0.426	0.041	1.028	0.100
17	0.709	0.069	0.409	0.039	1.010	0.099

$a = \frac{ml/kPa}{ml}$; $b = \frac{ml/cm\ H_2O}{ml}$.

$\frac{Cst}{FRC_{box}}\left(\frac{ml/cm\ H_2O}{ml}\right) = 0.0988 - 0.00172 \cdot x$;

SD $y \cdot x = \pm 0.0149$.

Formula: $y = a + b \cdot x$;

$y = \frac{Cst}{FRC_{box}}\left(\frac{ml/kPa}{ml}\ or\ \frac{ml/cm\ H_2O}{ml}\right)$; x = age (years);

$\frac{Cst}{FRC_{box}}\left(\frac{ml/kPa}{ml}\right) = 1.0074 - 0.0175 \cdot age\ (years)$;

SD $y \cdot x = \pm 0.1519$; n = 130; r = −0.26.

Table 155. Static lung compliance per milliliter of FRC_{box} $\left(\frac{Cst}{FRC_{box}}\right)$ in relation to body surface in boys and girls

Body surface m^2	$\frac{Cst}{FRC_{box}}$ mean		lower limits		upper limits	
	a	b	a	b	a	b
0.60	0.916	0.0899	0.616	0.0602	1.215	0.1195
0.70	0.901	0.0884	0.601	0.0587	1.200	0.1180
0.80	0.885	0.0869	0.586	0.0572	1.185	0.1165
0.90	0.870	0.0854	0.571	0.0558	1.170	0.1151
1.00	0.855	0.0839	0.555	0.0543	1.155	0.1136
1.10	0.840	0.0824	0.540	0.0528	1.139	0.1121
1.20	0.825	0.0810	0.525	0.0513	1.124	0.1106
1.30	0.809	0.0795	0.510	0.0498	1.109	0.1091
1.40	0.794	0.0780	0.495	0.0483	1.094	0.1076
1.50	0.779	0.0755	0.480	0.0468	1.079	0.1061
1.60	0.764	0.0750	0.464	0.0454	1.064	0.1047
1.70	0.749	0.0735	0.449	0.0439	1.048	0.1032
1.80	0.734	0.0720	0.434	0.0424	1.033	0.1017
1.90	0.718	0.0705	0.419	0.0409	1.018	0.1002
2.00	0.703	0.0691	0.400	0.0394	1.006	0.0987

$a = \frac{ml/kPa}{ml}$; $b = \frac{ml/cm\ H_2O}{ml}$.

$\frac{Cst}{FRC_{box}}\left(\frac{ml/cm\ H_2O}{ml}\right) = 0.0988 - 0.0149 \cdot x$;

SD $y \cdot x = \pm 0.0149$.

Formula: $y = a + b \cdot x$;

$y = \frac{Cst}{FRC_{box}}\left(\frac{ml/kPa}{ml}\ or\ \frac{ml/cm\ H_2O}{ml}\right)$; x = body surface ($m^2$);

$\frac{Cst}{FRC_{box}}\left(\frac{ml/kPa}{ml}\right) = 1.0074 - 0.1519 \cdot body\ surface\ (m^2)$;

SD $y \cdot x = \pm 0.1514$; n = 130; r = −0.26.

Table 156. Dynamic lung compliance (Cdyn) in relation to body height in boys and girls

Height cm	Cdyn mean		lower limits		upper limits	
	a	b	a	b	a	b
115	492.22	48.26	329.05	32.26	736.31	72.21
116	504.77	49.49	337.44	33.08	755.08	74.05
118	530.49	52.02	354.62	34.77	793.56	77.83
120	557.06	54.62	372.39	36.51	833.30	81.72
122	584.48	57.31	390.72	38.31	874.32	85.75
124	612.78	60.09	409.64	40.16	916.65	89.90
126	641.95	62.95	429.14	42.07	960.30	94.18
128	672.03	65.90	449.25	44.04	1,005.28	98.59
130	703.02	68.94	469.96	46.07	1,051.64	103.14
132	734.92	72.06	491.29	48.17	1,099.37	107.82
134	767.77	75.28	513.25	50.32	1,148.50	112.64
136	801.56	78.60	535.84	52.53	1,199.05	117.59
138	836.31	82.01	559.07	54.81	1,251.03	122.69
140	872.04	85.51	582.95	57.15	1,304.47	127.94
142	908.75	89.11	607.50	59.56	1,359.40	133.32
144	946.47	92.81	632.71	62.03	1,415.81	138.85
146	985.19	96.61	658.60	64.57	1,473.74	144.54
148	1,024.94	100.50	685.17	67.18	1,533.21	150.37
150	1,065.73	104.50	712.44	69.85	1,594.22	156.35
152	1,107.57	108.61	740.41	72.59	1,656.81	162.49
154	1,150.47	112.81	769.09	75.40	1,720.99	168.79
156	1,194.46	117.13	798.49	78.29	1,786.77	175.24
158	1,239.52	121.55	828.62	81.24	1,854.19	181.85
160	1,285.69	126.07	859.48	84.27	1,923.26	188.62
162	1,332.97	130.71	891.09	87.37	1,993.98	195.56
164	1,381.38	135.46	923.45	90.54	2,066.40	202.66
166	1,430.93	140.32	956.57	93.79	2,140.52	209.93
168	1,481.63	145.29	990.47	97.11	2,216.36	217.37
170	1,533.50	150.38	1,025.14	100.51	2,293.94	224.98
172	1,586.54	155.58	1,060.60	103.99	2,373.29	232.76
174	1,640.77	160.90	1,096.85	107.54	2,454.41	240.72
176	1,696.20	166.33	1,133.91	111.17	2,537.33	248.85
178	1,752.85	171.89	1,171.78	114.89	2,622.08	257.16
180	1,810.73	177.56	1,210.47	118.68	2,708.65	265.65

Formula: $\log y = a + b \cdot \log x$;
y = Cdyn (ml/kPa or ml/cm H_2O); x = body height (cm);
log Cdyn (ml/kPa) = $-3.2989 + 2.9073 \cdot$ body height (cm);
SD $\log y \cdot x = \pm 0.0884$; n = 131; r = +0.82.
log Cdyn (ml/cm H_2O) = $-4.3074 + 2.9073 \cdot \log x$;
log SD $y \cdot x = \pm 0.0884$.
a = ml/kPa; b = ml/cm H_2O.

Table 157. Dynamic lung compliance (Cdyn) in relation to age in boys and girls

Age years	Cdyn mean		lower limits		upper limits	
	a	b	a	b	a	b
6	473.85	46.48	300.73	29.49	746.61	73.24
7	576.92	56.59	366.15	35.91	909.02	89.18
8	684.17	67.11	434.22	42.58	1,078.00	105.76
9	795.20	78.00	504.68	49.49	1,252.94	122.92
10	909.70	89.23	577.35	56.62	1,433.35	140.62
11	1,027.42	100.78	652.07	63.95	1,618.84	158.82
12	1,148.15	112.62	728.69	71.46	1,809.06	177.49
13	1,271.69	124.74	807.10	79.15	2,003.72	196.59
14	1,397.90	137.12	887.20	87.01	2,202.57	216.10
15	1,526.62	149.75	968.90	95.02	2,405.40	236.00
16	1,657.75	162.62	1,052.12	103.19	2,612.00	256.27
17	1,791.17	175.70	1,136.79	111.49	2,822.22	276.90

Formula: $\log y = a + b \cdot \log x$;
y = Cdyn (ml/kPa or ml/cm H_2O); x = age (years);
log Cdyn (ml/kPa) = $1.6821 + 1.2768 \cdot \log$ age (years);
SD $\log y \cdot x = \pm 0.0998$; n = 131; r = +0.77.
log Cdyn (ml/cm H_2O) = $0.6736 + 1.2768 \cdot \log x$;
SD $\log y \cdot x = \pm 0.0998$.
a = ml/kPa; b = ml/cm H_2O.

Table 158. Dynamic lung compliance (Cdyn) in relation to body surface in boys and girls

Body surface m²	Cdyn mean		lower limits		upper limits	
	a	b	a	b	a	b
0.60	369.76	36.2	235.42	23.0	580.76	56.9
0.70	455.80	44.6	290.21	28.4	715.89	70.2
0.80	546.36	53.5	347.86	34.1	858.12	84.1
0.90	641.04	62.8	408.16	40.0	1,006.86	98.7
1.00	739.60	72.5	470.90	46.1	1,161.63	113.9
1.10	841.73	82.5	535.92	52.5	1,322.03	129.6
1.20	947.23	92.8	603.09	59.1	1,487.73	145.9
1.30	1,055.92	103.5	672.30	65.9	1,658.44	162.7
1.40	1,167.64	114.5	743.43	72.8	1,833.91	179.9
1.50	1,282.25	125.7	816.40	80.0	2,013.92	197.5
1.60	1,399.62	137.2	891.13	87.3	2,198.26	215.6
1.70	1,519.64	149.0	967.54	94.8	2,386.77	234.1
1.80	1,642.21	161.0	1,045.58	102.5	2,579.28	253.0
1.90	1,767.24	173.3	1,119.68	110.3	2,789.31	272.3
2.00	1,894.64	185.8	1,200.41	118.2	2,990.38	291.9

Formula: $\log y = a + b \cdot \log x$;
y = Cdyn (ml/kPa or ml/cm H_2O); x = body surface (m²);
log Cdyn (ml/kPa) =
    $2.8690 + 1.3571 \cdot \log$ body surface (m²);
SD $\log y \cdot x = \pm 0.0991$; n = 131; r = +0.77.
log Cdyn (ml/cm H_2O) = $1.8605 + 1.3571 \cdot \log x$;
SD $\log y \cdot x = \pm 0.0991$.
a = ml/kPa; b = ml/cm H_2O.

Table 159. Dynamic lung compliance (Cdyn) in relation to vital capacity (VC) in boys and girls

VC ml	Cdyn					
	mean		lower limits		upper limits	
	a	b	a	b	a	b
1,250	399.83	39.23	28.63	2.81	771.04	75.65
1,500	504.86	49.54	133.65	13.11	876.06	85.96
2,000	714.91	70.15	343.70	33.72	1,086.11	106.57
2,500	924.96	90.75	553.75	54.33	1,296.16	127.17
3,000	1,135.01	111.36	763.80	74.94	1,506.22	147.78
3,500	1,345.06	131,97	973,85	95.55	1,716.26	168.71
4,000	1,555.11	152.58	1,183.90	116.16	1,926.31	189.31
4,500	1,765.16	173.19	1,393.95	136.77	2,136.37	209.61
5,000	1,975.21	193.80	1,604.00	157.38	2,346.41	230.22
5,250	2,080.24	204.10	1,704.99	167.68	2,455.47	240.52

Formula: $y = a + b \cdot x$;
y = Cdyn (ml/kPa or ml/cm H_2O); x = VC (ml);
Cdyn (ml/kPa) = $-125.2863 + 0.4201 \cdot$ VC (ml);
SD $y \cdot x = \pm 187.62$ n = 131; r = +0.89.
Cdyn (ml/cm H_2O) = $-12.2864 + 0.0412 \cdot x$;
SD $y \cdot x = \pm 18.40$.
a = ml/kPa; b = ml/cm H_2O.

Table 161. Dynamic lung compliance (Cdyn) in relation to functional residual capacity measured in a body plethysmograph (FRC_{box}) in boys and girls

FRC_{box} ml	Cdyn					
	mean		lower limits		upper limits	
	a	b	a	b	a	b
900	470.77	46.22	50.90	5.03	890.57	87.41
1,000	533.58	52.39	113.77	11.20	953.38	93.58
1,500	847.63	83.22	427.82	42.03	1,267.43	124.41
2,000	1,161.68	114.05	741.87	72.86	1,581.48	155.24
2,500	1,475.73	144.88	1,055.92	103.70	1,895.53	186.07
3,000	1,789.78	175.72	1,369.97	134.53	2,209.58	216.91
3,500	2,103.83	206.55	1,684.02	165.36	2,523.63	247.74

Formula: $y = a + b \cdot x$;
y = Cdyn (ml/kPa or ml/cm H_2O); x = FRC_{box} (ml);
Cdyn (ml/kPa) = $-94.5184 + 0.6281 \cdot FRC_{box}$ (ml);
SD $y \cdot x = \pm 211.99$; n = 120; r = +0.86.
Cdyn (ml/cm H_2O) = $-9.2691 + 0.0616 \cdot x$;
SD $y \cdot x = \pm 20.79$.
a = ml/kPa; b = ml/cm H_2O.

Table 160. Dynamic lung compliance (Cdyn) in relation to total lung capacity measured in a body plethysmograph (TLC_{box}) in boys and girls

TLC_{box} ml	Cdyn					
	mean		lower limits		upper limits	
	a	b	a	b	a	b
1,750	370.76	36.49	–	–	742.92	72.99
2,000	456.66	44.93	84.51	8.43	828.82	81.44
2,500	628.46	61.82	256.31	25.32	1,000.62	98.32
3,000	800.26	78.71	428.11	42.21	1,172.42	115.21
3,500	972.06	95.59	599.91	59.09	1,344.22	132.10
4,000	1,143.86	112.48	771.71	75.98	1,516.02	148.98
4,500	1,315.66	129.37	943.51	92.87	1,687.82	165.87
5,000	1,487.46	146.25	1,115.31	109.75	1,859.62	182.76
5,500	1,659.26	163.14	1,287.11	126.64	2,031.42	199.64
6,000	1,831.06	180.03	1,458.91	143.52	2,203.22	216.53
6,500	2,002.86	196.91	1,630.71	160.41	2,375.02	233.41
6,620	2,044.09	200.97	1,668.24	164.46	2,419.95	237.47

Formula: $y = a + b \cdot x$;
y = Cdyn (ml/kPa or ml/cm H_2O); x = TLC_{box} (ml);
Cdyn (ml/kPa) = $-230.5322 + 0.3436 \cdot TLC_{box}$ (ml);
SD $y \cdot x = \pm 187.93$; n = 120; r = +0.89.
Cdyn (ml/cm H_2O) = $-22.6075 + 0.0337 \cdot x$;
SD $y \cdot x = \pm 18.43$.
a = ml/kPa; b = ml/cm H_2O.

Table 162. Dynamic lung compliance (Cdyn) in relation to residual volume measured in a body plethysmograph (RV_{box}) in boys and girls

RV_{box} ml	Cdyn					
	mean		lower limits		upper limits	
	a	b	a	b	a	b
417	563.1	55.24	–	–	1,172.2	114.96
500	650.1	63.76	41.08	4.02	1,259.1	123.49
750	911.9	89.45	302.80	29.72	1,520.9	149.17
1,000	1,173.7	115.14	564.68	55.40	1,782.7	174.85
1,250	1,435.5	140.81	826.48	81.08	2,044.5	200.53
1,500	1,697.3	166.49	1,088.2	106.76	2,306.3	226.22
1,750	1,959.1	192.17	1,350.0	132.44	2,568.1	251.90
1,870	2,084.7	204.50	1,469.6	144.77	2,699.8	264.22

Formula: $y = a + b \cdot x$;
y = Cdyn (ml/kPa or ml/cm H_2O); x = RV_{box} (ml);
Cdyn (ml/kPa) = $126.5110 + 1.0472 \cdot RV_{box}$ (ml);
SD $y \cdot x = \pm 307.54$; n = 120; r = +0.68.
Cdyn = $12.4065 + 0.1027 \cdot x$;
SD $y \cdot x = \pm 30.16$.
a = ml/kPa; b = ml/cm H_2O.

Table 163. Dynamic lung compliance (Cdyn) in relation to total lung capacity measured by helium-dilution method (TLC$_{He}$) in boys and girls

TLC$_{He}$ ml	Cdyn					
	mean		lower limits		upper limits	
	a	b	a	b	a	b
1,930	487.98	47.98	123.28	12.20	852.68	83.76
2,000	511.68	50.31	146.98	14.53	876.38	86.09
2,500	680.93	66.94	316.23	31.16	1,045.63	102.72
3,000	850.18	83.57	485.48	47.79	1,214.88	119.35
3,500	1,019.43	100.20	654.73	64.42	1,384.13	135.98
4,000	1,188.68	116.83	823.98	81.05	1,553.38	152.61
4,500	1,357.93	133.46	993.23	97.68	1,722.63	169.24
5,000	1,527.18	150.10	1,162.48	114.31	1,891.88	185.88
5,500	1,696.43	166.73	1,331.73	130.95	2,061.13	202.51
6,000	1,865.68	183.36	1,500.98	147.58	2,230.38	219.14
6,500	2,034.93	199.99	1,670.23	164.21	2,399.63	235.77
6,640	2,082.32	204.65	1,714.42	168.86	2,450.88	240.43

Formula: $y = a + b \cdot x$;
y = Cdyn (ml/kPa); x = TLC$_{He}$ (ml);
Cdyn (ml/kPa or ml/cm H_2O) =
  $-165.3184 + 0.3385 \cdot$ TLC$_{He}$ (ml);
SD $y \cdot x = \pm 183.95$; $n = 108$; $r = +0.89$.
Cdyn (ml/cm H_2O) = $-16.2122 + 0.0332 \cdot x$;
SD $y \cdot x = \pm 18.04$.
a = ml/kPa; b = ml/cm H_2O.

Table 165. Dynamic lung compliance (Cdyn) in relation to residual volume measured by helium-dilution method (RV$_{He}$) in boys and girls

RV$_{He}$ ml	Cdyn					
	mean		lower limits		upper limits	
	a	b	a	b	a	b
500	808.40	79.29	193.62	19.00	1,423.18	139.59
750	1,035.02	101.53	420.24	41.24	1,649.81	161.82
1,000	1,261.65	123.77	646.87	63.47	1,876.43	184.06
1,250	1,488.27	146.00	873.49	85.71	2,103.06	206.29
1,500	1,714.90	168.24	1,100.12	107.94	2,329.68	228.53
1,640	1,841.81	181.13	1,221.63	120.84	2,461.99	241.43

Formula: $y = a + b \cdot x$;
y = Cdyn (ml/kPa or ml/cm H_2O); x = RV$_{He}$ (ml);
Cdyn (ml/kPa) = $355.1548 + 0.9065 \cdot$ RV$_{He}$ (ml);
SD $y \cdot x = \pm 310.09$; $n = 108$; $r = +0.66$
Cdyn (ml/cm H_2O) = $34.8288 + 0.0889 \cdot x$;
SD $y \cdot x = \pm 30.41$.
a = ml/kPa; b = ml/cm H_2O.

Table 164. Dynamic lung compliance (Cdyn) in relation to functional residual capacity measured by helium-dilution method (FRC$_{He}$) in boys and girls

FRC$_{He}$ ml	Cdyn					
	mean		lower limits		upper limits	
	a	b	a	b	a	b
930	589.50	57.88	156.66	15.42	1,022.34	100.35
1,000	630.97	61.96	198.18	19.49	1,063.81	104.42
1,500	927.17	91.05	494.33	48.58	1,360.01	133.51
2,000	1,223.37	120.14	790.53	77.67	1,656.21	162.60
2,500	1,519.57	149.23	1,086.73	106.76	1,952.41	191.69
3,000	1,815.77	178.32	1,382.93	135.85	2,248.61	220.78
3,500	2,111.97	207.41	1,679.13	164.94	2,544.81	249.87

Formula: $y = a + b \cdot x$;
y = Cdyn (ml/kPa or ml/cm H_2O); x = FRC$_{He}$ (ml);
Cdyn (ml/kPa) = $38.5727 + 0.5924 \cdot$ FRC$_{He}$ (ml);
SD $y \cdot x = \pm 218.32$; $n = 108$; $r = +0.85$.
Cdyn (ml/cm H_2O) = $3.7827 + 0.0581 \cdot x$;
SD $y \cdot x = \pm 21.41$.
a = ml/kPa; b = ml/cm H_2O.

Table 166. Mean values of 'specific' dynamic lung compliance

Parameter	Mean ± SD		Number of subjects	r	p
	ml/ kPa/ml	ml/ cm H_2O/l			
Cdyn FRC	0.581 ±0.115	0.057 ±0.0113	130	+0.12	>0.05
Cdyn TLC	0.286 ±0.050	0.028 ±0.0049	130	+0.16	>0.05
Cdyn VC	0.377 ±0.066	0.037 ±0.0065	130	+0.07	>0.05

r = Correlation coefficient of 'specific' Cdyn to body height;
p = statistical significance of r.

Table 167. Maximum expiratory flow rate at 25% of vital capacity ($\dot{V}_{max\ 25\%\ VC}$, $MEF_{25\%\ VC}$) in relation to body height in boys and girls

Height cm	$\dot{V}_{max\ 25\%\ VC}$, liters/s		
	mean	lower limits	upper limits
115	0.94	0.63	1.41
116	0.96	0.64	1.44
118	1.00	0.67	1.49
120	1.04	0.69	1.55
122	1.08	0.72	1.61
124	1.11	0.75	1.66
126	1.16	0.77	1.73
128	1.20	0.80	1.79
130	1.24	0.83	1.85
132	1.28	0.86	1.91
134	1.32	0.89	1.98
136	1.37	0.92	2.04
138	1.41	0.95	2.11
140	1.46	0.98	2.18
142	1.51	1.01	2.25
144	1.55	1.04	2.32
146	1.60	1.07	2.39
148	1.65	1.11	2.46
150	1.70	1.14	2.54
152	1.75	1.17	2.61
154	1.80	1.21	2.69
156	1.86	1.24	2.77
158	1.91	1.28	2.85
160	1.96	1.31	2.93
162	2.02	1.35	3.01
164	2.07	1.39	3.09
166	2.13	1.43	3.18
168	2.19	1.47	3.26
170	2.25	1.50	3.35
172	2.30	1.54	3.44
174	2.36	1.58	3.53
176	2.42	1.62	3.62
178	2.49	1.67	3.71
180	2.55	1.71	3.80

Formula: $\log y = a + b \cdot \log x$;
$y = \dot{V}_{max\ 25\%\ VC}$ (l/s); x = body height (cm);
$\log \dot{V}_{max\ 25\%\ VC}$ (l/s) $= -4.5808 + 2.2116 \cdot \log$ height (cm);
SD $\log y \cdot x = \pm 0.0874$; n = 101; r = +0.76.

Table 168. Maximum expiratory flow rate at 25% of vital capacity ($\dot{V}_{max\ 25\%\ VC}$, $MEF_{25\%\ VC}$) in relation to age in boys and girls

Age years	$\dot{V}_{max\ 25\%\ VC}$, liters/s		
	mean	lower limits	upper limits
6	0.97	0.62	1.51
7	1.10	0.70	1.73
8	1.24	0.79	1.94
9	1.37	0.88	2.15
10	1.51	0.96	2.36
11	1.64	1.04	2.56
12	1.76	1.13	2.76
13	1.89	1.21	2.96
14	2.02	1.29	3.16
15	2.14	1.37	3.35
16	2.27	1.45	3.54
17	2.39	1.53	3.74

Formula: $\log y = a + b \cdot \log x$;
$y = \dot{V}_{max\ 25\%\ VC}$ (l/s); x = age (years);
$\log \dot{V}_{max\ 25\%\ VC}$ (l/s) $= -0.6876 + 0.8668 \cdot \log$ age (years);
SD $\log y \cdot x = \pm 0.0977$; n = 101; r = +0.63.

Table 169. Maximum expiratory flow rate at 25% of vital capacity ($\dot{V}_{max\ 25\%\ VC}$, $MEF_{25\%\ VC}$) in relation to body surface in boys and girls

Surface, m²	$\dot{V}_{max\ 25\%\ VC}$, liters/s		
	mean	lower limits	upper limits
0.6	0.72	0.48	1.09
0.7	0.85	0.56	1.29
0.8	0.99	0.65	1.50
0.9	1.13	0.75	1.71
1.0	1.27	0.84	1.92
1.1	1.41	0.93	2.13
1.2	1.55	1.03	2.34
1.3	1.69	1.12	2.56
1.4	1.84	1.22	2.78
1.5	1.99	1.31	3.00
1.6	2.13	1.41	3.22
1.7	2.26	1.51	3.44
1.8	2.43	1.61	3.67
1.9	2.58	1.71	3.89
2.0	2.73	1.81	4.12

Formula: $\log y = a + b \cdot \log x$;
$y = \dot{V}_{max\ 25\%\ VC}$ (l/s); x = body surface;
$\log \dot{V}_{max\ 25\%\ VC}$ (l/s) $= 0.1048 + 1.1101 \cdot \log$ body surface (m²);
SD $\log y = \pm 0.0900$; n = 101; r = +0.70.

Table 170. Maximal expiratory flow rate at 50% of vital capacity ($\dot{V}_{max\,50\%\,VC}$, $MEF_{50\%\,VC}$) relation to body height in boys and girls

Height cm	$\dot{V}_{max\,50\%\,VC}$ liters/s		
	mean	lower limits	upper limits
115	1.86	1.35	2.55
116	1.89	1.38	2.59
118	1.96	1.43	2.69
120	2.04	1.48	2.79
122	2.11	1.54	2.90
124	2.19	1.59	3.00
126	2.27	1.65	3.11
128	2.34	1.71	3.21
130	2.43	1.77	3.33
132	2.51	1.83	3.44
134	2.59	1.89	3.55
136	2.68	1.95	3.67
138	2.76	2.01	3.79
140	2.85	2.08	3.91
142	2.94	2.14	4.03
144	3.03	2.21	4.16
146	3.12	2.28	4.28
148	3.22	2.35	4.41
150	3.31	2.42	4.54
152	3.41	2.49	4.68
154	3.51	2.56	4.81
156	3.61	2.63	4.95
158	3.71	2.71	5.09
160	3.81	2.78	5.23
162	3.92	2.86	5.37
164	4.02	2.94	5.52
166	4.13	3.01	5.67
168	4.24	3.09	5.82
170	4.35	3.17	5.97
172	4.47	3.26	6.12
174	4.58	3.34	6.28
176	4.69	3.42	6.44
178	4.81	3.51	6.60
180	4.93	3.60	6.76

Formula: $\log y = a + b \cdot \log x$;
$y = \dot{V}_{max\,50\%\,VC}$ (l/s); x = body height (cm);
$\log \dot{V}_{max\,50\%\,VC}$ (l/s) = $-4.2168 + 2.1771 \cdot \log$ height (cm);
SD $\log y \cdot x = \pm 0.0689$; $n = 101$; $r = +0.79$.

Table 171. Maximum expiratory flow rate at 50% of vital capacity ($\dot{V}_{max\,50\%\,VC}$, $MEF_{50\%\,VC}$) in relation to age in boys and girls

Age years	$\dot{V}_{max\,50\%\,VC}$, liters/s		
	mean	lower limits	upper limits
6	1.90	1.31	2.75
7	2.16	1.49	3.13
8	2.43	1.67	3.52
9	2.68	1.85	3.89
10	2.94	2.03	4.26
11	3.19	2.20	4.62
12	3.44	2.37	4.98
13	3.68	2.54	5.33
14	3.92	2.71	5.68
15	4.16	2.87	6.03
16	4.40	3.03	6.37
17	4.63	3.20	6.71

Formula: $\log y = a + b \cdot \log x$;
$y = \dot{V}_{max\,50\%\,VC}$ (l/s); x = age (years);
$\log \dot{V}_{max\,50\%\,VC}$ (l/s) = $-0.3877 + 0.8564 \cdot \log$ age (years);
SD $\log y \cdot x = \pm 0.0810$; $n = 101$; $r = +0.70$.

Table 172. Maximum expiratory flow rate at 50% of vital capacity ($\dot{V}_{max\,50\%\,VC}$, $MEF_{50\,VC}$) in relation to body surface in boys and girls

Body surface m²	$\dot{V}_{max\,50\%\,VC}$, liters/s		
	mean	lower limits	upper limits
0.6	1.40	1.02	1.93
0.7	1.66	1.21	2.29
0.8	1.94	1.40	2.66
0.9	2.20	1.59	3.03
1.0	2.47	1.79	3.40
1.1	2.74	1.99	3.78
1.2	3.02	2.19	4.16
1.3	3.30	2.40	4.55
1.4	3.59	2.60	4.94
1.5	3.87	2.81	5.33
1.6	4.16	3.02	5.72
1.7	4.45	3.23	6.12
1.8	4.74	3.44	6.52
1.9	5.03	3.65	6.92
2.0	5.32	3.87	7.33

Formula: $\log y = a + b \cdot \log x$;
$y = \dot{V}_{max\,50\%\,VC}$ (l/s); x = body surface (m²);
$\log \dot{V}_{max\,50\%\,VC}$ (l/s) = $0.3934 + 1.1065 \cdot \log$ surface (m²);
SD $\log y \cdot x = \pm 0.0699$; $n = 101$; $r = +0.79$.

Table 173. Maximum expiratory flow rate at 75% of vital capacity ($\dot{V}_{max\,75\%\,VC}$, $MEF_{75\%\,VC}$) in relation to body height in boys and girls

Height cm	$\dot{V}_{max\,75\%\,VC}$, liters/s		
	mean	lower limits	upper limits
115	2.64	1.91	3.65
116	2.69	1.95	3.72
118	2.79	2.02	3.86
120	2.89	2.09	4.00
122	3.00	2.17	4.15
124	3.11	2.25	4.30
126	3.22	2.33	4.45
128	3.33	2.41	4.60
130	3.44	2.49	4.76
132	3.56	2.57	4.92
134	3.67	2.66	5.08
136	3.79	2.74	5.24
138	3.91	2.83	5.41
140	4.04	2.92	5.58
142	4.16	3.01	5.75
144	4.29	3.10	5.93
146	4.42	3.20	6.11
148	4.55	3.29	6.29
150	4.68	3.39	6.47
152	4.82	3.49	6.66
154	4.96	3.59	6.85
156	5.10	3.69	7.05
158	5.24	3.79	7.24
160	5.38	3.90	7.44
162	5.53	4.00	7.64
164	5.68	4.11	7.85
166	5.83	4.22	8.06
168	5.98	4.33	8.27
170	6.14	4.44	8.48
172	6.29	4.55	8.70
174	6.45	4.67	8.92
176	6.61	4.78	9.14
178	6.78	4.90	9.36
180	6.94	5.02	9.59

Formula: $\log y = a + b \cdot \log x$;
$y = \dot{V}_{max\,75\%\,VC}$ (l/s); x = body height (cm);
$\log \dot{V}_{max\,75\%\,VC}$ (l/s) = $-4.0164 + 2.1541 \cdot \log$ height (cm);
SD $\log y \cdot x = \pm 0.0704$; n = 77; r = +0.81.

Table 174. Maximum expiratory flow rate at 75% of vital capacity ($\dot{V}_{max\,75\%\,VC}$, $MEF_{75\%\,VC}$) in relation to age in boys and girls

Age years	$\dot{V}_{max\,75\%\,VC}$, liters/s		
	mean	lower limits	upper limits
6	2.58	1.84	3.63
7	2.98	2.12	4.19
8	3.37	2.40	4.74
9	3.76	2.68	5.28
10	4.15	2.96	5.83
11	4.53	3.23	6.36
12	4.91	3.50	6.90
13	5.29	3.77	7.43
14	5.67	4.04	7.96
15	6.04	4.30	8.48
16	6.41	4.57	9.00
17	6.78	4.83	9.52

Formula: $\log y = a + b \cdot \log x$;
$y = \dot{V}_{max\,75\%\,VC}$ (l/s); x = age (years);
$\log \dot{V}_{max\,75\%\,VC}$ (l/s) = $-0.3072 + 0.9257 \cdot \log$ age (years);
SD $\log y \cdot x = \pm 0.0738$; n = 77; r = +0.79.

Table 175. Maximum expiratory flow rate at 75% of vital capacity ($\dot{V}_{max\,75\%\,VC}$, $MEF_{75\%\,VC}$) in relation to body surface in boys and girls

Body surface m^2	$\dot{V}_{max\,75\%\,VC}$, liters/s		
	mean	lower limits	upper limits
0.6	2.01	1.44	2.79
0.7	2.23	1.71	3.31
0.8	2.75	1.98	3.83
0.9	3.13	2.25	4.36
1.0	3.52	2.53	4.89
1.1	3.90	2.81	5.43
1.2	4.30	3.09	5.97
1.3	4.69	3.37	6.52
1.4	5.09	3.66	7.07
1.5	5.49	3.95	7.63
1.6	5.89	4.24	8.19
1.7	6.29	4.53	8.75
1.8	6.70	4.82	9.31
1.9	7.11	5.11	9.88
2.0	7.52	5.41	10.45

Formula: $\log y = a + b \cdot \log x$;
$y = \dot{V}_{max\,75\%\,VC}$ (l/s); x = body surface (m^2);
$\log \dot{V}_{max\,75\%\,VC}$ (l/s) = $0.5467 + 1.0957 \cdot \log$ body surface (m^2);
SD $\log y \cdot x = \pm 0.0717$; n = 77; r = +0.80.

Table 176. Maximum expiratory flow rate at 50% of total lung capacity ($\dot{V}_{max\,50\%\,TLC}$, $MEF_{50\%\,TLC}$) in relation to body height in boys and girls

Height cm	$\dot{V}_{max\,50\%\,TLC}$, liters/s		
	mean	lower limits	upper limits
115	1.32	0.88	1.97
116	1.34	0.90	2.00
118	1.39	0.93	2.08
120	1.45	0.97	2.16
122	1.50	1.00	2.23
124	1.55	1.04	2.31
126	1.61	1.08	2.39
128	1.66	1.11	2.48
130	1.72	1.15	2.56
132	1.78	1.19	2.65
134	1.83	1.23	2.73
136	1.89	1.27	2.82
138	1.95	1.31	2.91
140	2.02	1.35	3.00
142	2.08	1.39	3.10
144	2.14	1.44	3.19
146	2.21	1.48	3.29
148	2.27	1.52	3.39
150	2.34	1.57	3.49
152	2.41	1.62	3.59
154	2.48	1.66	3.69
156	2.55	1.71	3.79
158	2.62	1.76	3.90
160	2.69	1.80	4.01
162	2.76	1.85	4.11
164	2.84	1.90	4.22
166	2.91	1.95	4.34
168	2.99	2.00	4.45
170	3.06	2.06	4.56
172	3.14	2.11	4.68
174	3.22	2.16	4.80
176	3.30	2.22	4.92
178	3.38	2.27	5.04
180	3.47	2.33	5.16

Formula: $\log y = a + b \cdot \log x$;
$y = \dot{V}_{max\,50\%\,TLC}$ (l/s); x = body height (cm);
$\log \dot{V}_{max\,50\%\,TLC}$ (l/s) = $-4.3104 + 2.1508 \cdot \log$ height (cm);
SD $\log y \cdot x = \pm 0.0871$; n = 101; r = +0.71.

Table 177. Maximum expiratory flow rate at 50% of total lung capacity ($\dot{V}_{max\,50\%\,TLC}$, $MEF_{50\%\,TLC}$) in relation to age in boys and girls

Age years	$\dot{V}_{max\,50\%\,TLC}$, liters/s		
	mean	lower limits	upper limits
6	1.36	0.87	2.12
7	1.54	0.99	2.41
8	1.73	1.10	2.70
9	1.90	1.22	2.98
10	2.08	1.33	3.25
11	2.25	1.44	3.52
12	2.42	1.55	3.79
13	2.59	1.66	4.05
14	2.76	1.76	4.31
15	2.92	1.87	4.56
16	3.08	1.97	4.82
17	3.24	2.07	5.07

Formula: $\log y = a + b \cdot \log x$;
$y = \dot{V}_{max\,50\%\,TLC}$ (l/s); x = age (years);
$\log \dot{V}_{max\,50\%\,TLC}$ (l/s) = $-0.5149 + 0.8340 \cdot \log$ age (years);
SD $\log y \cdot x = \pm 0.0976$; n = 101; r = +0.62.

Table 178. Maximum expiratory flow rate at 50% of total lung capacity ($\dot{V}_{max\,50\%\,TLC}$, $MEF_{50\%\,TLC}$) in relation to body surface in boys and girls

Body surface m^2	$\dot{V}_{max\,50\%\,TLC}$, liters/s		
	mean	lower limits	upper limits
0.6	0.99	0.66	1.48
0.7	1.18	0.79	1.75
0.8	1.36	0.91	2.03
0.9	1.55	1.04	2.31
1.0	1.74	1.17	2.60
1.1	1.94	1.30	2.89
1.2	2.14	1.43	3.18
1.3	2.33	1.57	3.47
1.4	2.53	1.70	3.77
1.5	2.73	1.84	4.07
1.6	2.94	1.97	4.37
1.7	3.14	2.11	4.67
1.8	3.34	2.25	4.98
1.9	3.55	2.38	5.28
2.0	3.76	2.52	5.59

Formula: $\log y = a + b \cdot \log x$;
$y = \dot{V}_{max\,50\%\,TLC}$ (l/s); x = body surface (m^2);
$\log \dot{V}_{max\,50\%\,TLC}$ (l/s) = $0.2429 + 1.1045 \cdot \log$ body surface (m^2);
SD $\log y \cdot x = \pm 0.0869$; n = 101; r = +0.71.

Table 179. Maximum expiratory flow rate at 60% of total lung capacity ($\dot{V}_{max\,60\%\,TLC}$, MEF$_{60\%\,TLC}$) in relation to body height in boys and girls

Height cm	$\dot{V}_{max\,60\%\,TLC}$, liters/s		
	mean	lower limits	upper limits
115	1.80	1.31	2.46
116	1.83	1.34	2.51
118	1.90	1.39	2.61
120	1.97	1.44	2.70
122	2.05	1.49	2.81
124	2.12	1.55	2.91
126	2.20	1.61	3.01
128	2.28	1.66	3.12
130	2.36	1.72	3.23
132	2.44	1.78	3.34
134	2.52	1.84	3.45
136	2.61	1.90	3.57
138	2.69	1.96	3.69
140	2.78	2.03	3.81
142	2.87	2.09	3.93
144	2.96	2.16	4.05
146	3.05	2.23	4.18
148	3.14	2.29	4.30
150	3.24	2.36	4.43
152	3.33	2.43	4.57
154	3.43	2.51	4.70
156	3.53	2.58	4.84
158	3.63	2.65	4.97
160	3.74	2.73	5.11
162	3.84	2.80	5.26
164	3.95	2.88	5.40
166	4.05	2.96	5.55
168	4.16	3.04	5.70
170	4.27	3.12	5.85
172	4.38	3.20	6.00
174	4.50	3.28	6.16
176	4.61	3.37	6.32
178	4.73	3.45	6.48
180	4.85	3.54	6.64

Formula: log y = a + b·log x;
y = $\dot{V}_{max\,60\%\,TLC}$ (l/s); x = body height (cm);
log $\dot{V}_{max\,60\%\,TLC}$ (l/s) = −4.3030 + 2.2122·log height (cm);
SD log y·x = ±0.0687; n = 101; r = +0.80.

Table 180. Maximum expiratory flow rate at 60% of total lung capacity ($\dot{V}_{max\,60\%\,TLC}$, MEF$_{60\%\,TLC}$) in relation to age in boys and girls

Age years	$\dot{V}_{max\,60\%\,TLC}$, liters/s		
	mean	lower limits	upper limits
6	1.82	1.26	2.63
7	2.09	1.45	3.02
8	2.35	1.63	3.39
9	2.61	1.81	3.76
10	2.86	1.98	4.13
11	3.11	2.16	4.49
12	3.36	2.33	4.85
13	3.61	2.50	5.21
14	3.85	2.67	5.56
15	4.09	2.84	5.91
16	4.33	3.00	6.25
17	4.57	3.17	6.60

Formula: log y = a + b·log x;
y = $\dot{V}_{max\,60\%\,TLC}$ (l/s); x = age (years);
log $\dot{V}_{max\,60\%\,TLC}$ (l/s) = −0.4235 + 0.8810·log age (years);
SD log y·x = ±0.0801; n = 101; r = +0.71.

Table 181. Maximum expiratory flow rate at 60% of total lung capacity ($\dot{V}_{max\,60\%\,TLC}$, MEF$_{60\%\,TLC}$) in relation to body surface in boys and girls

Body surface m²	$\dot{V}_{max\,60\%\,TLC}$, liters/s		
	mean	lower limits	upper limits
0.6	1.35	0.98	1.86
0.7	1.61	1.17	2.21
0.8	1.87	1.36	2.57
0.9	2.13	1.55	2.04
1.0	2.40	1.74	3.31
1.1	2.67	1.94	3.68
1.2	2.95	2.14	4.06
1.3	3.23	2.34	4.44
1.4	3.51	2.55	4.83
1.5	3.79	2.75	5.32
1.6	4.08	2.96	5.61
1.7	4.36	3.17	6.01
1.8	4.65	3.38	6.40
1.9	4.95	3.59	6.80
2.0	5.24	3.81	7.21

Formula: log y = a + b·log x;
y = $\dot{V}_{max\,60\%\,TLC}$ (l/s); x = body surface (m²);
log $\dot{V}_{max\,60\%\,TLC}$ (l/s) = 0.3814 + 1.1234·log body surface (m²);
SD log y·x = ±0.0698; n = 101; r = +0.79.

Table 182. Peak expiratory flow rate (PEFR) in relation to body height in boys and girls

Height cm	PEFR, liters/s		
	mean	lower limits	upper limits
115	2.85	2.05	3.96
116	2.91	2.09	4.04
118	3.03	2.18	4.21
120	3.15	2.26	4.38
122	3.27	2.35	4.55
124	3.40	2.44	4.73
126	3.53	2.54	4.91
128	3.66	2.63	5.09
130	3.80	2.73	5.28
132	3.94	2.83	5.47
134	4.08	2.93	5.67
136	4.22	3.04	5.87
138	4.37	3.14	6.08
140	4.52	3.25	6.28
142	4.67	3.36	6.50
144	4.83	3.47	6.71
146	4.99	3.59	6.93
148	5.15	3.70	7.16
150	5.31	3.82	7.39
152	5.48	3.94	7.62
154	5.65	4.07	7.86
156	5.83	4.19	8.10
158	6.00	4.32	8.34
160	6.18	4.45	8.59
162	6.36	4.58	8.85
164	6.55	4.71	9.11
166	6.74	4.85	9.37
168	6.93	4.99	9.64
170	7.13	5.13	9.91
172	7.32	5.27	10.18
174	7.53	5.41	10.46
176	7.73	5.56	10.75
178	7.94	5.71	11.03
180	8.15	5.86	11.33

Formula: log y = a + b·log x;
y = PEFR (l/s); x = body height (cm);
log PEFR (l/s) = −4.3722 + 2.3422·log body height (cm);
SD log y·x = ±0.0717; n = 76; r = +0.83.

Table 183. Peak expiratory flow rate (PEFR) in relation to age in boys and girls

Age years	PEFR, liters/s		
	mean	lower limits	upper limits
6	2.76	1.96	3.89
7	3.23	2.29	4.56
8	3.70	2.63	5.22
9	4.18	2.96	5.88
10	4.65	3.30	6.55
11	5.12	3.63	7.22
12	5.60	3.97	7.89
13	6.07	4.31	8.56
14	6.55	4.65	9.23
15	7.02	4.98	9.90
16	7.50	5.32	10.57
17	7.98	5.66	11.24

Formula: log y = a + b·log x;
y = PEFR (l/s); x = age (years);
log PEFR (l/s) = −0.3490 + 1.0168·log age (years);
SD log y·x = ±0.0746; n = 76; r = +0.81.

Table 184. Peak expiratory flow rate (PEFR) in relation to body surface in boys and girls

Body surface m²	PEFR, liters/s		
	mean	lower limits	upper limits
0.6	2.08	1.50	2.89
0.7	2.51	1.81	3.49
0.8	2.95	2.13	4.10
0.9	3.41	2.45	4.73
1.0	3.87	2.79	5.37
1.1	4.34	3.13	6.03
1.2	4.83	3.48	6.70
1.3	5.32	3.83	7.38
1.4	5.82	4.19	8.07
1.5	6.32	4.55	8.78
1.6	6.84	4.92	9.49
1.7	7.36	5.30	10.21
1.8	7.88	5.68	10.95
1.9	8.42	6.06	11.69
2.0	8.96	6.45	12.43

Formula: log y = a + b·log x;
y = PEFR (l/s); x = body surface (m²);
log PEFR (l/s) = 0.5882 + 1.2095·log body surface (m²);
SD log y·x = ±0.0714; n = 76; r = +0.82.

Table 185. Maximum expiratory flow rate at 25% VC expressed per liter of TLC_{box} $\left(\frac{\dot{V}_{max\,25\,\%\,VC}}{TLC_{box}}\right)$ in relation to body height in boys and girls

Height cm	$\frac{\dot{V}_{max\,25\,\%\,VC}}{TLC_{box}}$ $\left(\frac{l/s}{l}\right)$		
	mean	lower limits	upper limits
115	0.510	0.326	0.694
116	0.509	0.325	0.693
118	0.506	0.322	0.690
120	0.503	0.319	0.687
122	0.500	0.316	0.684
124	0.497	0.313	0.681
126	0.494	0.310	0.678
128	0.491	0.307	0.676
130	0.489	0.304	0.673
132	0.486	0.302	0.670
134	0.483	0.299	0.667
136	0.480	0.296	0.664
138	0.477	0.293	0.661
140	0.474	0.290	0.658
142	0.471	0.287	0.655
144	0.468	0.284	0.653
146	0.466	0.281	0.650
148	0.463	0.279	0.647
150	0.460	0.276	0.644
152	0.457	0.273	0.641
154	0.454	0.270	0.638
156	0.451	0.267	0.635
158	0.448	0.264	0.632
160	0.445	0.261	0.629
162	0.442	0.258	0.627
164	0.440	0.255	0.624
166	0.437	0.253	0.621
168	0.434	0.250	0.618
170	0.431	0.247	0.615
172	0.428	0.244	0.612
174	0.425	0.241	0.609
176	0.422	0.238	0.606
178	0.419	0.235	0.603
180	0.417	0.232	0.601

Formula: $y = a + b \cdot x$;

$y = \frac{\dot{V}_{max\,25\,\%\,VC}}{TLC_{box}} \left(\frac{l/s}{l}\right)$; x = body height (cm);

$\frac{\dot{V}_{max\,25\,\%\,VC}}{TLC_{box}} \left(\frac{l/s}{l}\right) = 0.6764 - 0.00144 \cdot$ height (cm);

SD $y \cdot x = \pm 0.0927$; n = 101; r = −0.21.

Table 186. Maximum expiratory flow rate at 25% VC expressed per liter of TLC_{box} $\left(\frac{\dot{V}_{max\,25\,\%\,VC}}{TLC_{box}}\right)$ in relation to age in boys and girls

Age years	$\frac{\dot{V}_{max\,25\,\%\,VC}}{TLC_{box}}$ $\left(\frac{l/s}{l}\right)$		
	mean	lower limits	upper limits
6	0.499	0.313	0.685
7	0.492	0.306	0.678
8	0.485	0.299	0.671
9	0.478	0.292	0.664
10	0.471	0.285	0.657
11	0.464	0.278	0.650
12	0.457	0.271	0.643
13	0.450	0.264	0.636
14	0.443	0.257	0.629
15	0.436	0.250	0.622
16	0.429	0.243	0.615
17	0.422	0.236	0.608

Formula: $y = a + b \cdot x$;

$y = \frac{\dot{V}_{max\,25\,\%\,VC}}{TLC_{box}} \left(\frac{l/s}{l}\right)$; x = age (years);

$\frac{\dot{V}_{max\,25\,\%\,VC}}{TLC_{box}} \left(\frac{l/s}{l}\right) = 0.5419 - 0.00701 \cdot$ age (years);

SD $y \cdot x = \pm 0.0936$; n = 101; r = −0.16.

Table 187. Maximum expiratory flow rate at 25% VC expressed per liter of TLC_{box} $\left(\frac{\dot{V}_{max\,25\,\%\,VC}}{TLC_{box}}\right)$ in relation to body surface in boys and girls

Body surface m^2	$\frac{\dot{V}_{max\,25\,\%\,VC}}{TLC_{box}}$ $\left(\frac{l/s}{l}\right)$		
	mean	lower limits	upper limits
0.60	0.508	0.322	0.694
0.70	0.501	0.316	0.687
0.80	0.495	0.309	0.680
0.90	0.488	0.302	0.674
1.00	0.481	0.296	0.667
1.10	0.475	0.289	0.660
1.20	0.468	0.282	0.654
1.30	0.461	0.275	0.647
1.40	0.455	0.269	0.640
1.50	0.448	0.262	0.634
1.60	0.441	0.255	0.627
1.70	0.434	0.249	0.620
1.80	0.428	0.242	0.614
1.90	0.421	0.235	0.607
2.00	0.414	0.229	0.600

Formula: $y = a + b \cdot x$;

$y = \frac{\dot{V}_{max\,25\,\%\,VC}}{TLC_{box}} \left(\frac{l/s}{l}\right)$; x = body surface ($m^2$);

$\frac{\dot{V}_{max\,25\,\%\,VC}}{TLC_{box}} \left(\frac{l/s}{l}\right) = 0.5487 - 0.0669 \cdot$ body surface (m^2);

SD $y \cdot x = \pm 0.0936$; n = 101; r = −0.16.

Table 188. Maximum expiratory flow rate at 50% of vital capacity expressed per liter of TLC_{box} $\left(\frac{\dot{V}_{max\ 50\ \%\ VC}}{TLC_{box}}\right)$ in relation to body height in boys and girls

Height cm	$\frac{\dot{V}_{max\ 50\ \%\ VC}}{TLC_{box}}\left(\frac{l/s}{l}\right)$		
	mean	lower limits	upper limits
115	0.996	0.710	1.282
116	0.993	0.707	1.278
118	0.986	0.701	1.272
120	0.980	0.694	1.266
122	0.974	0.688	1.259
124	0.967	0.682	1.253
126	0.961	0.675	1.246
128	0.954	0.669	1.240
130	0.948	0.662	1.234
132	0.942	0.656	1.227
134	0.935	0.650	1.221
136	0.929	0.643	1.215
138	0.923	0.637	1.208
140	0.916	0.631	1.202
142	0.910	0.624	1.195
144	0.903	0.618	1.189
146	0.897	0.611	1.183
148	0.891	0.605	1.176
150	0.884	0.599	1.170
152	0.878	0.592	1.163
154	0.871	0.586	1.157
156	0.865	0.579	1.151
158	0.859	0.573	1.144
160	0.852	0.567	1.138
162	0.846	0.560	1.131
164	0.839	0.554	1.125
166	0.833	0.547	1.119
168	0.827	0.541	1.112
170	0.820	0.535	1.106
172	0.814	0.528	1.100
174	0.808	0.522	1.093
176	0.801	0.516	1.087
178	0.795	0.509	1.080
180	0.788	0.503	1.074

Formula: $y = a + b \cdot x$;

$y = \frac{\dot{V}_{max\ 50\ \%\ VC}}{TLC_{box}}\left(\frac{l/s}{l}\right)$; x = body height (cm);

$\frac{\dot{V}_{max\ 50\ \%\ VC}}{TLC_{box}}\left(\frac{l/s}{l}\right) = 1.3638 - 0.00319 \cdot height$ (cm);

SD $y \cdot x = \pm 0.144$; n = 101; r = −0.29.

Table 189. Maximum expiratory flow rate at 50% of vital capacity expressed per liter of TLC_{box} $\left(\frac{\dot{V}_{max\ 50\ \%\ VC}}{TLC_{box}}\right)$ in relation to age in boys and girls

Age years	$\frac{\dot{V}_{max\ 50\ \%\ VC}}{TLC_{box}}\left(\frac{l/s}{l}\right)$		
	mean	lower limits	upper limits
6	0.974	0.682	1.265
7	0.958	0.667	1.249
8	0.942	0.661	1.233
9	0.926	0.653	1.217
10	0.910	0.619	1.201
11	0.894	0.603	1.185
12	0.879	0.587	1.170
13	0.863	0.572	1.154
14	0.847	0.556	1.138
15	0.831	0.540	1.122
16	0.815	0.524	1.106
17	0.799	0.508	1.090

Formula: $y = a + b \cdot x$;

$y = \frac{\dot{V}_{max\ 50\ \%\ VC}}{TLC_{box}}\left(\frac{l/s}{l}\right)$; x = age (years);

$\frac{\dot{V}_{max\ 50\ \%\ VC}}{TLC_{box}}\left(\frac{l/s}{l}\right) = 1.0691 - 0.01584 \cdot age$ (years);

SD $y \cdot x = \pm 0.1466$; n = 101; r = −0.23.

Table 190. Maximum expiratory flow rate at 50% of vital capacity expressed per liter of TLC_{box} $\left(\frac{\dot{V}_{max\ 50\ \%\ VC}}{TLC_{box}}\right)$ in relation to body surface in boys and girls

Body surface m²	$\frac{\dot{V}_{max\ 50\ \%\ VC}}{TLC_{box}}\left(\frac{l/s}{l}\right)$		
	mean	lower limits	upper limits
0.60	0.986	0.695	1.278
0.70	0.972	0.681	1.264
0.80	0.958	0.667	1.250
0.90	0.944	0.652	1.236
1.00	0.930	0.638	1.222
1.10	0.916	0.624	1.207
1.20	0.902	0.610	1.193
1.30	0.888	0.596	1.179
1.40	0.873	0.582	1.165
1.50	0.859	0.568	1.151
1.60	0.845	0.553	1.137
1.70	0.831	0.539	1.123
1.80	0.817	0.526	1.108
1.90	0.803	0.511	1.094
2.00	0.789	0.497	1.080

Formula: $y = a + b \cdot x$;

$y = \frac{\dot{V}_{max\ 50\ \%\ VC}}{TLC_{box}}\left(\frac{l/s}{l}\right)$; x = body surface (m²);

$\frac{\dot{V}_{max\ 50\ \%\ VC}}{TLC_{box}}\left(\frac{l/s}{l}\right) = 1.0718 - 0.1413 \cdot body\ surface$ (m²);

SD $y \cdot x = \pm 0.1469$; n = 101; r = −0.22.

Table 191. Maximum expiratory flow rate at 75% VC expressed per liter of TLC_{box} $\left(\frac{\dot{V}_{max\,75\%\,VC}}{TLC_{box}}\right)$ in relation to body height in boys and girls

Height cm	$\frac{\dot{V}_{max\,75\%\,VC}}{TLC_{box}}$ $\left(\frac{l/s}{l}\right)$		
	mean	lower limits	upper limits
115	1.409	1.008	1.810
116	1.405	1.004	1.806
118	1.396	0.995	1.797
120	1.387	0.987	1.788
122	1.379	0.978	1.780
124	1.370	0.969	1.771
126	1.361	0.961	1.762
128	1.353	0.952	1.754
130	1.344	0.943	1.745
132	1.335	0.935	1.736
134	1.327	0.962	1.728
136	1.318	0.917	1.719
138	1.309	0.909	1.710
140	1.301	0.900	1.702
142	1.292	0.891	1.693
144	1.283	0.883	1.684
146	1.275	0.874	1.676
148	1.266	0.865	1.667
150	1.257	0.857	1.658
152	1.249	0.848	1.650
154	1.240	0.839	1.641
156	1.231	0.831	1.632
158	1.223	0.822	1.623
160	1.214	0.813	1.615
162	1.205	0.805	1.606
164	1.197	0.796	1.597
166	1.185	0.787	1.589
168	1.179	0.779	1.580
170	1.171	0.770	1.571
172	1.162	0.761	1.563
174	1.153	0.753	1.554
176	1.145	0.744	1.545
178	1.136	0.735	1.537
180	1.127	0.727	1.528

Formula: $y = a + b \cdot x$;

$y = \frac{\dot{V}_{max\,75\%\,VC}}{TLC_{box}}\left(\frac{l/s}{l}\right)$; x = body height (cm);

$\frac{\dot{V}_{max\,75\%\,VC}}{TLC_{box}}\left(\frac{l/s}{l}\right) = 1.9083 - 0.00433 \cdot$ body height (cm);

SD $y \cdot x = \pm 0.201$; n = 77; r = -0.31.

Table 192. Maximum expiratory flow rate at 75% VC expressed per liter of TLC_{box} $\left(\frac{\dot{V}_{max\,75\%\,VC}}{TLC_{box}}\right)$ in relation to age in boys and girls

Age years	$\frac{\dot{V}_{max\,75\%\,VC}}{TLC_{box}}$ $\left(\frac{l/s}{l}\right)$		
	mean	lower limits	upper limits
6	1.342	0.926	1.758
7	1.327	0.912	1.743
8	1.313	0.897	1.728
9	1.298	0.882	1.714
10	1.284	0.868	1.699
11	1.269	0.853	1.685
12	1.254	0.839	1.670
13	1.240	0.824	1.655
14	1.225	0.810	1.641
15	1.211	0.795	1.625
16	1.196	0.780	1.612
17	1.181	0.766	1.597

Formula: $y = a + b \cdot x$;

$y = \frac{\dot{V}_{max\,75\%\,VC}}{TLC_{box}}\left(\frac{l/s}{l}\right)$; x = age (years);

$\frac{\dot{V}_{max\,75\%\,VC}}{TLC_{box}}\left(\frac{l/s}{l}\right) = 1.4297 - 0.01457 \cdot$ age (years);

SD $y \cdot x = \pm 0.2086$; n = 77; r = -0.16.

Table 193. Maximum expiratory flow rate at 75% VC expressed per liter of TLC_{box} $\left(\frac{\dot{V}_{max\,75\%\,VC}}{TLC_{box}}\right)$ in relation to body surface in boys and girls

Body surface m²	$\frac{\dot{V}_{max\,75\%\,VC}}{TLC_{box}}$ $\left(\frac{l/s}{l}\right)$		
	mean	lower limits	upper limits
0.60	1.414	1.007	1.821
0.70	1.392	0.985	1.799
0.80	1.370	0.963	1.777
0.90	1.348	0.941	1.755
1.00	1.326	0.920	1.733
1.10	1.305	0.898	1.711
1.20	1.283	0.876	1.690
1.30	1.261	0.854	1.668
1.40	1.239	0.832	1.646
1.50	1.217	0.810	1.624
1.60	1.196	0.789	1.602
1.70	1.174	0.767	1.581
1.80	1.152	0.745	1.559
1.90	1.130	0.723	1.537
2.00	1.108	0.701	1.515

Formula: $y = a + b \cdot x$;

$y = \frac{\dot{V}_{max\,75\%\,VC}}{TLC_{box}}\left(\frac{l/s}{l}\right)$; x = body surface (m²);

$\frac{\dot{V}_{max\,75\%\,VC}}{TLC_{box}}\left(\frac{l/s}{l}\right) = 1.5450 - 0.2181 \cdot$ body surface (m²);

SD $y \cdot x = \pm 0.2041$; n = 77; r = -0.26.

Table 194. Maximum expiratory flow rate at 50% TLC expressed per liter of TLC_{box} $\left(\frac{\dot{V}_{max\ 50\ \%\ TLC}}{TLC_{box}}\right)$ in relation to body height in boys and girls

Height cm	$\frac{\dot{V}_{max\ 50\ \%\ TLC}}{TLC_{box}}\left(\frac{l/s}{l}\right)$		
	mean	lower limits	upper limits
115	0.696	0.421	0.971
116	0.695	0.420	0.970
118	0.692	0.417	0.967
120	0.689	0.414	0.964
122	0.686	0.411	0.961
124	0.683	0.408	0.958
126	0.680	0.405	0.955
128	0.677	0.402	0.952
130	0.673	0.398	0.948
132	0.670	0.395	0.945
134	0.667	0.392	0.942
136	0.664	0.389	0.939
138	0.661	0.386	0.936
140	0.658	0.383	0.933
142	0.655	0.380	0.930
144	0.652	0.377	0.927
146	0.649	0.374	0.924
148	0.646	0.371	0.921
150	0.643	0.368	0.918
152	0.640	0.365	0.915
154	0.637	0.362	0.912
156	0.634	0.359	0.909
158	0.631	0.356	0.906
160	0.627	0.352	0.902
162	0.624	0.349	0.899
164	0.621	0.346	0.896
166	0.618	0.343	0.893
168	0.615	0.340	0.890
170	0.612	0.337	0.887
172	0.609	0.334	0.884
174	0.606	0.331	0.881
176	0.603	0.328	0.878
178	0.600	0.325	0.875
180	0.597	0.322	0.872

Formula: $y = a + b \cdot x$;

$y = \frac{\dot{V}_{max\ 50\ \%\ TLC}}{TLC_{box}}\left(\frac{l/s}{l}\right)$; x = body height (cm);

$\frac{\dot{V}_{max\ 50\ \%\ TLC}}{TLC_{box}}\left(\frac{l/s}{l}\right) = 0.8731 - 0.00152 \cdot$ body height (cm);

SD $y \cdot x = \pm 0.138$; n = 101; r = −0.20.

Table 195. Maximum expiratory flow rate at 50% TLC expressed per liter of TLC_{box} $\left(\frac{\dot{V}_{max\ 50\ \%\ TLC}}{TLC_{box}}\right)$ in relation to age in boys and girls

Age years	$\frac{\dot{V}_{max\ 50\ \%\ TLC}}{TLC_{box}}\left(\frac{l/s}{l}\right)$		
	mean	lower limits	upper limits
6	0.692	0.416	0.967
7	0.683	0.407	0.959
8	0.674	0.398	0.950
9	0.665	0.390	0.941
10	0.657	0.381	0.932
11	0.648	0.372	0.924
12	0.639	0.364	0.915
13	0.631	0.355	0.906
14	0.622	0.346	0.898
15	0.613	0.337	0.889
16	0.604	0.329	0.880
17	0.596	0.320	0.871

Formula: $y = a + b \cdot x$;

$y = \frac{\dot{V}_{max\ 50\ \%\ TLC}}{TLC_{box}}\left(\frac{l/s}{l}\right)$; x = age (years);

$\frac{\dot{V}_{max\ 50\ \%\ TLC}}{TLC_{box}}\left(\frac{l/s}{l}\right) = 0.7443 - 0.00870 \cdot$ age (years);

SD $y \cdot x = \pm 0.1389$; n = 101; r = −0.13.

Table 196. Maximum expiratory flow rate at 50% TLC expressed per liter of TLC_{box} $\left(\frac{\dot{V}_{max\ 50\ \%\ TLC}}{TLC_{box}}\right)$ in relation to body surface in boys and girls

Body surface m²	$\frac{\dot{V}_{max\ 50\ \%\ TLC}}{TLC_{box}}\left(\frac{l/s}{l}\right)$		
	mean	lower limits	upper limits
0.60	0.680	0.403	0.957
0.70	0.675	0.398	0.952
0.80	0.670	0.393	0.947
0.90	0.665	0.388	0.942
1.00	0.660	0.383	0.937
1.10	0.655	0.378	0.932
1.20	0.650	0.373	0.927
1.30	0.645	0.367	0.922
1.40	0.640	0.362	0.917
1.50	0.634	0.357	0.912
1.60	0.629	0.352	0.907
1.70	0.624	0.347	0.902
1.80	0.619	0.342	0.896
1.90	0.614	0.337	0.891
2.00	0.609	0.332	0.886

Formula: $y = a + b \cdot x$;

$y = \frac{\dot{V}_{max\ 50\ \%\ TLC}}{TLC_{box}}\left(\frac{l/s}{l}\right)$; x = body surface (m²);

$\frac{\dot{V}_{max\ 50\ \%\ TLC}}{TLC_{box}}\left(\frac{l/s}{l}\right) = 0.7112 - 0.0508 \cdot$ body surface (m²);

SD $y \cdot x = \pm 0.1396$; n = 101; r = −0.10.

Table 197. Maximum expiratory flow rate at 60% TLC expressed per liter of TLC $_{box}$ $\left(\frac{\dot{V}_{max\,60\,\%\,TLC}}{TLC_{box}}\right)$ in relation to body height in boys and girls

Height cm	$\frac{\dot{V}_{max\,60\,\%\,TLC}}{TLC_{box}} \left(\frac{l/s}{l}\right)$		
	mean	lower limits	upper limits
115	0.959	0.655	1.263
116	0.956	0.652	1.260
118	0.950	0.647	1.254
120	0.944	0.641	1.248
122	0.939	0.635	1.242
124	0.933	0.629	1.236
126	0.927	0.623	1.231
128	0.921	0.617	1.225
130	0.915	0.611	1.219
132	0.909	0.605	1.213
134	0.903	0.600	1.207
136	0.897	0.594	1.201
138	0.892	0.588	1.195
140	0.886	0.582	1.189
142	0.880	0.576	1.183
144	0.874	0.570	1.178
146	0.868	0.564	1.172
148	0.862	0.558	1.166
150	0.856	0.553	1.160
152	0.850	0.547	1.154
154	0.844	0.541	1.148
156	0.839	0.535	1.142
158	0.833	0.529	1.136
160	0.827	0.523	1.131
162	0.821	0.517	1.125
164	0.815	0.511	1.119
166	0.809	0.505	1.113
168	0.803	0.500	1.107
170	0.797	0.494	1.101
172	0.792	0.488	1.095
174	0.786	0.482	1.089
176	0.780	0.476	1.083
178	0.774	0.470	1.078
180	0.768	0.464	1.072

Formula: $y = a + b \cdot x$;
$y = \frac{\dot{V}_{max\,60\,\%\,TLC}}{TLC_{box}} \left(\frac{l/s}{l}\right)$; x = body height (cm);
$\frac{\dot{V}_{max\,60\,\%\,TLC}}{TLC_{box}} \left(\frac{l/s}{l}\right) = 1.2978 - 0.00294 \cdot$ body height (cm);
SD $y \cdot x = \pm 0.153$; n = 101; r = -0.26.

Table 198. Maximum expiratory flow rate at 60% TLC expressed per liter of TLC$_{box}$ $\left(\frac{\dot{V}_{max\,60\,\%\,TLC}}{TLC_{box}}\right)$ in relation to age in boys and girls

Age years	$\frac{\dot{V}_{max\,60\,\%\,TLC}}{TLC_{box}} \left(\frac{l/s}{l}\right)$		
	mean	lower limits	upper limits
6	0.934	0.626	1.243
7	0.921	0.612	1.229
8	0.907	0.598	1.216
9	0.893	0.584	1.202
10	0.879	0.570	1.188
11	0.865	0.557	1.174
12	0.852	0.543	1.160
13	0.838	0.529	1.146
14	0.824	0.515	1.133
15	0.810	0.501	1.119
16	0.796	0.488	1.105
17	0.782	0.474	1.091

Formula: $y = a + b \cdot x$;
$y = \frac{\dot{V}_{max\,60\,\%\,TLC}}{TLC_{box}} \left(\frac{l/s}{l}\right)$; x = age (years);
$\frac{\dot{V}_{max\,60\,\%\,TLC}}{TLC_{box}} \left(\frac{l/s}{l}\right) = 1.0177 - 0.0138 \cdot$ age (years);
SD $y \cdot x = \pm 0.1555$; n = 101; r = -0.19.

Table 199. Maximum expiratory flow rate at 60% TLC expressed per liter of TLC$_{box}$ $\left(\frac{\dot{V}_{max\,60\,\%\,TLC}}{TLC_{box}}\right)$ in relation to body surface in boys and girls

Body surface m²	$\frac{\dot{V}_{max\,60\,\%\,TLC}}{TLC_{box}} \left(\frac{l/s}{l}\right)$		
	mean	lower limits	upper limits
0.60	0.946	0.637	1.255
0.70	0.933	0.624	1.243
0.80	0.921	0.612	1.230
0.90	0.909	0.600	1.218
1.00	0.896	0.587	1.206
1.10	0.884	0.575	1.193
1.20	0.872	0.563	1.181
1.30	0.859	0.550	1.168
1.40	0.847	0.538	1.156
1.50	0.835	0.526	1.144
1.60	0.822	0.513	1.131
1.70	0.810	0.501	1.119
1.80	0.798	0.489	1.107
1.90	0.785	0.476	1.094
2.00	0.773	0.464	1.082

Formula: $y = a + b \cdot x$;
$y = \frac{\dot{V}_{max\,60\,\%\,TLC}}{TLC_{box}} \left(\frac{l/s}{l}\right)$; x = body surface (m²);
$\frac{\dot{V}_{max\,60\,\%\,TLC}}{TLC_{box}} \left(\frac{l/s}{l}\right) = 1.0204 - 0.1235 \cdot$ body surface (m²);
SD $y \cdot x = \pm 0.1557$; n = 101; r = -0.18.

Table 200. Maximum expiratory flow rate at 25% VC expressed per liter of FVC $\left(\frac{\dot{V}_{max\ 25\ \%\ VC}}{FVC}\right)$ in relation to body height in boys and girls

Height cm	$\frac{\dot{V}_{max\ 25\ \%\ VC}}{FVC}\left(\frac{l/s}{l}\right)$		
	mean	lower limits	upper limits
115	0.731	0.472	0.989
116	0.728	0.469	0.986
118	0.721	0.463	0.980
120	0.715	0.457	0.973
122	0.709	0.450	0.967
124	0.702	0.444	0.961
126	0.696	0.438	0.954
128	0.690	0.431	0.948
130	0.683	0.425	0.942
132	0.677	0.419	0.935
134	0.671	0.412	0.929
136	0.664	0.406	0.923
138	0.658	0.400	0.916
140	0.652	0.393	0.910
142	0.645	0.387	0.904
144	0.639	0.381	0.897
146	0.633	0.374	0.891
148	0.626	0.368	0.885
150	0.620	0.362	0.878
152	0.615	0.355	0.872
154	0.607	0.349	0.866
156	0.601	0.348	0.859
158	0.595	0.336	0.853
160	0.588	0.330	0.847
162	0.582	0.323	0.840
164	0.575	0.317	0.834
166	0.569	0.311	0.827
168	0.563	0.304	0.821
170	0.556	0.298	0.815
172	0.550	0.292	0.808
174	0.544	0.285	0.802
176	0.537	0.279	0.796
178	0.531	0.273	0.789
180	0.525	0.266	0.783

Formula: $y = a + b \cdot x$;

$y = \frac{\dot{V}_{max\ 25\ \%\ VC}}{FVC}\left(\frac{l/s}{l}\right)$; x = body height (cm);

$\frac{\dot{V}_{max\ 25\ \%\ VC}}{FVC}\left(\frac{l/s}{l}\right) = 1.0958 - 0.003170 \cdot$ body height (cm);

SD $y \cdot x = \pm 0.130$; n = 101; r = -0.32.

Table 201. Maximum expiratory flow rate at 50% VC expressed per liter of FVC $\left(\frac{\dot{V}_{max\ 50\ \%\ VC}}{FVC}\right)$ in relation to body height in boys and girls

Height cm	$\frac{\dot{V}_{max\ 50\ \%\ VC}}{FVC}\left(\frac{l/s}{l}\right)$		
	mean	lower limits	upper limits
115	1.429	1.039	1.819
116	1.422	1.032	1.812
118	1.409	1.019	1.799
120	1.396	1.006	1.786
122	1.382	0.992	1.772
124	1.369	0.976	1.759
126	1.356	0.966	1.746
128	1.343	0.953	1.733
130	1.329	0.939	1.719
132	1.316	0.926	1.706
134	1.303	0.913	1.693
136	1.289	0.899	1.679
138	1.276	0.886	1.666
140	1.263	0.873	1.653
142	1.249	0.859	1.639
144	1.236	0.846	1.626
146	1.223	0.833	1.613
148	1.210	0.820	1.600
150	1.196	0.806	1.586
152	1.183	0.793	1.573
154	1.170	0.780	1.560
156	1.156	0.766	1.546
158	1.143	0.753	1.533
160	1.130	0.740	1.520
162	1.116	0.726	1.506
164	1.103	0.713	1.493
166	1.090	0.700	1.480
168	1.077	0.687	1.466
170	1.063	0.673	1.453
172	1.050	0.660	1.440
174	1.037	0.647	1.427
176	1.023	0.633	1.413
178	1.010	0.620	1.400
180	0.997	0.607	1.387

Formula: $y = a + b \cdot x$;

$y = \frac{\dot{V}_{max\ 50\ \%\ VC}}{FVC}\left(\frac{l/s}{l}\right)$; x = body height (cm);

$\frac{\dot{V}_{max\ 50\ \%\ VC}}{FVC}\left(\frac{l/s}{l}\right) = 2.1943 - 0.00665 \cdot$ body height (cm);

SD $y \cdot x = \pm 0.196$; n = 101; r = -0.43.

Table 202. Maximum expiratory flow rate at 75% of VC expressed per liter of FVC $\left(\frac{\dot{V}_{max\,75\%\,VC}}{FVC}\right)$ in relation to body height in boys and girls

Height cm	$\frac{\dot{V}_{max\,75\%\,VC}}{FVC}\left(\frac{l/s}{l}\right)$		
	mean	lower limits	upper limits
115	2.038	1.552	2.523
116	2.028	1.543	2.514
118	2.009	1.524	2.495
120	1.990	1.505	2.476
122	1.971	1.486	2.457
124	1.952	1.466	2.438
126	1.933	1.447	2.418
128	1.914	1.428	2.399
130	1.895	1.409	2.380
132	1.876	1.390	2.361
134	1.856	1.371	2.342
136	1.837	1.352	2.323
138	1.818	1.333	2.304
140	1.799	1.314	2.285
142	1.780	1.294	2.266
144	1.761	1.275	2.246
146	1.742	1.256	2.227
148	1.723	1.237	2.208
150	1.704	1.218	2.189
152	1.684	1.199	2.170
154	1.665	1.180	2.151
156	1.646	1.161	2.132
158	1.627	1.142	2.113
160	1.608	1.123	2.094
162	1.589	1.103	2.074
164	1.570	1.084	2.055
166	1.551	1.065	2.036
168	1.532	1.046	2.017
170	1.513	1.027	1.998
172	1.493	1.008	1.979
174	1.474	0.989	1.960
176	1.455	0.970	1.941
178	1.436	0.951	1.922
180	1.417	0.931	1.903

Formula: $y = a + b \cdot x$;

$y = \frac{\dot{V}_{max\,75\%\,VC}}{FVC}\left(\frac{l/s}{l}\right)$; x = body height (cm);

$\frac{\dot{V}_{max\,75\%\,VC}}{FVC}\left(\frac{l/s}{l}\right) = 3.1370 - 0.00955 \cdot$ body height (cm);

SD $y \cdot x = \pm 0.243$; n = 77; r = -0.51.

Table 203. Maximum expiratory flow rate at 50% TLC expressed per liter of FVC $\left(\frac{\dot{V}_{max\,50\%\,TLC}}{FVC}\right)$ in relation to body height in boys and girls

Height cm	$\frac{\dot{V}_{max\,50\%\,TLC}}{FVC}\left(\frac{l/s}{l}\right)$		
	mean	lower limits	upper limits
115	1.014	0.689	1.340
116	1.010	0.684	1.336
118	1.000	0.674	1.326
120	0.991	0.665	1.317
122	0.982	0.656	1.307
124	0.972	0.646	1.298
126	0.963	0.637	1.289
128	0.953	0.627	1.279
130	0.944	0.618	1.270
132	0.934	0.609	1.260
134	0.925	0.599	1.251
136	0.916	0.590	1.242
138	0.906	0.580	1.232
140	0.897	0.571	1.223
142	0.887	0.562	1.213
144	0.878	0.552	1.204
146	0.869	0.543	1.194
148	0.859	0.533	1.185
150	0.850	0.524	1.176
152	0.840	0.515	1.166
154	0.831	0.505	1.157
156	0.822	0.496	1.147
158	0.812	0.486	1.138
160	0.803	0.477	1.129
162	0.793	0.468	1.119
164	0.784	0.458	1.110
166	0.775	0.449	1.100
168	0.765	0.439	1.091
170	0.756	0.430	1.082
172	0.746	0.421	1.072
174	0.737	0.411	1.063
176	0.728	0.402	1.053
178	0.718	0.392	1.044
180	0.709	0.383	1.035

Formula: $y = a + b \cdot x$;

$y = \frac{\dot{V}_{max\,50\%\,TLC}}{FVC}\left(\frac{l/s}{l}\right)$; x = body height (cm);

$\frac{\dot{V}_{max\,50\%\,TLC}}{FVC}\left(\frac{l/s}{l}\right) = 1.5556 - 0.00470 \cdot$ body height (cm);

SD $y \cdot x = \pm 0.164$; n = 101; r = -0.37.

Table 204. Maximum expiratory flow rate at 60% TLC expressed per liter of FVC $\left(\frac{\dot{V}_{max\,60\%\,TLC}}{FVC}\right)$ in relation to body height in boys and girls

Height cm	$\frac{\dot{V}_{max\,60\%\,TLC}}{FVC}\left(\frac{l/s}{l}\right)$		
	mean	lower limits	upper limits
115	1.379	1.006	1.751
116	1.373	1.000	1.745
118	1.361	0.988	1.737
120	1.349	0.976	1.721
122	1.337	0.964	1.709
124	1.325	0.952	1.697
126	1.313	0.940	1.685
128	1.301	0.928	1.673
130	1.289	0.916	1.661
132	1.277	0.904	1.649
134	1.264	0.892	1.637
136	1.252	0.880	1.625
138	1.240	0.868	1.613
140	1.228	0.856	1.601
142	1.216	0.844	1.589
144	1.204	0.832	1.577
146	1.192	0.820	1.565
148	1.180	0.808	1.553
150	1.168	0.796	1.541
152	1.156	0.784	1.529
154	1.144	0.772	1.517
156	1.132	0.759	1.505
158	1.120	0.747	1.493
160	1.108	0.735	1.481
162	1.096	0.723	1.468
164	1.084	0.711	1.456
166	1.072	0.699	1.444
168	1.060	0.687	1.432
170	1.048	0.675	1.420
172	1.036	0.663	1.408
174	1.024	0.651	1.396
176	1.012	0.639	1.381
178	1.000	0.627	1.372
180	0.988	0.615	1.360

Formula: $y = a + b \cdot x$;
$y = \frac{\dot{V}_{max\,60\%\,TLC}}{FVC}\left(\frac{l/s}{l}\right)$; x = body height (cm);
$\frac{\dot{V}_{max\,60\%\,TLC}}{FVC}\left(\frac{l/s}{l}\right) = 2.0717 - 0.00602 \cdot$ body height (cm);
SD $y \cdot x = \pm 0.187$; n = 101; r = −0.41.

Table 205. Peak expiratory flow rate expressed per liter of FVC $\left(\frac{PEFR}{FVC}\right)$ in relation to body height in boys and girls

Height cm	$\frac{PEFR}{FVC}\left(\frac{l/s}{l}\right)$		
	mean	lower limits	upper limits
115	2.215	1.654	2.775
116	2.206	1.646	2.767
118	2.190	1.629	2.750
120	2.173	1.613	2.734
122	2.157	1.596	2.717
124	2.140	1.580	2.701
126	2.124	1.564	2.684
128	2.107	1.547	2.668
130	2.091	1.531	2.651
132	2.074	1.514	2.635
134	2.058	1.498	2.618
136	2.041	1.481	2.602
138	2.025	1.465	2.585
140	2.009	1.448	2.569
142	1.992	1.432	2.552
144	1.976	1.415	2.535
146	1.959	1.399	2.519
148	1.943	1.382	2.503
150	1.926	1.366	2.486
152	1.910	1.349	2.470
154	1.893	1.333	2.454
156	1.877	1.316	2.437
158	1.860	1.300	2.421
160	1.844	1.283	2.404
162	1.827	1.267	2.388
164	1.811	1.250	2.371
166	1.794	1.234	2.355
168	1.778	1.217	2.338
170	1.761	1.201	2.322
172	1.745	1.184	2.305
174	1.728	1.168	2.289
176	1.712	1.151	2.272
178	1.695	1.135	2.256
180	1.679	1.118	2.239

Formula: $y = a + b \cdot x$;
$y = \frac{PEFR}{FVC}\left(\frac{l/s}{l}\right)$; x = body height (cm);
$\frac{PEFR}{FVC}\left(\frac{l/s}{l}\right) = 3.1628 - 0.00824 \cdot$ body height (cm);
SD $y \cdot x = \pm 0.281$; n = 76; r = −0.41.

Table 206. Upstream airway conductance at 25% VC expressed per liter of TLC_{box} $\left(\frac{Gus_{25\% VC}}{TLC_{box}}\right)$ in relation to body height in boys and girls

Height cm	$Gus_{25\% VC}$					
	mean		lower limits		upper limits	
	a	b	a	b	a	b
115	2.777	0.272	1.122	0.110	6.874	0.674
116	2.722	0.266	1.100	0.107	6.737	0.660
118	2.616	0.256	1.057	0.103	6.476	0.635
120	2.516	0.246	1.017	0.099	6.228	0.610
122	2.422	0.237	0.978	0.095	5.994	0.587
124	2.332	0.228	0.942	0.092	5.772	0.566
126	2.247	0.220	0.908	0.089	5.562	0.545
128	2.167	0.212	0.875	0.085	5.363	0.526
130	2.090	0.204	0.844	0.082	5.173	0.507
132	2.017	0.197	0.815	0.079	4.994	0.489
134	1.948	0.191	0.787	0.077	4.822	0.473
136	1.883	0.184	0.760	0.074	4.660	0.457
138	1.820	0.178	0.735	0.072	4.505	0.441
140	1.760	0.172	0.711	0.069	4.357	0.427
142	1.703	0.167	0.688	0.067	4.216	0.413
144	1.649	0.161	0.666	0.065	4.081	0.400
146	1.597	0.156	0.645	0.063	3.953	0.387
148	1.547	0.151	0.625	0.061	3.830	0.375
150	1.500	0.147	0.606	0.059	3.713	0.364
152	1.455	0.142	0.588	0.057	3.601	0.353
154	1.411	0.138	0.570	0.055	3.493	0.342
156	1.370	0.134	0.553	0.054	3.390	0.332
158	1.330	0.130	0.537	0.052	3.292	0.322
160	1.292	0.126	0.522	0.051	3.197	0.313
162	1.255	0.123	0.507	0.049	3.106	0.304
164	1.220	0.119	0.493	0.048	3.019	0.296
166	1.186	0.116	0.479	0.046	2.935	0.287
168	1.153	0.113	0.466	0.045	2.855	0.280
170	1.122	0.110	0.453	0.044	2.778	0.272
172	1.092	0.107	0.441	0.043	2.703	0.265
174	1.063	0.104	0.429	0.042	2.632	0.258
176	1.035	0.101	0.418	0.041	2.563	0.251
178	1.009	0.098	0.407	0.039	2.497	0.244
180	0.983	0.096	0.397	0.038	2.433	0.238

Formula: $\log y = a + b \cdot \log x$;
$y = Gus_{25\% VC}$ (TLC/s/kPa or TLC/s/cm H_2O);
x = body height (cm);
$\log Gus_{25\% VC}$ (TLC/s/kPa) =
    $5.22018 - 2.3179 \cdot \log$ height (cm);
SD $\log y \cdot x = \pm 0.1944$; n = 69; r = −0.46.
$\log Gus_{25\% VC}$ (TLC/s/cm H_2O) = $4.2117 - 2.3179 \cdot \log x$;
$\log$ SD $y \cdot x = \pm 0.1944$.
a = TLC/s/kPa; b = TLC/s/cm H_2O.

Table 207. Upstream airway conductance at 50% VC expressed per liter of TLC_{box} $\left(\frac{Gus_{50\% VC}}{TLC_{box}}\right)$ in relation to body height in boys and girls

Height cm	$Gus_{50\% VC}$					
	mean		lower limits		upper limits	
	a	b	a	b	a	b
115	1.930	0.189	1.118	0.109	3.330	0.327
116	1.896	0.186	1.098	0.108	3.271	0.321
118	1.830	0.179	1.061	0.104	3.151	0.310
120	1.768	0.173	1.025	0.100	3.052	0.300
122	1.709	0.168	0.991	0.097	2.950	0.290
124	1.653	0.162	0.958	0.094	2.853	0.280
126	1.600	0.157	0.927	0.091	2.761	0.271
128	1.549	0.152	0.898	0.088	2.674	0.262
130	1.501	0.147	0.870	0.085	2.590	0.254
132	1.454	0.143	0.843	0.082	2.510	0.246
134	1.410	0.138	0.817	0.080	2.434	0.239
136	1.368	0.134	0.793	0.077	2.361	0.232
138	1.328	0.130	0.769	0.075	2.291	0.225
140	1.289	0.126	0.747	0.073	2.225	0.218
142	1.252	0.123	0.725	0.071	2.161	0.212
144	1.217	0.119	0.705	0.069	2.100	0.206
146	1.183	0.116	0.685	0.067	2.041	0.200
148	1.150	0.113	0.666	0.065	1.985	0.195
150	1.119	0.110	0.648	0.063	1.931	0.189
152	1.089	0.107	0.631	0.062	1.880	0.184
154	1.060	0.104	0.614	0.060	1.830	0.179
156	1.033	0.101	0.598	0.058	1.782	0.175
158	1.006	0.098	0.583	0.057	1.736	0.170
160	0.980	0.096	0.568	0.055	1.692	0.166
162	0.956	0.093	0.554	0.054	1.649	0.162
164	0.932	0.091	0.540	0.053	1.608	0.158
166	0.909	0.089	0.527	0.051	1.569	0.154
168	0.887	0.087	0.514	0.050	1.531	0.150
170	0.866	0.085	0.502	0.049	1.494	0.146
172	0.845	0.083	0.490	0.048	1.459	0.143
174	0.825	0.081	0.478	0.047	1.425	0.140
176	0.806	0.079	0.467	0.045	1.392	0.136
178	0.788	0.077	0.456	0.044	1.360	0.133
180	0.770	0.075	0.446	0.043	1.329	0.130

Formula: $\log y = a + b \cdot \log x$;
$y = Gus_{50\% VC}$ (TLC/s/kPa or TLC/s/cm H_2O);
x = body height (cm);
$\log Gus_{50\% VC}$ (TLC/s/kPa) =
    $4.51008 - 2.05003 \cdot \log$ height (cm);
SD $\log y \cdot x = \pm 0.1187$; n = 69; r = −0.62.
$\log Gus_{50\% VC}$ (TLC/s/cm H_2O) = $3.5026 - 2.05003 \cdot \log x$;
SD $\log y \cdot x = \pm 0.1187$.
a = TLC/s/kPa; b = TLC/s/cm H_2O.

Table 208. Upstream airway conductance at 75% VC expressed per liter of TLC_{box} $\left(\frac{Gus_{75\%\,vc}}{TLC_{box}}\right)$ in relation to body height in boys and girls

Height cm	$Gus_{75\%\,VC}$					
	mean		lower limits		upper limits	
	a	b	a	b	a	b
115	1.508	0.147	0.965	0.094	2.358	0.231
116	1.485	0.145	0.950	0.093	2.322	0.227
118	1.440	0.141	0.921	0.090	2.251	0.220
120	1.396	0.137	0.893	0.087	2.183	0.214
122	1.355	0.132	0.867	0.085	2.119	0.207
124	1.316	0.129	0.842	0.082	2.057	0.201
126	1.278	0.125	0.818	0.080	1.999	0.196
128	1.242	0.121	0.795	0.077	1.942	0.190
130	1.208	0.118	0.772	0.075	1.889	0.185
132	1.175	0.115	0.751	0.073	1.837	0.180
134	1.143	0.112	0.731	0.071	1.788	0.175
136	1.113	0.109	0.712	0.069	1.740	0.170
138	1.084	0.106	0.693	0.068	1.695	0.166
140	1.056	0.103	0.675	0.066	1.651	0.162
142	1.029	0.100	0.658	0.064	1.609	0.157
144	1.004	0.098	0.642	0.062	1.569	0.153
146	0.979	0.096	0.626	0.061	1.530	0.150
148	0.955	0.093	0.611	0.059	1.493	0.146
150	0.932	0.091	0.596	0.058	1.457	0.143
152	0.910	0.089	0.582	0.057	1.423	0.139
154	0.889	0.087	0.568	0.055	1.389	0.136
156	0.868	0.085	0.555	0.054	1.357	0.133
158	0.848	0.083	0.542	0.053	1.326	0.130
160	0.829	0.081	0.530	0.052	1.296	0.127
162	0.811	0.079	0.518	0.050	1.268	0.124
164	0.793	0.077	0.507	0.049	1.240	0.121
166	0.776	0.076	0.496	0.048	1.213	0.119
168	0.759	0.074	0.485	0.047	1.187	0.116
170	0.743	0.072	0.475	0.046	1.161	0.114
172	0.727	0.071	0.465	0.045	1.137	0.111
174	0.712	0.069	0.455	0.044	1.114	0.109
176	0.698	0.068	0.446	0.043	1.091	0.107
178	0.683	0.067	0.437	0.042	1.069	0.104
180	0.670	0.065	0.428	0.041	1.047	0.102

Formula: $\log y = a + b \cdot \log x$;
$y = Gus_{75\%\,VC}$ ($TLC/s/kPa$ or $TLC/s/cm\ H_2O$);
x = body height (cm);
$\log Gus_{75\%\,VC}$ ($TLC/s/kPa$) =
    $3.91138 - 1.8114 \cdot \log$ body height;
SD $\log y \cdot x = \pm 0.0967$; n = 54; r = -0.68.
$\log Gus_{75\%\,VC}$ ($TLC/s/cm\ H_2O$) = $2.9029 - 1.8114 \cdot \log x$;
SD $\log y \cdot x = \pm 0.0967$.
a = $TLC/s/kPa$; b = $TLC/s/cm\ H_2O$.

Table 209. Upstream airway conductance at 50% of TLC expressed per liter of TLC_{box} $\left(\frac{Gus_{50\%\,TLC}}{TLC_{box}}\right)$ in relation to body height in boys and girls

Height cm	$Gus_{50\%\,TLC}$					
	mean		lower limits		upper limits	
	a	b	a	b	a	b
115	2.728	0.267	1.365	0.133	5.453	0.534
116	2.664	0.261	1.333	0.130	5.325	0.521
118	2.542	0.249	1.272	0.124	5.082	0.498
120	2.428	0.238	1.215	0.119	4.854	0.476
122	2.321	0.227	1.161	0.113	4.639	0.455
124	2.220	0.217	1.110	0.108	4.438	0.435
126	2.125	0.208	1.063	0.104	4.248	0.416
128	2.035	0.199	1.018	0.099	4.069	0.399
130	1.951	0.191	0.976	0.095	3.900	0.382
132	1.871	0.183	0.936	0.091	3.740	0.366
134	1.796	0.176	0.898	0.088	3.590	0.352
136	1.724	0.169	0.862	0.084	3.447	0.338
138	1.657	0.162	0.829	0.081	3.312	0.324
140	1.593	0.156	0.797	0.078	3.184	0.312
142	1.532	0.150	0.766	0.075	3.063	0.300
144	1.475	0.144	0.738	0.072	2.948	0.289
146	1.420	0.139	0.710	0.069	2.839	0.278
148	1.368	0.134	0.684	0.067	2.735	0.268
150	1.319	0.129	0.660	0.064	2.637	0.258
152	1.272	0.124	0.636	0.062	2.543	0.249
154	1.227	0.120	0.614	0.060	2.454	0.240
156	1.185	0.116	0.593	0.058	2.369	0.232
158	1.144	0.112	0.572	0.056	2.288	0.224
160	1.106	0.108	0.553	0.054	2.210	0.216
162	1.069	0.104	0.534	0.052	2.136	0.209
164	1.033	0.101	0.517	0.050	2.066	0.202
166	1.000	0.098	0.500	0.049	1.998	0.196
168	0.967	0.094	0.484	0.047	1.934	0.189
170	0.937	0.091	0.468	0.045	1.872	0.183
172	0.907	0.088	0.454	0.044	1.814	0.177
174	0.879	0.086	0.439	0.043	1.757	0.172
176	0.852	0.083	0.426	0.041	1.703	0.167
178	0.826	0.081	0.413	0.040	1.651	0.161
180	0.801	0.078	0.401	0.039	1.601	0.157

Formula: $\log y = a + b \cdot \log x$;
$y = Gus_{50\%\,TLC}$ ($TLC/s/kPa$ or $TLC/s/cm\ H_2O$);
x = body height (cm);
$\log Gus_{50\%\,TLC}$ ($TLC/s/kPa$) =
    $6.07048 - 2.7343 \cdot \log$ height;
SD $\log y \cdot x = \pm 0.1502$; n = 69; r = -0.64.
$\log Gus_{50\%\,TLC}$ ($TLC/s/cm\ H_2O$) = $5.0621 - 2.7343 \cdot \log x$;
SD $\log y \cdot x = \pm 0.1502$.
a = $TLC/s/kPa$; b = $TLC/s/cm\ H_2O$.

Table 210. Upstream airway conductance at 60 % of TLC_{box} expressed per liter of TLC_{box} $\left(\frac{Gus_{60\% TLC}}{TLC_{box}}\right)$ in relation to body height in boys and girls

Height cm	$Gus_{60\% TLC}$					
	mean		lower limits		upper limits	
	a	b	a	b	a	b
115	2.134	0.209	1.191	0.116	3.825	0.375
116	2.092	0.205	1.168	0.114	3.750	0.367
118	2.012	0.197	1.123	0.110	3.606	0.353
120	1.937	0.189	1.081	0.106	3.470	0.340
122	1.865	0.182	1.041	0.102	3.342	0.327
124	1.797	0.176	1.003	0.098	3.220	0.315
126	1.732	0.169	0.967	0.094	3.105	0.304
128	1.671	0.163	0.933	0.091	2.995	0.293
130	1.613	0.158	0.900	0.088	2.891	0.283
132	1.558	0.152	0.869	0.085	2.792	0.273
134	1.505	0.147	0.840	0.082	2.698	0.264
136	1.455	0.142	0.812	0.079	2.608	0.255
138	1.408	0.138	0.785	0.077	2.522	0.247
140	1.362	0.133	0.760	0.074	2.441	0.239
142	1.319	0.129	0.736	0.072	2.363	0.231
144	1.277	0.125	0.713	0.069	2.289	0.224
146	1.238	0.121	0.691	0.067	2.218	0.217
148	1.200	0.117	0.669	0.065	2.150	0.210
150	1.164	0.114	0.649	0.063	2.085	0.204
152	1.129	0.110	0.630	0.061	2.023	0.198
154	1.096	0.107	0.611	0.059	1.964	0.192
156	1.064	0.104	0.594	0.058	1.907	0.187
158	1.033	0.101	0.577	0.056	1.852	0.181
160	1.004	0.098	0.560	0.054	1.800	0.176
162	0.976	0.095	0.545	0.053	1.749	0.171
164	0.949	0.093	0.529	0.051	1.701	0.166
166	0.923	0.090	0.515	0.050	1.654	0.162
168	0.898	0.088	0.501	0.049	1.610	0.157
170	0.874	0.085	0.488	0.047	1.567	0.153
172	0.851	0.083	0.475	0.046	1.526	0.149
174	0.829	0.081	0.462	0.045	1.486	0.145
176	0.808	0.079	0.451	0.044	1.448	0.142
178	0.787	0.077	0.439	0.043	1.411	0.138
180	0.767	0.075	0.428	0.042	1.375	0.134

Formula: $\log y = a + b \cdot \log x$;
$y = Gus_{60\% TLC}$ ($TLC/s/kPa$ or $TLC/s/cm\ H_2O$);
x = body height (cm);
$\log Gus_{60\% TLC}$ ($TLC/s/kPa$) =
    $5.03288 - 2.2825 \cdot$ height (cm);
SD $\log y \cdot x = \pm 0.1269$; $n = 69$; $r = -0.64$.
$\log Gus_{60\% TLC}$ ($TLC/s/cm\ H_2O$) = $4.0245 - 2.2825 \cdot \log x$;
SD $\log y \cdot x = \pm 0.1269$.
$a = TLC/s/kPa$; $b = TLC/s/cm\ H_2O$.

Table 211. Forced vital capacity (FVC) in relation to body height in boys and girls

Height cm	FVC, ml		
	mean	lower limits	upper limits
115	1,307	1,079	1,582
116	1,340	1,106	1,622
118	1,407	1,162	1,704
120	1,477	1,219	1,789
122	1,549	1,279	1,876
124	1,623	1,340	1,966
126	1,700	1,403	2,059
128	1,779	1,469	2,154
130	1,860	1,536	2,252
132	1,943	1,605	2,354
134	2,029	1,676	2,458
136	2,118	1,749	2,565
138	2,209	1,824	2,675
140	2,302	1,901	2,788
142	2,398	1,980	2,905
144	2,497	2,062	3,024
146	2,598	2,145	3,146
148	2,702	2,231	3,272
150	2,808	2,319	3,401
152	2,917	2,409	3,533
154	3,029	2,501	3,669
156	3,144	2,596	3,808
158	3,262	2,693	3,950
160	3,382	2,792	4,096
162	3,505	2,894	4,245
164	3,631	2,998	4,398
166	3,760	3,105	4,554
168	3,892	3,214	4,714
170	4,027	3,325	4,877
172	4,165	3,439	5,044
174	4,306	3,555	5,215
176	4,450	3,674	5,389
178	4,597	3,796	5,567
180	4,747	3,920	5,750

Formula: log y = a + b·log x;
y = FVC (ml); x = body height (cm);
log FVC (ml) = −2.816 + 2.879·log height (cm);
SD log y·x = ±0.0419; n = 111; r = +0.94.

Table 212. Forced vital capacity (FVC) in relation to age in boys and girls

Age years	FVC, ml		
	mean	lower limits	upper limits
6	1,342	972	1,852
7	1,600	1,159	2,208
8	1,863	1,350	2,571
9	2,131	1,544	2,940
10	2,403	1,741	3,316
11	2,679	1,941	3,696
12	2,958	2,144	4,082
13	3,241	2,348	4,472
14	3,526	2,555	4,866
15	3,815	2,765	5,264
16	4,106	2,976	5,666
17	4,400	3,189	6,071

Formula: log y = a + b·log x;
y = FVC (ml); x = age (years);
log FVC (ml) = 2.2409 + 1.1398·log age (years);
SD log y·x = ±0.0705; n = 111; r = +0.82.

Table 213. Forced vital capacity (FVC) in relation to body surface in boys and girls

Body surface m²	FVC, ml		
	mean	lower limits	upper limits
0.6	933	739	1,178
0.7	1,160	919	1,465
0.8	1,402	1,110	1,770
0.9	1,657	1,312	2,092
1.0	1,923	1,523	2,429
1.1	2,202	1,744	2,780
1.2	2,490	1,972	3,144
1.3	2,789	2,209	3,522
1.4	3,098	2,454	3,912
1.5	3,416	2,706	4,313
1.6	3,743	2,965	4,726
1.7	4,079	3,231	5,150
1.8	4,423	3,503	5,584
1.9	4,775	3,782	6,029
2.0	5,135	4,067	6,483

Formula: log y = a + b·log x;
y = FVC (ml); x = body surface (m²);
log FVC (ml) = 3.2842 + 1.4163·log body surface;
SD log y·x = ±0.0510; n = 111; r = +0.91.

Table 214. Forced vital capacity (FVC) in relation to body height in boys

Height cm	FVC, ml		
	mean	lower limits	upper limits
115	1,338	1,158	1,545
116	1,372	1,188	1,585
118	1,443	1,249	1,667
120	1,516	1,313	1,751
122	1,592	1,378	1,838
124	1,669	1,445	1,928
126	1,750	1,515	2,021
128	1,833	1,587	2,116
130	1,918	1,661	2,215
132	2,006	1,737	2,317
134	2,096	1,815	2,421
136	2,190	1,896	2,529
138	2,286	1,979	2,640
140	2,384	2,064	2,754
142	2,486	2,152	2,871
144	2,590	2,242	2,991
146	2,697	2,335	3,115
148	2,807	2,430	3,242
150	2,920	2,528	3,372
152	3,035	2,628	3,506
154	3,154	2,731	3,643
156	3,276	2,837	3,783
158	3,401	2,945	3,928
160	3,529	3,056	4,075
162	3,660	3,169	4,227
164	3,794	3,285	4,382
166	3,932	3,404	4,541
168	4,072	3,526	4,703
170	4,216	3,651	4,870
172	4,364	3,778	5,040
174	4,514	3,909	5,214
176	4,669	4,042	5,392
178	4,826	4,179	5,574
180	4,987	4,318	5,759

Formula: $\log y = a + b \cdot \log x$;
y = FVC (ml); x = body height (cm);
$\log$ FVC (ml) = $-2.9236 + 2.9360 \cdot \log$ height (cm);
SD $\log y \cdot x = \pm 0.0312$; n = 60; r = +0.96.

Table 215. Forced vital capacity (FVC) in relation to age in boys

Age years	FVC, ml		
	mean	lower limits	upper limits
6	1,394	1,040	1,869
7	1,659	1,238	2,223
8	1,928	1,438	2,584
9	2,201	1,643	2,950
10	2,479	1,849	3,322
11	2,760	2,059	3,698
12	3,044	2,271	4,079
13	3,331	2,485	4,464
14	3,621	2,702	4,853
15	3,913	2,920	5,245
16	4,208	3,140	5,640
17	4,506	3,362	6,038

Formula: $\log y = a + b \cdot \log x$;
y = FVC (ml); x = age (years);
$\log$ FVC (ml) = $2.2682 + 1.1260 \cdot \log$ age (years);
SD $\log y \cdot x = \pm 0.0635$; n = 60; r = +0.83.

Table 216. Forced vital capacity (FVC) in relation to body surface in boys

Body surface m²	FVC, ml		
	mean	lower limits	upper limits
0.6	978	775	1,234
0.7	1,218	965	1,536
0.8	1,472	1,168	1,857
0.9	1,739	1,379	2,195
1.0	2,020	1,601	2,549
1.1	2,313	1,833	2,918
1.2	2,616	2,074	3,301
1.3	2,931	2,323	3,698
1.4	3,256	2,581	4,108
1.5	3,591	2,846	4,531
1.6	3,936	3,120	4,965
1.7	4,289	3,400	5,411
1.8	4,652	3,687	5,869
1.9	5,023	3,981	6,337
2.0	5,402	4,282	6,815

Formula: $\log y = a + b \cdot \log x$;
y = FVC (ml); x = body surface (m²);
$\log$ FVC (ml) = $3.3054 + 1.4188 \cdot \log$ body surface (m²);
SD $\log y \cdot x = \pm 0.0504$; n = 60; r = +0.89.

Table 217. Forced vital capacity (FVC) in relation to body height in girls

Height cm	FVC, ml		
	mean	lower limits	upper limits
115	1,268	1,031	1,560
116	1,300	1,056	1,599
118	1,364	1,108	1,678
120	1,430	1,162	1,759
122	1,498	1,218	1,843
124	1,568	1,275	1,930
126	1,641	1,334	2,019
128	1,715	1,394	2,110
130	1,792	1,456	2,205
132	1,871	1,520	2,302
134	1,952	1,586	2,401
136	2,035	1,654	2,504
138	2,120	1,723	2,609
140	2,208	1,795	2,717
142	2,298	1,868	2,828
144	2,391	1,943	2,941
146	2,485	2,020	3,058
148	2,583	2,099	3,178
150	2,682	2,180	3,300
152	2,784	2,263	3,426
154	2,889	2,348	3,554
156	2,996	2,435	3,686
158	3,105	2,524	3,821
160	3,217	2,615	3,958
162	3,332	2,708	4,099
164	3,449	2,804	4,244
166	3,569	2,901	4,391
168	3,692	3,001	4,542
170	3,817	3,102	4,696
172	3,945	3,206	4,853
174	4,075	3,313	5,014
176	4,209	3,421	5,178
178	4,345	3,532	5,346
180	4,484	3,645	5,517

Formula: $\log y = a + b \cdot \log x$;
y = FVC (ml); x = body height (cm);
log FVC (ml) = $-2.7040 + 2.8181 \cdot \log$ height (cm);
SD log y·x = ± 0.0447; n = 51; r = +0.94.

Table 218. Forced vital capacity (FVC) in relation to age in girls

Age years	FVC, ml		
	mean	lower limits	upper limits
6	1,302	914	1,856
7	1,551	1,088	2,210
8	1,804	1,266	2,571
9	2,062	1,446	2,938
10	2,323	1,630	3,311
11	2,588	1,816	3,688
12	2,856	2,004	4,070
13	3,127	2,194	4,456
14	3,401	2,386	4,847
15	3,677	2,580	5,241
16	3,956	2,776	5,638
17	4,237	2,973	6,039

Formula: $\log y = a + b \cdot \log x$;
y = FVC (ml); x = age (years);
log FVC (ml) = $2.2335 + 1.1325 \cdot \log$ age (years);
SD log y·x = ± 0.0765; n = 51; r = +0.83.

Table 219. Forced vital capacity (FVC) in relation to body surface in girls

Body surface m²	FVC, ml			
	mean		lower limits	upper limits
0.6	872		727	1,048
0.7	1,087		905	1,305
0.8	1,316		1,095	1,580
0.9	1,557	↔	1,296	1,869
1.0	1,809	↔	1,507	2,172
1.1	2,073	↔	1,727	2,489
1.2	1,955	↔	2,347	2,818
1.3	2,192	↔	2,632	3,160
1.4	2,437	↔	2,925	3,512
1.5	2,689	↔	3,228	3,876
1.6	2,948	↔	3,540	4,250
1.7	3,215	↔	3,860	4,634
1.8	3,488	↔	4,188	5,028
1.9	3,768	↔	4,524	5,431
2.0	4,868	↔	4,054	5,844

Formula: $\log y = a + b \cdot \log x$;
y = FVC (ml); x = body surface (m²);
log FVC (ml) = $3.2576 + 1.4274 \cdot \log$ body surface (m²);
SD log y·x = ± 0.0398; n = 51; r = +0.95.

Table 220. Forced expiratory volume in the first second (FEV$_1$) in relation to body height in boys and girls

Height cm	FEV$_1$, ml		
	mean	lower limits	upper limits
115	1,123	916	1,377
116	1,151	938	1,411
118	1,207	984	1,480
120	1,265	1,032	1,552
122	1,325	1,081	1,626
124	1,387	1,131	1,702
126	1,451	1,183	1,780
128	1,517	1,237	1,860
130	1,584	1,292	1,943
132	1,653	1,348	2,028
134	1,725	1,406	2,115
136	1,798	1,466	2,205
138	1,873	1,527	2,297
140	1,950	1,590	2,392
142	2,030	1,655	2,489
144	2,111	1,721	2,589
146	2,194	1,789	2,691
148	2,280	1,859	2,796
150	2,367	1,930	2,903
152	2,457	2,003	3,013
154	2,549	2,078	3,126
156	2,642	2,155	3,241
158	2,739	2,233	3,359
160	2,837	2,313	3,479
162	2,938	2,395	3,603
164	3,041	2,479	3,729
166	3,146	2,565	3,858
168	3,253	2,653	3,990
170	3,363	2,742	4,125
172	3,475	2,834	4,262
174	3,590	2,927	4,403
176	3,707	3,023	4,546
178	3,826	3,120	4,693
180	3,948	3,219	4,842

Formula: $\log y = a + b \cdot \log x$;
$y = \text{FEV}_1$ (ml); $x = $ body height (cm);
$\log \text{FEV}_1$ (ml) $= -2.731 + 2.805 \cdot \log$ height (cm);
SD $\log y \cdot x = \pm 0.0447$; $n = 111$; $r = +0.93$.

Table 221. Forced expiratory volume in the first second (FEV$_1$) in relation to age in boys and girls

Age years	FEV$_1$, ml		
	mean	lower limits	upper limits
6	1,148	833	1,583
7	1,364	989	1,881
8	1,584	1,149	2,183
9	1,806	1,310	2,490
10	2,032	1,474	2,801
11	2,260	1,640	3,116
12	2,491	1,807	3,434
13	2,724	1,976	3,755
14	2,959	2,147	4,079
15	3,196	2,318	4,406
16	3,435	2,492	4,735
17	3,676	2,666	5,067

Formula: $\log y = a + b \cdot \log x$;
$y = \text{FEV}_1$ (ml); $x = $ age (years);
$\log \text{FEV}_1$ (ml) $= 2.1911 + 1.1168 \cdot \log$ age (years);
SD $\log y \cdot x = \pm 0.0703$; $n = 111$; $r = +0.82$.

Table 222. Forced expiratory volume in the first second (FEV$_1$) in relation to body surface in boys and girls

Body surface m^2	FEV$_1$, ml		
	mean	lower limits	upper limits
0.6	815	635	1,046
0.7	1,007	784	1,292
0.8	1,209	942	1,552
0.9	1,421	1,107	1,823
1.0	1,641	1,279	2,106
1.1	1,870	1,457	2,400
1.2	2,107	1,642	2,704
1.3	2,351	1,832	3,018
1.4	2,602	2,028	3,340
1.5	2,860	2,229	3,671
1.6	3,125	2,435	4,011
1.7	3,396	2,646	4,358
1.8	3,672	2,861	4,713
1.9	3,954	3,081	5,075
2.0	4,242	3,305	5,445

Formula: $\log y = a + b \cdot \log x$;
$y = \text{FEV}_1$ (ml); $x = $ body surface (m^2);
$\log \text{FEV}_1$ (ml) $= 3.2152 + 1.3698 \cdot \log$ body surface (m^2);
SD $\log y \cdot x = \pm 0.0546$; $n = 111$; $r = +0.90$.

Table 223. Percentage of forced expiratory volume in the first second from forced vital capacity (% FEV$_1$/FVC) in relation to body height in boys and girls

Height cm	FEV$_1$/FVC, %		
	mean	lower limits	upper limits
115	85.88	76.87	94.89
116	85.84	76.83	94.84
118	85.76	76.75	94.76
120	85.67	76.67	94.68
122	85.59	76.59	94.60
124	85.51	76.50	94.52
126	85.43	76.42	94.43
128	85.35	76.34	94.35
130	85.26	76.26	94.27
132	85.18	76.18	94.19
134	85.10	76.09	94.11
136	85.02	76.01	94.02
138	84.94	75.93	93.94
140	84.85	75.85	93.86
142	84.77	75.77	93.78
144	84.69	75.68	93.70
146	84.61	75.60	93.61
148	84.53	75.52	93.53
150	84.44	75.44	93.45
152	84.36	75.36	93.37
154	84.28	75.27	93.28
156	84.20	75.19	93.20
158	84.11	75.11	93.12
160	84.03	75.03	93.04
162	83.95	74.95	92.96
164	83.87	74.86	92.87
166	83.79	74.78	92.79
168	83.70	74.70	92.71
170	83.62	74.62	92.63
172	83.54	74.53	92.55
174	83.46	74.45	92.46
176	83.38	74.37	92.38
178	83.29	74.29	92.30
180	83.21	74.21	92.22

Formula: $y = a + b \cdot x$;

y = FEV$_1$/FVC (%); x = body height (cm);

FEV$_1$/FVC (%) = 90.6043 − 0.04104·body height (cm);

SD $y \cdot x = \pm 4.54$; $n = 111$; $r = -0.12$.

Table 224. Forced expiratory volume in the first second (FEV₁) in relation to body height in boys

Height cm	FEV₁, ml mean	lower limits	upper limits
115	1,135	952	1,352
116	1,163	976	1,386
118	1,222	1,025	1,456
120	1,282	1,076	1,528
122	1,345	1,128	1,602
124	1,409	1,182	1,679
126	1,475	1,238	1,758
128	1,544	1,295	1,839
130	1,614	1,354	1,923
132	1,686	1,415	2,009
134	1,761	1,478	2,098
136	1,837	1,542	2,189
138	1,916	1,608	2,283
140	1,997	1,676	2,380
142	2,080	1,746	2,479
144	2,165	1,817	2,580
146	2,253	1,891	2,685
148	2,343	1,966	2,792
150	2,435	2,043	2,901
152	2,529	2,123	3,014
154	2,626	2,204	3,129
156	2,725	2,287	3,248
158	2,827	2,372	3,369
160	2,931	2,460	3,493
162	3,038	2,549	3,620
164	3,147	2,641	3,749
166	3,258	2,734	3,882
168	3,372	2,830	4,018
170	3,489	2,928	4,157
172	3,608	3,028	4,299
174	3,730	3,130	4,445
176	3,854	3,235	4,593
178	3,982	3,342	4,744
180	4,112	3,451	4,899

Formula: $\log y = a + b \cdot \log x$;
$y = FEV_1$ (ml); x = body height (cm);
$\log FEV_1$ (ml) $= -2.8652 + 2.8729 \cdot \log$ body height (cm);
SD $\log y \cdot x = \pm 0.0380$; $n = 60$; $r = +0.94$.

Table 225. Forced expiratory volume in the first second (FEV₁) in relation to age in boys

Age years	FEV₁, ml mean	lower limits	upper limits
6	1,165	869	1,561
7	1,385	1,033	1,857
8	1,610	1,201	2,158
9	1,838	1,371	2,463
10	2,069	1,543	2,773
11	2,303	1,718	3,086
12	2,539	1,890	3,403
13	2,778	2,073	3,724
14	3,020	2,253	4,047
15	3,263	2,435	4,374
16	3,509	2,618	4,703
17	3,756	2,803	5,035

Formula: $\log y = a + b \cdot \log x$;
$y = FEV_1$ (ml); x = age (years);
$\log FEV_1$ (ml) $= 2.1917 + 1.1240 \cdot \log$ age (years);
SD $\log y \cdot x = \pm 0.0635$; $n = 60$; $r = +0.83$.

Table 226. Forced expiratory volume in the first second (FEV₁) in relation to body surface in boys

Body surface m²	FEV₁, ml mean	lower limits	upper limits
0.6	846	652	1,097
0.7	1,045	806	1,355
0.8	1,255	968	1,628
0.9	1,475	1,138	1,913
1.0	1,705	1,315	2,211
1.1	1,943	1,498	2,520
1.2	2,190	1,688	2,839
1.3	2,444	1,884	3,169
1.4	2,705	2,086	3,508
1.5	2,974	2,293	3,856
1.6	3,249	2,506	4,213
1.7	3,531	2,723	4,579
1.8	3,819	2,945	4,952
1.9	4,113	3,172	5,333
2.0	4,413	3,403	5,722

Formula: $\log y = a + b \cdot \log x$;
$y = FEV_1$ (ml); x = body surface (m²);
$\log FEV_1$ (ml) $= 3.2318 + 1.3717 \cdot \log$ body surface (m²);
SD $\log y \cdot x = \pm 0.0563$; $n = 60$; $r = +0.87$.

Table 227. Forced expiratory volume in the first second (FEV₁) in relation to body height in girls

Height cm	FEV₁, ml		
	mean	lower limits	upper limits
115	1,105	883	1,382
116	1,131	905	1,415
118	1,186	948	1,483
120	1,242	993	1,553
122	1,299	1,039	1,625
124	1,358	1,086	1,699
126	1,419	1,135	1,775
128	1,482	1,185	1,853
130	1,546	1,236	1,934
132	1,612	1,289	2,016
134	1,680	1,344	2,101
136	1,750	1,399	2,188
138	1,821	1,457	2,278
140	1,895	1,515	2,369
142	1,970	1,575	2,463
144	2,047	1,637	2,560
146	2,126	1,700	2,658
148	2,207	1,765	2,759
150	2,289	1,831	2,863
152	2,374	1,898	2,969
154	2,461	1,968	3,077
156	2,549	2,039	3,188
158	2,640	2,111	3,301
160	2,732	2,185	3,417
162	2,827	2,261	3,535
164	2,924	2,338	3,656
166	3,023	2,417	3,780
168	3,124	2,498	3,906
170	3,227	2,580	4,035
172	3,332	2,664	4,166
174	3,439	2,750	4,300
176	3,549	2,838	4,437
178	3,660	2,927	4,577
180	3,774	3,018	4,719

Formula: $\log y = a + b \cdot \log x$;
$y = FEV_1$ (ml); x = body height (cm);
$\log FEV_1$ (ml) = $-2.6056 + 2.7413 \cdot \log$ body height (cm);
SD $\log y \cdot x = \pm 0.0483$; n = 51; r = +0.93.

Table 227a. Forced expiratory volume in the first second (FEV₁) in relation to age in girls

Age years	FEV₁, ml		
	mean	lower limits	upper limits
6	1,136	792	1,627
7	1,345	939	1,928
8	1,558	1,087	2,233
9	1,773	1,237	2,541
10	1,991	1,389	2,853
11	2,211	1,543	3,158
12	2,433	1,698	3,486
13	2,659	1,854	3,807
14	2,882	2,011	4,130
15	3,109	2,170	4,455
16	3,337	2,329	4,782
17	3,567	2,489	5,112

Formula: $\log y = a + b \cdot \log x$;
$y = FEV_1$ (ml); x = age (years);
$\log FEV_1$ (ml) = $2.2003 + 1.0988 \cdot \log$ age (years);
SD $\log y \cdot x = \pm 0.0777$; n = 51; r = +0.81.

Table 228. Forced expiratory volume in the first second (FEV₁) in relation to body surface in girls

Body surface m²	FEV₁, ml		
	mean	lower limits	upper limits
0.6	774	624	959
0.7	957	772	1,186
0.8	1,150	929	1,425
0.9	1,353	1,092	1,677
1.0	1,565	1,263	1,939
1.1	1,785	1,441	2,211
1.2	2,012	1,624	2,493
1.3	2,247	1,814	2,784
1.4	2,489	2,009	3,083
1.5	2,737	2,209	3,391
1.6	2,992	2,415	3,706
1.7	3,253	2,626	4,030
1.8	3,519	2,841	4,360
1.9	3,792	3,061	4,697
2.0	4,070	3,285	5,041

Formula: $\log y = a + b \cdot \log x$;
$y = FEV_1$ (ml); x = body surface (m²);
$\log FEV_1$ (ml) = $3.1946 + 1.3784 \cdot \log$ body surface (m²);
SD $\log y \cdot x = \pm 0.0462$; n = 51; r = +0.93.

Table 229. Maximum mid-expiratory flow (MMEF$_{25-75\% \text{ VC}}$) in relation to body height in boys and girls

Height cm	MMEF$_{25-75\% \text{ VC}}$, liters/s		
	mean	lower limits	upper limits
115	1.57	1.11	2.20
116	1.60	1.13	2.25
118	1.66	1.18	2.34
120	1.73	1.23	2.43
122	1.80	1.28	2.53
124	1.87	1.33	2.63
126	1.94	1.38	2.73
128	2.02	1.43	2.84
130	2.09	1.49	2.94
132	2.17	1.54	3.05
134	2.25	1.60	3.16
136	2.33	1.65	3.27
138	2.41	1.71	3.39
140	2.49	1.77	3.50
142	2.58	1.83	3.62
144	2.66	1.89	3.75
146	2.75	1.95	3.87
148	2.84	2.02	4.00
150	2.93	2.08	4.12
152	3.02	2.15	4.26
154	3.12	2.22	4.39
156	3.22	2.29	4.52
158	3.31	2.36	4.66
160	3.41	2.43	4.80
162	3.52	2.50	4.95
164	3.62	2.57	5.09
166	3.72	2.65	5.24
168	3.83	2.72	5.39
170	3.94	2.80	5.54
172	4.05	2.88	5.70
174	4.16	2.96	5.86
176	4.28	3.04	6.02
178	4.39	3.12	6.18
180	4.51	3.21	6.34

Formula: log y = a + b·log x;
y = MMEF$_{25-75\% \text{ VC}}$ (l/s); x = body height (cm);
log MMEF$_{25-75\% \text{ VC}}$ (l/s) = −4.6651 + 2.3588·log height (cm);
SD log y·x = ±0.0746; n = 108; r = +0.78.

Table 230. Maximum mid-expiratory flow (MMEF$_{25-75\% \text{ VC}}$) in relation to age in boys and girls

Age years	MMEF$_{25-75\% \text{ VC}}$, liters/s		
	mean	lower limits	upper limits
6	1.57	1.07	2.31
7	1.83	1.24	2.68
8	2.08	1.41	3.05
9	2.33	1.59	3.42
10	2.58	1.76	3.79
11	2.83	1.93	4.16
12	3.08	2.10	4.52
13	3.33	2.26	4.88
14	3.57	2.43	5.25
15	3.82	2.60	5.61
16	4.06	2.77	5.97
17	4.31	2.93	6.33

Formula: log y = a + b·log x;
y = MMEF$_{25-75\% \text{ VC}}$ (l/s); x = age (years);
log MMEF$_{25-75\% \text{ VC}}$ (l/s) = −0.5529 + 0.9654·log age (years);
SD log y·x = ±0.0840; n = 108; r = +0.72.

Table 231. Maximum mid-expiratory flow (MMEF$_{25-75\% \text{ VC}}$) in relation to body surface in boys and girls

Body surface m^2	MMEF$_{25-75\% \text{ VC}}$, liters/s		
	mean	lower limits	upper limits
0.6	1.15	0.82	1.61
0.7	1.39	0.99	1.94
0.8	1.63	1.17	2.28
0.9	1.88	1.35	2.62
1.0	2.13	1.53	2.98
1.1	2.39	1.71	3.34
1.2	2.66	1.90	3.71
1.3	2.93	2.10	4.08
1.4	3.20	2.29	4.47
1.5	3.48	2.49	4.85
1.6	3.76	2.69	5.24
1.7	4.04	2.89	5.64
1.8	4.33	3.10	6.04
1.9	4.62	3.31	6.45
2.0	4.91	3.52	6.86

Formula: log y = a + b·log x;
y = MMEF$_{25-75\% \text{ VC}}$ (l/s); x = body surface (m^2);
log MMEF$_{25-75\% \text{ VC}}$ (l/s) =
    0.3301 + 1.2013·log body surface (m^2);
SD log y·x = ±0.0729; n = 108; r = +0.79.

Table 232. Maximum mid-expiratory flow expressed per liter of TLC_{box} $\left(\frac{MMEF_{25-75\ \%\ VC}}{TLC_{box}}\right)$ in relation to body height in boys and girls

Height cm	$\frac{MMEF_{25-75\ \%\ VC}}{TLC_{box}}$ $\left(\frac{l/s}{l}\right)$		
	mean	lower limits	upper limits
115	0.800	0.535	1.064
116	0.799	0.535	1.063
118	0.798	0.533	1.062
120	0.796	0.532	1.061
122	0.795	0.531	1.060
124	0.794	0.530	1.058
126	0.793	0.528	1.057
128	0.791	0.527	1.056
130	0.790	0.526	1.054
132	0.789	0.524	1.053
134	0.788	0.523	1.052
136	0.786	0.522	1.051
138	0.785	0.521	1.049
140	0.784	0.519	1.048
142	0.782	0.518	1.047
144	0.781	0.517	1.046
146	0.780	0.516	1.044
148	0.779	0.514	1.043
150	0.777	0.513	1.042
152	0.776	0.512	1.040
154	0.775	0.510	1.039
156	0.774	0.509	1.038
158	0.772	0.508	1.037
160	0.771	0.507	1.035
162	0.770	0.505	1.034
164	0.768	0.504	1.033
166	0.767	0.503	1.032
168	0.766	0.501	1.030
170	0.765	0.500	1.029
172	0.763	0.499	1.028
174	0.762	0.498	1.026
176	0.761	0.496	1.025
178	0.760	0.495	1.024
180	0.758	0.494	1.023

Formula: $y = a + b \cdot x$;

$y = \frac{MMEF_{25-75\ \%\ VC}}{TLC_{box}}$ $\left(\frac{l/s}{l}\right)$; x = body height (cm);

$\frac{MMEF_{25-75\ \%\ VC}}{TLC_{box}}$ $\left(\frac{l/s}{l}\right) = 0.8734 - 0.00064 \cdot height\ (cm)$;

SD $y \cdot x = \pm 0.133$; n = 97; r = -0.19.

Table 233. Maximum mid-expiratory flow expressed per liter of FVC $\left(\frac{MMEF_{25-75\ \%\ VC}}{FVC}\right)$ in relation to body height in boys and girls

Height cm	$\frac{MMEF_{25-75\ \%\ VC}}{FVC}$ $\left(\frac{l/s}{l}\right)$		
	mean	lower limits	upper limits
115	1.202	0.821	1.583
116	1.198	0.817	1.579
118	1.190	0.809	1.572
120	1.183	0.802	1.564
122	1.175	0.794	1.556
124	1.167	0.786	1.549
126	1.160	0.779	1.541
128	1.152	0.771	1.534
130	1.144	0.763	1.526
132	1.137	0.756	1.518
134	1.129	0.748	1.510
136	1.120	0.740	1.503
138	1.111	0.733	1.494
140	1.106	0.725	1.487
142	1.099	0.717	1.480
144	1.091	0.710	1.472
146	1.083	0.702	1.464
148	1.076	0.694	1.457
150	1.068	0.687	1.449
152	1.060	0.679	1.442
154	1.053	0.671	1.434
156	1.045	0.664	1.426
158	1.037	0.656	1.419
160	1.030	0.649	1.411
162	1.022	0.641	1.403
164	1.014	0.633	1.396
166	1.007	0.626	1.388
168	0.999	0.618	1.380
170	0.991	0.610	1.373
172	0.984	0.603	1.365
174	0.976	5.595	1.357
176	0.969	0.587	1.350
178	0.961	0.580	1.342
180	0.953	0.572	1.334

Formula: $y = a + b \cdot x$;

$y = \frac{MMEF_{25-75\ \%\ VC}}{FVC}$ $\left(\frac{l/s}{l}\right)$; x = body height (cm);

$\frac{MMEF_{25-75\ \%\ VC}}{FVC}$ $\left(\frac{l/s}{l}\right) = 1.6422 - 0.00382 \cdot height\ (cm)$;

SD $y \cdot x = \pm 0.191$; n = 108; r = -0.26.

Table 234. Airway resistance at FRC level (Raw_{FRC}) in relation to FRC_{box} in boys and girls

FRC ml	Raw_{FRC}					
	mean		lower limits		upper limits	
	a	b	a	b	a	b
1,000	0.497	5.06	0.327	3.33	0.756	7.70
1.250	0.405	4.12	0.266	2.71	0.616	6.28
1,500	0.342	3.49	0.225	2.29	0.521	5.31
1,750	0.297	3.03	0.195	1.99	0.452	4.61
2,000	0.263	2.68	0.173	1.76	0.400	4.07
2,250	0.236	2.40	0.155	1.58	0.359	3.66
2,500	0.214	2.18	0.141	1.43	0.326	3.32
2,750	0.196	2.00	0.129	1.31	0.298	3.04
3,000	0.181	1.84	0.119	1.21	0.275	2.81
3,250	0.168	1.71	0.110	1.12	0.256	2.61
3,500	0.157	1.60	0.103	1.05	0.239	2.44

Formula: $\log y = a + b \cdot \log x$;
$y = Raw_{FRC}$ (kPa/l/s or cm H_2O/l/s); $x = FRC$ (ml);
$\log Raw_{FRC}$ (kPa/l/s) $= 2.45052 - 0.9180 \cdot \log FRC$ (ml);
SD $\log y \cdot x = \pm 0.0921$; $n = 149$; $r = -0.77$.
$\log Raw_{FRC}$ (cm H_2O/l/s) $= 3.4590 - 0.9180 \cdot \log x$;
$\log$ SD $y \cdot x = \pm 0.0921$.
a = kPa/l/s; b = cm H_2O/l/s.

Table 235. Airway conductance at FRC level (Gaw_{FRC}) in relation to FRC_{box} in boys and girls

FRC ml	Gaw_{FRC}					
	mean		lower limits		upper limits	
	a	b	a	b	a	b
1,000	2.159	0.211	0.639	0.062	3.679	0.360
1,100	2.330	0.229	0.810	0.078	3.850	0.380
1,200	2.500	0.245	0.980	0.095	4.020	0.394
1,300	2.671	0.261	1.151	0.111	4.191	0.411
1,400	2.841	0.278	1.322	0.129	4.361	0.427
1,500	3.012	0.295	1.492	0.144	4.532	0.445
1,600	3.182	0.312	1.663	0.162	4.702	0.461
1,700	3.353	0.328	1.833	0.178	4.873	0.479
1,800	3.523	0.345	2.004	0.196	5.043	0.494
1,900	3.694	0.362	2.174	0.211	5.214	0.513
2,000	3.864	0.378	2.345	0.229	5.384	0.528
2,100	4.035	0.395	2.515	0.244	5.555	0.546
2,200	4.206	0.412	2.686	0.263	5.725	0.561
2,300	4.376	0.429	2.856	0.278	5.896	0.579
2,400	4.547	0.445	3.027	0.296	6.066	0.594
2,500	4.717	0.462	3.197	0.311	6.237	0.613
2,600	4.888	0.479	3.368	0.330	6.407	0.628
2,700	5.058	0.496	3.538	0.345	6.578	0.646
2,800	5.229	0.512	3.709	0.363	6.748	0.661
2,900	5.399	0.529	3.879	0.378	6.919	0.680
3,000	5.570	0.546	4.050	0.397	7.090	0.695
3,100	5.740	0.562	4.220	0.412	7.260	0.713
3,200	5.911	0.579	4.391	0.428	7.431	0.730
3,300	6.081	0.596	4.562	0.445	7.601	0.747
3,400	6.252	0.613	4.732	0.462	7.772	0.763
3,500	6.422	0.629	4.903	0.478	7.942	0.780

Formula: $y = a + b \cdot x$;
$y = Gaw_{FRC}$ (l/s/kPa or l/s/cm H_2O); $x = FRC$ (ml);
Gaw_{FRC} (l/s/kPa) $= 0.45438 + 1.70527 \cdot 10^{-3} \cdot FRC$ (ml);
SD $y \cdot x = \pm 0.769$; $n = 149$; $r = +0.77$.
Gaw_{FRC} (l/s/cm H_2O) $= 0.04456 + 0.16723 \cdot 10^{-3} \cdot x$;
SD $y \cdot x = \pm 0.0754$.
a = l/s/kPa; b = l/s/cm H_2O.

Table 236. Airway resistance at FRC level (Raw$_{FRC}$) in relation to body height in boys and girls

Height cm	Raw$_{FRC}$ mean		lower limits		upper limits	
	a	b	a	b	a	b
115	0.566	5.77	0.375	3.82	0.853	8.70
116	0.553	5.64	0.367	3.74	0.834	8.50
118	0.529	5.39	0.350	3.57	0.797	8.13
120	0.505	5.15	0.335	3.42	0.762	7.77
122	0.484	4.93	0.321	3.27	0.729	7.44
124	0.463	4.72	0.307	3.13	0.699	7.12
126	0.444	4.53	0.294	3.00	0.669	6.83
128	0.426	4.34	0.282	2.88	0.642	6.55
130	0.409	4.16	0.271	2.76	0.616	6.28
132	0.392	4.00	0.260	2.65	0.592	6.03
134	0.377	3.84	0.250	2.55	0.568	5.80
136	0.362	3.69	0.240	2.45	0.546	5.57
138	0.349	3.55	0.231	2.35	0.526	5.36
140	0.335	3.42	0.222	2.27	0.506	5.16
142	0.323	3.29	0.214	2.18	0.487	4.97
144	0.311	3.17	0.206	2.10	0.469	4.79
146	0.300	3.06	0.199	2.03	0.453	4.61
148	0.289	2.95	0.192	1.95	0.436	4.45
150	0.279	2.85	0.185	1.89	0.421	4.29
152	0.270	2.75	0.179	1.82	0.407	4.15
154	0.260	2.65	0.173	1.76	0.393	4.00
156	0.252	2.56	0.167	1.70	0.379	3.87
158	0.243	2.48	0.161	1.64	0.367	3.74
160	0.235	2.40	0.156	1.59	0.355	3.62
162	0.228	2.32	0.151	1.54	0.343	3.50
164	0.220	2.24	0.146	1.49	0.332	3.39
166	0.213	2.17	0.141	1.44	0.322	3.28
168	0.207	2.11	0.137	1.39	0.312	3.18
170	0.200	2.04	0.133	1.35	0.302	3.08
172	0.194	1.98	0.129	1.31	0.293	2.98
174	0.188	1.92	0.125	1.27	0.284	2.89
176	0.182	1.86	0.121	1.23	0.275	2.81
178	0.177	1.80	0.117	1.20	0.267	2.72
180	0.172	1.75	0.114	1.16	0.259	2.64

Formula: log y = a + b·log x;
y = Raw$_{FRC}$ (kPa/l/s or cm H$_2$O/l/s); x = body height (cm);
log Raw$_{FRC}$ (kPa/l/s) = 5.22592 − 2.6558·log height (cm);
SD log y·x = ±0.0902; n = 149; r = −0.78.
log Raw$_{FRC}$ (cm H$_2$O/l/s) = 6.2344 − 2.6558·log x;
SD log y·x = ±0.0902.
a = kPa/l/s; b = cm H$_2$O/l/s.

Table 237. Airway resistance at FRC level (Raw$_{FRC}$) in relation to age in boys and girls

Age years	Raw$_{FRC}$ mean		lower limits		upper limits	
	a	b	a	b	a	b
6	0.559	5.70	0.347	3.54	0.900	9.18
7	0.473	4.82	0.294	3.00	0.762	7.77
8	0.409	4.17	0.254	2.59	0.659	6.72
9	0.360	3.67	0.224	2.28	0.580	5.91
10	0.321	3.28	0.200	2.03	0.517	5.28
11	0.290	2.95	0.180	1.83	0.467	4.76
12	0.264	2.69	0.164	1.67	0.425	4.33
13	0.242	2.46	0.150	1.53	0.389	3.97
14	0.223	2.27	0.138	1.41	0.359	3.66
15	0.207	2.11	0.128	1.31	0.333	3.40
16	0.193	1.97	0.120	1.22	0.311	3.17
17	0.181	1.84	0.112	1.14	0.291	2.97

Formula: log y = a + b·log x;
y = Raw$_{FRC}$ (kPa/l/s or cm H$_2$O/l/s); x = age (years);
log Raw$_{FRC}$ (kPa/l/s) = 0.59092 − 1.0833·log age (years);
SD log y·x = ±0.1045; n = 149; r = −0.69.
log Raw$_{FRC}$ (cm H$_2$O/l/s) = 1.5994 − 1.0833·log x;
SD log y·x = ±0.1045.
a = kPa/l/s; b = cm H$_2$O/l/s.

Table 238. Airway resistance at FRC level (Raw$_{FRC}$) in relation to body surface in boys and girls

Body surface m^2	Raw$_{FRC}$ mean		lower limits		upper limits	
	a	b	a	b	a	b
0.6	0.726	7.40	0.463	4.72	1.137	11.60
0.7	0.601	6.13	0.383	3.91	0.941	9.60
0.8	0.510	5.20	0.325	3.32	0.798	8.14
0.9	0.441	4.50	0.281	2.87	0.691	7.05
1.0	0.387	3.95	0.247	2.52	0.607	6.19
1.1	0.344	3.51	0.220	2.24	0.540	5.50
1.2	0.309	3.16	0.197	2.01	0.485	4.95
1.3	0.280	2.86	0.179	1.82	0.439	4.48
1.4	0.256	2.61	0.163	1.66	0.401	4.09
1.5	0.235	2.40	0.150	1.53	0.368	3.76
1.6	0.217	2.21	0.138	1.41	0.340	3.47
1.7	0.201	2.05	0.128	1.31	0.316	3.22
1.8	0.188	1.91	0.120	1.22	0.294	3.00
1.9	0.176	1.79	0.112	1.14	0.275	2.81
2.0	0.165	1.68	0.105	1.07	0.259	2.64

Formula: log y = a + b·log x;
y = Raw$_{FRC}$ (kPa/l/s or cm H$_2$O/l/s); x = body surface (m^2);
log Raw$_{FRC}$ (kPa/l/s) =
    −0.41148 − 1.2293·log body surface (m^2);
SD log y·x = ±0.0986; n = 149; r = −0.73.
log Raw$_{FRC}$ (cm H$_2$O/l/s) = 0.5970 − 1.2293·log x;
SD log y·x = ±0.0986.
a = kPa/l/s; b = cm H$_2$O/l/s.

Table 239. Airway conductance at FRC level (Gaw_{FRC}) in relation to body height in boys and girls

Height cm	Gaw_{FRC}					
	mean		lower limits		upper limits	
	a	b	a	b	a	b
115	1.769	0.173	1.177	0.115	2.659	0.260
116	1.810	0.177	1.205	0.118	2.721	0.266
118	1.894	0.185	1.260	0.123	2.847	0.279
120	1.981	0.194	1.318	0.129	2.977	0.292
122	2.069	0.202	1.377	0.135	3.110	0.305
124	2.160	0.211	1.438	0.140	3.247	0.318
126	2.254	0.221	1.500	0.147	3.387	0.332
128	2.350	0.230	1.564	0.153	3.532	0.346
130	2.449	0.240	1.629	0.159	3.680	0.361
132	2.550	0.250	1.697	0.166	3.832	0.375
134	2.653	0.260	1.766	0.173	3.988	0.391
136	2.760	0.270	1.836	0.180	4.147	0.406
138	2.869	0.281	1.909	0.187	4.311	0.422
140	2.980	0.292	1.983	0.194	4.478	0.439
142	3.094	0.303	2.059	0.201	4.650	0.456
144	3.211	0.314	2.137	0.209	4.826	0.473
146	3.331	0.326	2.216	0.217	5.005	0.491
148	3.453	0.338	2.298	0.225	5.189	0.509
150	3.578	0.350	2.381	0.233	5.377	0.527
152	3.706	0.363	2.466	0.241	5.569	0.546
154	3.836	0.376	2.553	0.250	5.765	0.565
156	3.970	0.389	2.642	0.259	5.966	0.585
158	4.106	0.402	2.732	0.267	6.171	0.605
160	4.245	0.416	2.825	0.276	6.380	0.625
162	4.387	0.430	2.919	0.286	6.593	0.646
164	4.532	0.444	3.016	0.295	6.811	0.668
166	4.680	0.459	3.114	0.305	7.034	0.690
168	4.831	0.473	3.215	0.315	7.260	0.712
170	4.985	0.488	3.317	0.325	7.492	0.734
172	5.142	0.504	3.422	0.335	7.727	0.758
174	5.302	0.520	3.528	0.345	7.968	0.781
176	5.465	0.536	3.637	0.356	8.213	0.805
178	5.631	0.552	3.747	0.367	8.463	0.830
180	5.801	0.568	3.860	0.378	8.717	0.855

Formula: $\log y = a + b \cdot \log x$;
$y = Gaw_{FRC}$ (l/s/kPa or l/s/cm H_2O); x = body height (cm);
$\log Gaw_{FRC}$ (l/s/kPa) = $-5.21252 + 2.6498 \cdot \log$ height (cm);
SD $\log y \cdot x = \pm 0.0895$; n = 149; r = +0.78.
$\log Gaw_{FRC}$ (l/s/cm H_2O) = $-6.2210 + 2.6498 \cdot \log x$;
SD $\log y \cdot x = \pm 0.0895$.
a = l/s/kPa; b = l/s/cm H_2O.

Table 240. Airway conductance at FRC level (Gaw_{FRC}) in relation to age in boys and girls

Age years	Gaw_{FRC}					
	mean		lower limits		upper limits	
	a	b	a	b	a	b
6	1.789	0.175	1.116	0.109	2.868	0.281
7	2.114	0.207	1.319	0.129	3.389	0.332
8	2.443	0.239	1.524	0.149	3.916	0.384
9	2.775	0.272	1.731	0.169	4.448	0.436
10	3.110	0.304	1.940	0.190	4.985	0.489
11	3.448	0.338	2.150	0.210	5.527	0.542
12	3.788	0.371	2.363	0.231	6.072	0.595
13	4.131	0.405	2.577	0.252	6.622	0.649
14	4.475	0.438	2.792	0.273	7.174	0.703
15	4.822	0.472	3.008	0.294	7.731	0.758
16	5.171	0.507	3.226	0.316	8.290	0.813
17	5.522	0.541	3.444	0.337	8.852	0.868

Formula: $\log y = a + b \cdot \log x$;
$y = Gaw_{FRC}$ (l/s/kPa or l/s/cm H_2O); x = age (years);
$\log Gaw_{FRC}$ (l/s/kPa) = $-0.58912 + 1.0819 \cdot \log$ age (years);
SD $\log y \cdot x = \pm 0.1037$; n = 149; r = +0.69.
$\log Gaw_{FRC}$ (l/s/cm H_2O) = $-1.5976 + 1.0819 \cdot \log x$;
SD $\log y \cdot x = \pm 0.1037$.
a = l/s/kPa; b = l/s/cm H_2O.

Table 241. Airway conductance at FRC level (Gaw_{FRC}) in relation to body surface in boys and girls

Body surface m²	Gaw_{FRC}					
	mean		lower limits		upper limits	
	a	b	a	b	a	b
0.6	1.380	0.135	0.884	0.086	2.154	0.211
0.7	1.667	0.163	1.068	0.104	2.603	0.255
0.8	1.964	0.192	1.258	0.123	3.066	0.300
0.9	2.269	0.222	1.453	0.142	3.543	0.347
1.0	2.582	0.253	1.654	0.162	4.032	0.395
1.1	2.903	0.284	1.859	0.182	4.532	0.444
1.2	3.229	0.316	2.068	0.202	5.042	0.494
1.3	3.563	0.349	2.282	0.223	5.563	0.545
1.4	3.902	0.382	2.499	0.244	6.092	0.597
1.5	4.246	0.416	2.720	0.266	6.630	0.650
1.6	4.596	0.450	2.944	0.288	7.176	0.704
1.7	4.951	0.485	3.171	0.310	7.730	0.758
1.8	5.311	0.520	3.401	0.333	8.292	0.813
1.9	5.675	0.556	3.635	0.356	8.860	0.869
2.0	6.043	0.592	3.871	0.379	9.436	0.925

Formula: $\log y = a + b \cdot \log x$;
$y = Gaw_{FRC}$ (l/s/kPa or l/s/cm H_2O); x = body surface (m²);
$\log Gaw_{FRC}$ (l/s/kPa) =
    $0.41207 + 1.2266 \cdot \log$ body surface (m²);
SD $\log y \cdot x = \pm 0.0979$; n = 149; r = +0.73.
$\log Gaw_{FRC}$ (l/s/cm H_2O) = $-0.5964 + 1.2266 \cdot \log x$;
SD $\log y \cdot x = \pm 0.0979$.
a = l/s/kPa; b = l/s/cm H_2O.

Table 242. Lung (pulmonary) resistance (R_L) in relation to body height in boys and girls

Height cm	R_L mean a	b	lower limits a	b	upper limits a	b
115	0.5533	5.64	0.3006	3.06	1.0185	10.38
116	0.5413	5.51	0.2941	2.99	0.9964	10.16
118	0.5184	5.28	0.2816	2.87	0.9543	9.73
120	0.4969	5.06	0.2699	2.75	0.9146	9.32
122	0.4766	4.85	0.2589	2.63	0.8772	8.94
124	0.4574	4.66	0.2485	2.53	0.8419	8.58
126	0.4393	4.47	0.2386	2.43	0.8086	8.24
128	0.4221	4.30	0.2293	2.33	0.7770	7.92
130	0.4059	4.13	0.2205	2.24	0.7472	7.61
132	0.3905	3.98	0.2122	2.16	0.7189	7.33
134	0.3760	3.83	0.2043	2.08	0.6921	7.05
136	0.3622	3.69	0.1967	2.00	0.6667	6.79
138	0.3490	3.55	0.1896	1.93	0.6425	6.55
140	0.3366	3.43	0.1829	1.86	0.6196	6.31
142	0.3247	3.31	0.1764	1.79	0.5978	6.09
144	0.3135	3.19	0.1703	1.73	0.5770	5.88
146	0.3027	3.08	0.1645	1.67	0.5572	5.68
148	0.2925	2.98	0.1589	1.61	0.5384	5.49
150	0.2827	2.88	0.1536	1.56	0.5205	5.30
152	0.2734	2.78	0.1485	1.51	0.5033	5.13
154	0.2646	2.69	0.1437	1.46	0.4870	4.96
156	0.2561	2.61	0.1391	1.41	0.4714	4.80
158	0.2480	2.52	0.1347	1.37	0.4564	4.65
160	0.2402	2.44	0.1305	1.33	0.4421	4.50
162	0.2328	2.37	0.1265	1.28	0.4285	4.36
164	0.2257	2.30	0.1226	1.24	0.4154	4.23
166	0.2189	2.23	0.1189	1.21	0.4029	4.10
168	0.2123	2.16	0.1154	1.17	0.3909	3.98
170	0.2061	2.10	0.1120	1.14	0.3793	3.86
172	0.2001	2.03	0.1087	1.10	0.3683	3.75
174	0.1943	1.98	0.1056	1.07	0.3577	3.64
176	0.1888	1.92	0.1026	1.04	0.3475	3.54
178	0.1835	1.87	0.0997	1.01	0.3377	3.44
180	0.1784	1.81	0.0969	0.98	0.3283	3.34

Formula: $\log y = a + b \cdot \log x$;
$y = R_L$ (kPa/l/s or cm H_2O/l/s); x = body height (cm);
$\log R_L$ (kPa/l/s) = $4.94972 - 2.5267 \cdot \log$ height (cm);
SD $\log y \cdot x = \pm 0.1337$; n = 111; r = -0.64.
$\log R_L$ (cm H_2O/l/s) = $5.9582 - 2.5267 \cdot \log x$;
SD $\log y \cdot x = \pm 0.1337$.
a = kPa/l/s; b = cm H_2O/l/s.

Table 243. Pulmonary resistance (R_p) in relation to age in boys and girls

Age years	R_p mean a	b	lower limits a	b	upper limits a	b
6	0.5689	5.80	0.2996	3.05	1.0802	11.01
7	0.4804	4.89	0.2530	2.57	0.9121	9.30
8	0.4149	4.23	0.2185	2.22	0.7878	8.03
9	0.3646	3.71	0.1920	1.95	0.6923	7.06
10	0.3248	3.31	0.1711	1.74	0.6167	6.28
11	0.2926	2.98	0.1541	1.57	0.5555	5.66
12	0.2659	2.71	0.1400	1.42	0.5049	5.14
13	0.2436	2.48	0.1283	1.30	0.4625	4.71
14	0.2245	2.28	0.1183	1.20	0.4263	4.34
15	0.2082	2.12	0.1096	1.11	0.3953	4.03
16	0.1939	1.97	0.1021	1.04	0.3682	3.75
17	0.1815	1.84	0.0956	0.97	0.3445	3.51

Formula: $\log y = a + b \cdot \log x$;
$y = R_p$ (kPa/l/s or cm H_2O/l/s); x = age (years);
$\log R_p$ (kPa/l/s) = $0.60882 - 1.0972 \cdot \log$ age (years);
SD $\log y \cdot x = \pm 0.1405$; n = 111; r = -0.59.
$\log R_p$ (cm H_2O/l/s) = $1.6173 - 1.0972 \cdot x$;
SD $\log y \cdot x = \pm 0.1405$.
a = kPa/l/s; b = cm H_2O/l/s.

Table 244. Pulmonary resistance (R_p) in relation to body surface in boys and girls

Body surface m²	R_p mean a	b	lower limits a	b	upper limits a	b
0.6	0.7263	7.40	0.3876	3.95	1.3609	13.87
0.7	0.6030	6.14	0.3218	3.28	1.1299	11.52
0.8	0.5132	5.23	0.2739	2.79	0.9617	9.80
0.9	0.4452	4.53	0.2376	2.42	0.8342	8.50
1.0	0.3920	3.99	0.2092	2.13	0.7346	7.49
1.1	0.3494	3.56	0.1865	1.90	0.6548	6.67
1.2	0.3146	3.20	0.1679	1.71	0.5895	6.01
1.3	0.2856	2.91	0.1524	1.55	0.5352	5.45
1.4	0.2612	2.66	0.1394	1.42	0.4894	4.99
1.5	0.2403	2.45	0.1282	1.30	0.4503	4.59
1.6	0.2223	2.26	0.1186	1.20	0.4165	4.24
1.7	0.2066	2.10	0.1103	1.12	0.3871	3.94
1.8	0.1928	1.96	0.1029	1.04	0.3613	3.68
1.9	0.1806	1.84	0.0964	0.98	0.3385	3.45
2.0	0.1698	1.73	0.0906	0.92	0.3182	3.24

Formula: $\log y = a + b \cdot \log x$;
$y = R_p$ (kPa/l/s or cm H_2O/l/s); x = body surface (m²);
$\log R_p$ (kPa/l/s) = $-0.40668 - 1.2071 \cdot \log$ body surface (m²);
SD $\log y \cdot x = \pm 0.1376$; n = 111; r = -0.62.
$\log R_p$ (cm H_2O/l/s) = $0.6018 - 1.2071 \cdot \log x$;
SD $\log y \cdot x = \pm 0.1376$.
a = kPa/l/s; b = cm H_2O/l/s.

Table 245. Airway resistance in middle of tidal volume (at isovolume level) (Raw_{in-ex}) in relation to body height in boys and girls

Height cm	Raw_{in-ex}					
	mean		lower limits		upper limits	
	a	b	a	b	a	b
115	0.493	5.03	0.324	3.30	0.750	7.65
116	0.482	4.92	0.317	3.23	0.733	7.48
118	0.462	4.71	0.303	3.08	0.702	7.19
120	0.442	4.51	0.291	2.96	0.672	6.86
122	0.424	4.32	0.279	2.84	0.644	6.57
124	0.406	4.14	0.267	2.72	0.618	6.30
126	0.390	3.98	0.256	2.61	0.593	6.05
128	0.375	3.82	0.246	2.51	0.570	5.81
130	0.360	3.67	0.237	2.41	0.547	5.58
132	0.346	3.53	0.228	2.32	0.526	5.37
134	0.333	3.39	0.219	2.23	0.506	5.17
136	0.321	3.27	0.211	2.15	0.488	4.97
138	0.309	3.15	0.203	2.07	0.470	4.79
140	0.298	3.03	0.196	1.99	0.453	4.62
142	0.287	2.92	0.189	1.92	0.436	4.45
144	0.277	2.82	0.182	1.85	0.421	4.29
146	0.267	2.72	0.176	1.79	0.406	4.14
148	0.258	2.63	0.170	1.73	0.392	4.00
150	0.249	2.54	0.164	1.67	0.379	3.87
152	0.241	2.46	0.158	1.61	0.366	3.74
154	0.233	2.37	0.153	1.56	0.354	3.61
156	0.225	2.30	0.148	1.51	0.343	3.50
158	0.218	2.22	0.143	1.46	0.332	3.38
160	0.211	2.15	0.139	1.41	0.321	3.28
162	0.204	2.08	0.134	1.37	0.311	3.17
164	0.198	2.02	0.130	1.33	0.301	3.07
166	0.192	1.96	0.126	1.29	0.292	2.98
168	0.186	1.90	0.122	1.25	0.283	2.89
170	0.181	1.84	0.119	1.21	0.275	2.80
172	0.175	1.79	0.115	1.17	0.267	2.72
174	0.170	1.73	0.112	1.14	0.259	2.64
176	0.165	1.68	0.109	1.11	0.251	2.56
178	0.160	1.64	0.105	1.07	0.244	2.49
180	0.156	1.59	0.102	1.04	0.237	2.42

Formula: $\log y = a + b \cdot \log x$;
$y = Raw_{in-ex}$ (kPa/l/s or cm H_2O/l/s); x = body height (cm);
$\log Raw_{in-ex}$ (kPa/l/s) =
    $4.98032 - 2.5656 \cdot \log$ body height (cm);
SD $\log y \cdot x = \pm 0.0920$; n = 140; r = -0.77.
$\log Raw_{in-ex}$ (cm H_2O/l/s) = $5.9888 - 2.5656 \cdot \log x$;
SD $\log y \cdot x = \pm 0.0920$.
a = kPa/l/s; b = cm H_2O/l/s.

Table 246. Nitrogen washout time for 2% nitrogen concentration ($t_{2\% N_2}$) in expired gas in relation to body height in boys and girls

Height cm	$t_{2\% N_2}$, s		
	mean	lower limits	upper limits
114	64.99	–	139.96
116	67.16	–	142.12
118	69.32	–	144.28
120	71.48	–	146.45
122	73.65	–	148.61
124	75.81	0.84	150.78
126	77.97	3.01	152.78
128	80.14	5.17	155.10
130	82.30	7.33	157.27
132	84.46	9.50	159.43
134	86.63	11.66	161.59
136	88.79	13.82	163.76
138	90.95	15.99	165.92
140	93.12	18.15	168.08
142	95.28	20.31	170.25
144	97.44	22.48	172.41
146	99.61	24.64	174.57
148	101.77	26.80	176.74
150	103.94	28.97	178.30
152	106.10	31.13	181.06
154	108.26	33.30	183.23
156	110.43	35.46	185.39
158	112.59	37.62	187.56
160	114.75	39.79	189.72
162	116.92	41.95	191.88
164	119.08	44.11	194.04
166	121.24	46.28	196.21
168	123.41	48.44	198.37
170	125.57	50.60	200.59
172	127.73	52.77	202.70
174	129.90	54.93	204.86
176	132.06	57.09	207.03
178	134.22	59.26	209.19
180	136.39	61.42	211.35
182	138.55	63.58	213.52

Formula: $y = a + b \cdot x$;
$y = t_{2\% N_2}$ (s); x = body height (cm);
$t_{2\% N_2}$ (s) = $-58.3244 + 1.08176 \cdot$ height;
SD $y \cdot x = \pm 37.4832$; n = 86; r = +0.42.

Table 247. Nitrogen washout volume by oxygen for 2% nitrogen concentration ($V_{O_2i} - 2\% N_2$) in expired gas in relation to body height in boys and girls

Height cm	$V_{O_2i} - 2\% N_2$, liters		
	mean	lower limits	upper limits
114	8.65	1.44	15.87
116	9.08	1.86	16.30
118	9.51	2.29	16.72
120	9.93	2.71	17.14
122	10.36	3.14	17.57
124	10.78	3.57	18.00
126	11.21	3.99	18.42
128	11.64	4.42	18.85
130	12.06	4.84	19.27
132	12.49	5.27	19.70
134	12.91	5.70	20.13
136	13.34	6.12	20.55
138	13.77	6.55	20.97
140	14.19	6.97	21.40
142	14.62	7.40	21.83
144	15.04	7.83	22.26
146	15.47	8.25	22.68
148	15.90	8.68	23.11
150	16.32	9.10	23.53
152	16.75	9.53	23.95
154	17.17	9.96	24.39
156	17.60	10.38	24.81
158	18.03	10.81	25.24
160	18.45	11.23	25.66
162	18.88	11.66	26.10
164	19.30	12.09	26.52
166	19.73	13.73	26.95
168	20.16	12.94	27.37
170	20.58	13.36	27.80
172	21.01	13.79	28.23
174	21.34	14.22	28.65
176	21.86	14.64	29.08
178	22.29	15.07	29.50
180	22.71	15.49	29.93
182	23.14	15.92	30.36

Formula: $y = a + b \cdot x$;
$y = V_{O_2i} - 2\% N_2$ (l); x = body height (cm);
$V_{O_2i} - 2\% N_2$ (l) = $-15.6253 + 0.21301 \cdot$ body height (cm);
SD $y \cdot x = \pm 3.6088$; n = 86; r = +0.68.

Table 248. Nitrogen washout volume by oxygen for 2% nitrogen concentration in expired gas per liter of FRC ($V_{O_2}/FRC_{2\% N_2}$) (lung clearance index of Becklake) in relation to body height in boys and girls

Height cm	$V_{O_2}/FRC_{2\% N_2}$, l/l		
	mean	lower limits	upper limits
114	10.52	5.92	15.12
116	10.42	5.82	15.02
118	10.32	5.72	14.92
120	10.22	5.62	14.81
122	10.12	5.52	14.71
124	10.02	5.42	14.61
126	9.92	5.32	14.51
128	9.82	5.22	14.41
130	9.72	5.12	14.31
132	9.62	5.02	14.21
134	9.52	4.92	14.11
136	9.42	4.82	14.01
138	9.32	4.72	13.91
140	9.22	4.62	13.81
142	9.12	4.52	13.71
144	9.02	4.42	13.61
146	8.92	4.32	13.51
148	8.82	4.22	13.41
150	8.72	4.12	13.31
152	8.62	4.02	13.21
154	8.52	3.92	13.11
156	8.42	3.82	13.01
158	8.32	3.72	12.91
160	8.22	3.62	12.81
162	8.12	3.52	12.71
164	8.02	3.42	12.61
166	7.92	3.32	12.51
168	7.82	3.22	12.41
170	7.72	3.12	12.31
172	7.62	3.02	12.21
174	7.52	2.92	12.11
176	7.42	2.82	12.01
178	7.32	2.72	11.91
180	7.22	2.62	11.81
182	7.12	2.52	11.71

Formula: $y = a + b \cdot x$;
$y = V_{O_2}/FRC_{2\% N_2}$ (l/l); x = body height (cm);
$V_{O_2}/FRC_{2\% N_2}$ (l/l) = $16.2403 - 0.05013 \cdot$ body height (cm);
SD $y \cdot x = \pm 2.2979$; n = 81; r = -0.32.

Table 249. Total work of breathing (W_{tot}) in relation to body height in boys and girls

Height cm	W_{tot} mean		lower limits		upper limits	
	a	b	a	b	a	b
115	0.4865	0.0497	0.3577	0.0365	0.6152	0.0629
116	0.4818	0.0491	0.3530	0.0360	0.6106	0.0622
120	0.4632	0.0472	0.3344	0.0341	0.5919	0.0603
124	0.4445	0.0453	0.3157	0.0322	0.5733	0.0584
128	0.4259	0.0434	0.2971	0.0302	0.5546	0.0565
132	0.4072	0.0415	0.2784	0.0283	0.5360	0.0546
136	0.3886	0.0396	0.2598	0.0264	0.5173	0.0527
140	0.3699	0.0377	0.2411	0.0245	0.4987	0.0508
144	0.3513	0.0358	0.2225	0.0226	0.4800	0.0489
148	0.3326	0.0339	0.2038	0.0207	0.4614	0.0470
152	0.3140	0.0320	0.1852	0.0188	0.4427	0.0451
156	0.2953	0.0301	0.1665	0.0169	0.4241	0.0432
160	0.2767	0.0282	0.1479	0.0150	0.4054	0.0413
164	0.2580	0.0263	0.1292	0.0131	0.3868	0.0394
168	0.2394	0.0244	0.1106	0.0112	0.3681	0.0375
172	0.2207	0.0225	0.0919	0.0093	0.3495	0.0356
176	0.2021	0.0206	0.0733	0.0074	0.3308	0.0337
180	0.1834	0.0187	0.0547	0.0055	0.3122	0.0318
182	0.1741	0.0177	0.0451	0.0045	0.3031	0.0309

Formula: $y = a + b \cdot x$;
$y = W_{tot}$ (J/l or kpm/l); x = body height (cm);
W_{tot} (J/l) $= 1.02263 - 4.66225 \cdot 10^{-3} \cdot x$;
SD $y \cdot x = \pm 6.4498 \cdot 10^{-2}$; n = 73; r = -0.78.
W_{tot} (kpm/l) $= 0.10428 - 0.47542 \cdot 10^{-3} \cdot x$;
SD $y \cdot x = \pm 0.6577 \cdot 10^{-2}$.
a = J/l; b = kpm/l.

Table 251. Elastic work of breathing (W_{el}) in relation to body height in boys and girls

Height cm	W_{el} mean		lower limits		upper limits	
	a	b	a	b	a	b
115	0.2989	0.0304	0.1934	0.0197	0.4043	0.0411
116	0.2962	0.0302	0.1907	0.0194	0.4017	0.0409
120	0.2856	0.0291	0.1801	0.0183	0.3911	0.0398
124	0.2750	0.0280	0.1695	0.0172	0.3805	0.0388
128	0.2645	0.0269	0.1590	0.0162	0.3700	0.0377
132	0.2539	0.0258	0.1484	0.0152	0.3594	0.0366
136	0.2433	0.0248	0.1378	0.0140	0.3488	0.0355
140	0.2327	0.0237	0.1272	0.0129	0.3382	0.0344
144	0.2221	0.0226	0.1166	0.0118	0.3276	0.0334
148	0.2115	0.0215	0.1060	0.0108	0.3170	0.0323
152	0.2010	0.0204	0.0955	0.0097	0.3065	0.0312
156	0.1904	0.0194	0.0849	0.0086	0.2959	0.0301
160	0.1798	0.0183	0.0743	0.0075	0.2853	0.0290
164	0.1692	0.0172	0.0637	0.0065	0.2747	0.0280
168	0.1586	0.0161	0.0531	0.0054	0.2641	0.0269
172	0.1480	0.0151	0.0426	0.0043	0.2535	0.0258
176	0.1375	0.0140	0.0320	0.0032	0.2430	0.0247
180	0.1269	0.0129	0.0214	0.0021	0.2324	0.0237
182	0.1216	0.0124	0.0161	0.0016	0.2271	0.0232

Formula: $y = a + b \cdot x$;
$y = W_{el}$ (J/l or kpm/l); x = body height (cm);
W_{el} (J/l) $= 0.60311 - 2.64572 \cdot 10^{-3} \cdot x$;
SD $y \cdot x = \pm 5.2838 \cdot 10^{-2}$; n = 73; r = -0.65.
W_{el} (kpm/l) $= 0.06150 - 0.26979 \cdot 10^{-3} \cdot x$;
SD $y \cdot x = \pm 0.5388 \cdot 10^{-2}$.
a = J/l; b = kpm/l.

Table 250. Total work of breathing (W_{tot}) in relation to age in boys and girls

Age years	W_{tot} mean		lower limits		upper limits	
	a	b	a	b	a	b
6	0.4080	0.0416	0.2436	0.0248	0.5725	0.0583
8	0.3800	0.0387	0.2155	0.0219	0.5445	0.0555
10	0.3519	0.0358	0.1875	0.0191	0.5164	0.0526
12	0.3239	0.0330	0.1594	0.0162	0.4884	0.0498
14	0.2958	0.0301	0.1314	0.0133	0.4603	0.0469
16	0.2678	0.0273	0.1033	0.0185	0.4323	0.0440
18	0.2398	0.0244	0.0753	0.0076	0.4042	0.0412
20	0.2117	0.0215	0.0472	0.0048	0.3762	0.0383
22	0.1837	0.0187	0.0192	0.0019	0.3481	0.0355
24	0.1556	0.0158	–	–	0.3201	0.0326
26	0.1276	0.0130	–	–	0.2920	0.0297

Formula: $y = a + b \cdot x$;
$y = W_{tot}$ (J/l or kpm/l); x = age (years);
W_{tot} (J/l) $= 0.49219 - 1.40244 \cdot 10^{-2} \cdot x$;
SD $y \cdot x = \pm 8.23857 \cdot 10^{-2}$; n = 73; r = -0.60.
W_{tot} (kpm/l) $= 0.05019 - 0.14301 \cdot 10^{-2} \cdot x$;
SD $y \cdot x = \pm 0.8401 \cdot 10^{-2}$.
a = J/l; b = kpm/l.

Table 252. Elastic work of breathing (W_{el}) in relation to age in boys and girls

Age years	W_{el} mean		lower limits		upper limits	
	a	b	a	b	a	b
6	0.2533	0.0258	0.1320	0.0134	0.3746	0.0381
8	0.2377	0.0242	0.1165	0.0118	0.3590	0.0366
10	0.2221	0.0226	0.1009	0.0102	0.3434	0.0350
12	0.2065	0.0210	0.0853	0.0086	0.3278	0.0334
14	0.1909	0.0194	0.0697	0.0071	0.3122	0.0318
16	0.1753	0.0178	0.0541	0.0055	0.2966	0.0302
18	0.1597	0.0162	0.0385	0.0039	0.2810	0.0286
20	0.1442	0.0147	0.0229	0.0023	0.2654	0.0270
22	0.1286	0.0131	0.0073	0.0007	0.2498	0.0254
24	0.1130	0.0115	–	–	0.2342	0.0238
26	0.0974	0.0099	–	–	0.2188	0.0222

Formula: $y = a + b \cdot x$;
$y = W_{el}$ (J/l or kpm/l); x = age (years);
W_{el} (J/l) $= 0.30008 - 7.79644 \cdot 10^{-3} \cdot x$;
SD $y \cdot x = \pm 6.0732 \cdot 10^{-2}$; n = 73; r = -0.49.
W_{el} (kpm/l) $= 0.03060 - 0.79502 \cdot 10^{-3} \cdot x$;
SD $y \cdot x = \pm 0.6193 \cdot 10^{-2}$.
a = J/l; b = kpm/l.

Table 253. Dynamic (viscous) work of breathing (W_{dyn}) in relation to body height in boys and girls

Height cm	W_{dyn} mean		lower limits		upper limits	
	a	b	a	b	a	b
115	0.3734	0.0381	0.2592	0.0255	0.4875	0.0507
116	0.3694	0.0376	0.2552	0.0260	0.4835	0.0493
120	0.3535	0.0360	0.2393	0.0243	0.4676	0.0476
124	0.3376	0.0344	0.2234	0.0227	0.4517	0.0460
128	0.3216	0.0327	0.2075	0.0211	0.4358	0.0444
132	0.3057	0.0311	0.1916	0.0195	0.4199	0.0428
136	0.2898	0.0295	0.1757	0.0179	0.4040	0.0411
140	0.2739	0.0279	0.1597	0.0162	0.3881	0.0395
144	0.2580	0.0263	0.1438	0.0146	0.3722	0.0379
148	0.2421	0.0246	0.1279	0.0130	0.3563	0.0363
152	0.2262	0.0230	0.1120	0.0114	0.3403	0.0347
156	0.2103	0.0214	0.0961	0.0097	0.3244	0.0330
160	0.1943	0.0198	0.0802	0.0081	0.3085	0.0314
164	0.1784	0.0181	0.0643	0.0065	0.2926	0.0298
168	0.1625	0.0165	0.0484	0.0049	0.2767	0.0282
172	0.1466	0.0149	0.0324	0.0033	0.2608	0.0262
176	0.1307	0.0133	0.0165	0.0016	0.2449	0.0249
180	0.1148	0.0117	0.0060	0.0006	0.2290	0.0233
182	0.1068	0.0109	–	–	0.2112	0.0215

Formula: $y = a + b \cdot x$;
$y = W_{dyn}$ (J/l or kpm/l); x = body height (cm);
W_{dyn} (J/l) $= 0.83082 - 3.97795 \cdot 10^{-3} \cdot x$;
SD $y \cdot x = \pm 5.7182 \cdot 10^{-2}$; n = 73; r = –0.77.
W_{dyn} (kpm/l) $= 0.08472 - 0.40564 \cdot 10^{-3} \cdot x$;
SD $y \cdot x = \pm 0.5831 \cdot 10^{-2}$.
a = J/l; b = kpm/l.

Table 255. Inspiratory dynamic work of breathing (W_{in}) in relation to body height in boys and girls

Height cm	W_{in} mean		lower limits		upper limits	
	a	b	a	b	a	b
115	0.1918	0.0195	0.1280	0.0130	0.2555	0.0260
116	0.1897	0.0193	0.1259	0.0128	0.2534	0.0258
120	0.1812	0.0184	0.1175	0.0119	0.2450	0.0249
124	0.1728	0.0176	0.1090	0.0111	0.2366	0.0241
128	0.1644	0.0167	0.1006	0.0102	0.2282	0.0232
132	0.1560	0.0159	0.0922	0.0094	0.2197	0.0224
136	0.1475	0.0150	0.0838	0.0085	0.2113	0.0215
140	0.1391	0.0141	0.0754	0.0076	0.2029	0.0207
144	0.1307	0.0133	0.0669	0.0068	0.1945	0.0198
148	0.1223	0.0124	0.0585	0.0059	0.1861	0.0189
152	0.1139	0.0116	0.0501	0.0051	0.1776	0.0181
156	0.1054	0.0107	0.0417	0.0042	0.1692	0.0172
160	0.0970	0.0099	0.0333	0.0033	0.1608	0.0164
164	0.0886	0.0090	0.0248	0.0025	0.1524	0.0155
168	0.0802	0.0081	0.0164	0.0016	0.1440	0.0146
172	0.0718	0.0073	0.0080	0.0008	0.1355	0.0138
176	0.0633	0.0064	–	–	0.1271	0.0129
180	0.0549	0.0056	–	–	0.1187	0.0121
182	0.0507	0.0052	–	–	0.1145	0.0117

Formula: $y = a + b \cdot x$;
$y = W_{in}$ (J/l or kpm/l); x = body height (cm);
W_{in} (J/l) $= 0.43384 - 2.10508 \cdot 10^{-3} \cdot x$;
SD log $y \cdot x = \pm 3.19401 \cdot 10^{-2}$; n = 73; r = –0.75.
W_{in} (kpm/l) $= 0.04424 - 0.21466 \cdot 10^{-3} \cdot x$;
SD $y \cdot x = \pm 0.3257 \cdot 10^{-2}$.
a = J/l; b = kpm/l.

Table 254. Dynamic (viscous) work of breathing (W_{dyn}) in relation to age in boys and girls

Age years	W_{dyn} mean		lower limits		upper limits	
	a	b	a	b	a	b
6	0.3071	0.0313	0.1643	0.0167	0.4500	0.0458
8	0.2830	0.0288	0.1401	0.0142	0.4258	0.0434
10	0.2588	0.0263	0.1159	0.0118	0.4017	0.0409
12	0.2346	0.0239	0.0917	0.0093	0.3775	0.0384
14	0.2104	0.0214	0.0675	0.0068	0.3533	0.0360
16	0.1862	0.0189	0.0433	0.0044	0.3291	0.0335
18	0.1620	0.0165	0.0191	0.0019	0.3049	0.0310
20	0.1378	0.0140	–	–	0.2807	0.0286
22	0.1136	0.0115	–	–	0.2565	0.0261
24	0.0894	0.0091	–	–	0.2323	0.0236
26	0.0653	0.0066	–	–	0.2081	0.0212

Formula: $y = a + b \cdot x$;
$y = W_{dyn}$ (J/l or kpm/l); x = age (years);
W_{dyn} (J/l) $= 0.37971 - 1.20945 \cdot 10^{-2} \cdot x$;
SD $y \cdot x = \pm 7.1569 \cdot 10^{-2}$; n = 73; r = –0.60.
W_{dyn} (kpm/l) $= 0.03872 - 0.12333 \cdot 10^{-2} \cdot x$;
SD $y \cdot x = \pm 0.7298 \cdot 10^{-2}$.
a = J/l; b = kpm/l.

Table 256. Inspiratory dynamic work of breathing (W_{in}) in relation to age in boys and girls

Age years	W_{in} mean		lower limits		upper limits	
	a	b	a	b	a	b
6	0.1577	0.0160	0.0802	0.0081	0.2352	0.0239
8	0.1447	0.0147	0.0672	0.0068	0.2221	0.0226
10	0.1316	0.0134	0.0542	0.0055	0.2091	0.0213
12	0.1186	0.0120	0.0411	0.0041	0.1960	0.0199
14	0.1055	0.0107	0.0281	0.0028	0.1830	0.0186
16	0.0925	0.0094	0.0150	0.0015	0.1700	0.0173
18	0.0795	0.0080	0.0010	0.0001	0.1569	0.0159
20	0.0664	0.0067	–	–	0.1439	0.0146
22	0.0534	0.0054	–	–	0.1308	0.0133
24	0.0403	0.0040	–	–	0.1178	0.0119
26	0.0273	0.0027	–	–	0.1047	0.0106

Formula: $y = a + b \cdot x$;
$y = W_{in}$ (J/l or kpm/l); x = age (years);
W_{in} (J/l) $= 0.19682 - 6.52041 \cdot 10^{-3} \cdot x$;
SD $y \cdot x = \pm 3.8795 \cdot 10^{-2}$; n = 73; r = –0.60.
W_{in} (kpm/l) $= 0.02007 - 0.66649 \cdot 10^{-3} \cdot x$;
SD $y \cdot x = \pm 0.3956 \cdot 10^{-2}$.
a = J/l; b = kpm/l.

Table 257. Expiratory dynamic work of breathing (W_{ex}) in relation to body height in boys and girls

Height cm	W_{ex} mean		lower limits		upper limits	
	a	b	a	b	a	b
115	0.1818	0.0185	0.1054	0.0107	0.2581	0.0262
116	0.1799	0.0183	0.1035	0.0105	0.2562	0.0261
120	0.1723	0.0175	0.0960	0.0097	0.2487	0.0253
124	0.1648	0.0168	0.0885	0.0090	0.2412	0.0245
128	0.1573	0.0160	0.0809	0.0082	0.2336	0.0238
132	0.1497	0.0152	0.0734	0.0074	0.2261	0.0230
136	0.1422	0.0145	0.0659	0.0067	0.2186	0.0222
140	0.1347	0.0137	0.0538	0.0059	0.2110	0.0215
144	0.1272	0.0129	0.0508	0.0051	0.2035	0.0207
148	0.1196	0.0122	0.0433	0.0044	0.1960	0.0199
152	0.1121	0.0114	0.0357	0.0036	0.1884	0.0192
156	0.1046	0.0106	0.0282	0.0028	0.1809	0.0184
160	0.0970	0.0099	0.0207	0.0021	0.1734	0.0176
164	0.0895	0.0091	0.0131	0.0013	0.1658	0.0169
168	0.0820	0.0083	0.0050	0.0005	0.1583	0.0161
172	0.0744	0.0075	–	–	0.1508	0.0153
176	0.0669	0.0068	–	–	0.1432	0.0146
180	0.0594	0.0060	–	–	0.1357	0.0138
182	0.0556	0.0056	–	–	0.1321	0.0134

Formula: $y = a + b \cdot x$;
$y = W_{ex}$ (J/l or kpm/l); x = body height (cm);
W_{ex} (J/l) $= 0.39834 - 1.88326 \cdot 10^{-3} \cdot x$;
SD $y \cdot x = \pm 3.8236 \cdot 10^{-2}$; n = 73; r = −0.65.
W_{ex} (kpm/l) $= 0.04062 - 0.19204 \cdot 10^{-3} \cdot x$;
SD $y \cdot x = \pm 0.3899 \cdot 10^{-2}$.
a = J/l; b = kpm/l.

Table 259. Total work of breathing (W_{tot}) in relation to body height in boys and girls

Height cm	W_{tot} mean		lower limits		upper limits	
	a	b	a	b	a	b
115	3.257	0.332	1.480	0.151	5.050	0.515
116	3.236	0.330	1.431	0.146	5.030	0.513
120	3.149	0.321	1.353	0.138	4.942	0.504
124	3.063	0.312	1.265	0.129	4.854	0.495
128	2.977	0.303	1.176	0.120	4.766	0.486
132	2.890	0.294	1.088	0.111	4.677	0.477
136	2.804	0.285	1.000	0.102	4.599	0.469
140	2.717	0.277	0.921	0.094	4.511	0.460
144	2.631	0.268	0.833	0.085	4.422	0.451
148	2.545	0.259	0.745	0.076	4.138	0.442
152	2.458	0.250	0.657	0.067	4.246	0.433
156	2.372	0.241	0.568	0.058	4.157	0.424
160	2.286	0.233	0.490	0.050	4.079	0.416
164	2.199	0.224	0.402	0.041	3.991	0.407
168	2.113	0.215	0.313	0.032	3.903	0.398
172	2.026	0.206	0.225	0.023	3.814	0.389
176	1.940	0.197	0.137	0.014	3.726	0.380
180	1.854	0.189	0.058	0.006	3.648	0.372
182	1.811	0.184	0.009	0.001	3.549	0.362

Formula: $y = a + b \cdot x$;
$y = W_{tot}$ (J/min or kpm/min); x = body height (cm);
W_{tot} (J/min) $= 5.74137 - 2.15961 \cdot 10^{-2} \cdot x$;
SD $y \cdot x = \pm 0.8982$; n = 73; r = −0.38.
W_{tot} (kpm/min) $= 0.58546 - 0.22022 \cdot 10^{-2} \cdot x$;
SD $y \cdot x = \pm 0.0916$.
a = J/min; b = kpm/min.

Table 258. Expiratory dynamic work of breathing (W_{ex}) in relation to age in boys and girls

Age years	W_{ex} mean		lower limits		upper limits	
	a	b	a	b	a	b
6	0.1495	0.0152	0.0623	0.0068	0.2368	0.0241
8	0.1384	0.0141	0.0511	0.0052	0.2256	0.0230
10	0.1272	0.0129	0.0400	0.0040	0.2144	0.0218
12	0.1160	0.0118	0.0288	0.0029	0.2033	0.0207
14	0.1049	0.0107	0.0176	0.0018	0.1921	0.0196
16	0.0937	0.0095	0.0065	0.0006	0.1810	0.0184
18	0.0826	0.0084	–	–	0.1698	0.0173
20	0.0714	0.0072	–	–	0.1586	0.0161
22	0.0602	0.0061	–	–	0.1475	0.0150
24	0.0491	0.0050	–	–	0.1363	0.0139
26	0.0379	0.0038	–	–	0.1252	0.0127

Formula: $y = a + b \cdot x$;
$y = W_{ex}$ (J/l or kpm/l); x = age (years);
W_{ex} (J/l) $= 0.18299 - 5.57937 \cdot 10^{-3} \cdot x$;
SD $y \cdot x = \pm 4.3698 \cdot 10^{-2}$; n = 73; r = −0.49.
W_{ex} (kpm/l) $= 0.01866 - 0.56894 \cdot x$;
SD $y \cdot x = \pm 0.4456 \cdot 10^{-2}$.
a = J/l; b = kpm/l.

Table 260. Total work of breathing (W_{tot}) relation to age in boys and girls

Age years	W_{tot} mean		lower limits		upper limits	
	a	b	a	b	a	b
6	2.948	0.300	1.117	0.113	4.778	0.487
8	2.801	0.285	0.970	0.098	4.631	0.472
10	2.654	0.270	0.823	0.083	4.484	0.457
12	2.506	0.255	0.676	0.068	4.337	0.442
14	2.359	0.240	0.529	0.053	4.190	0.427
16	2.212	0.225	0.382	0.038	4.043	0.412
18	2.065	0.210	0.235	0.023	3.896	0.397
20	1.918	0.195	0.088	0.008	3.749	0.382
22	1.771	0.180	–	–	3.602	0.367
24	1.624	0.165	–	–	3.455	0.352
26	1.477	0.150	–	–	3.308	0.337

Formula: $y = a + b \cdot x$;
$y = W_{tot}$ (J/min or kpm/min); x = age (years);
W_{tot} (J/min) $= 3.38936 - 7.35358 \cdot 10^{-2} \cdot x$;
SD $y \cdot x = \pm 0.9169$; n = 73; r = −0.33.
W_{tot} (kpm/min) $= 0.34562 - 0.74986 \cdot 10^{-2} \cdot x$;
SD $y \cdot x = \pm 0.0935$.
a = J/min; b = kpm/min.

Table 261. Dynamic (viscous) work of breathing (W_{dyn}) in relation to body height in boys and girls

Height cm	W_{dyn} mean		lower limits		upper limits	
	a	b	a	b	a	b
115	2.480	0.253	0.976	0.100	3.983	0.406
116	2.460	0.250	0.957	0.097	3.964	0.404
120	2.383	0.243	0.880	0.089	3.887	0.396
124	2.306	0.235	0.802	0.081	3.810	0.388
128	2.229	0.227	0.725	0.073	3.732	0.380
132	2.152	0.219	0.648	0.065	3.655	0.372
136	2.074	0.211	0.571	0.058	3.578	0.365
140	1.997	0.203	0.494	0.050	3.501	0.357
144	1.920	0.195	0.416	0.042	3.424	0.349
148	1.843	0.187	0.339	0.034	3.347	0.341
152	1.766	0.180	0.254	0.026	3.269	0.333
156	1.689	0.172	0.176	0.018	3.192	0.325
160	1.611	0.164	0.100	0.010	3.115	0.317
164	1.534	0.156	0.019	0.002	3.038	0.310
168	1.457	0.148	–	–	2.961	0.302
172	1.380	0.140	–	–	2.883	0.294
176	1.303	0.132	–	–	2.806	0.286
180	1.225	0.124	–	–	2.729	0.278
182	1.187	0.121	–	–	2.693	0.274

Formula: $y = a + b \cdot x$;
$y = W_{dyn}$ (J/min or kpm/min); x = body height (cm);
W_{dyn} (J/min) = $4.69952 - 1.92984 \cdot 10^{-2} \cdot x$;
SD $y \cdot x = \pm 0.7531$; n = 73; r = –0.40.
W_{dyn} (kpm/min) = $0.47922 - 0.19679 \cdot 10^{-2} \cdot x$;
SD $y \cdot x = \pm 0.0768$.
a = J/min; b = kpm/min.

Table 263. Inspiratory dynamic work of breathing (W_{in}) in relation to body height in boys and girls

Height cm	W_{in} mean		lower limits		upper limits	
	a	b	a	b	a	b
115	1.248	0.127	0.500	0.051	1.996	0.203
116	1.237	0.126	0.480	0.049	1.985	0.202
120	1.196	0.121	0.448	0.045	1.943	0.198
124	1.154	0.117	0.406	0.041	1.902	0.194
128	1.112	0.113	0.353	0.036	1.860	0.189
132	1.070	0.109	0.313	0.032	1.818	0.185
136	1.028	0.104	0.274	0.028	1.776	0.181
140	0.986	0.100	0.238	0.024	1.734	0.177
144	0.944	0.096	0.186	0.019	1.692	0.172
148	0.902	0.092	0.147	0.015	1.650	0.168
152	0.860	0.087	0.110	0.011	1.608	0.164
156	0.818	0.083	0.068	0.007	1.566	0.159
160	0.776	0.079	0.019	0.002	1.524	0.155
164	0.734	0.074	–	–	1.482	0.151
168	0.692	0.070	–	–	1.440	0.147
172	0.650	0.066	–	–	1.398	0.142
176	0.608	0.062	–	–	1.356	0.138
180	0.567	0.057	–	–	1.314	0.134
182	0.546	0.055	–	–	1.295	0.132

Formula: $y = a + b \cdot x$;
$y = W_{in}$ (J/min or kpm/min); x = body height (cm);
W_{in} (J/min) = $2.45400 - 1.04833 \cdot 10^{-2} \cdot x$;
SD $y \cdot x = \pm 0.3746$; n = 73; r = –0.43.
W_{in} (kpm/min) = $0.25024 - 0.10690 \cdot 10^{-2} \cdot x$;
SD $y \cdot x = \pm 0.0382$.
a = J/min; b = kpm/min.

Table 262. Dynamic (viscous) work of breathing (W_{dyn}) in relation to age in boys and girls

Age years	W_{dyn} mean		lower limits		upper limits	
	a	b	a	b	a	b
6	2.206	0.224	0.667	0.068	3.743	0.381
8	2.073	0.211	0.530	0.054	3.610	0.368
10	1.941	0.197	0.404	0.041	3.478	0.354
12	1.809	0.184	0.264	0.027	3.346	0.341
14	1.677	0.171	0.137	0.014	3.214	0.327
16	1.544	0.157	0.058	0.006	3.081	0.314
18	1.412	0.144	–	–	2.949	0.300
20	1.280	0.130	–	–	2.817	0.287
22	1.147	0.117	–	–	2.684	0.273
24	1.015	0.103	–	–	2.552	0.260
26	0.883	0.090	–	–	2.420	0.246

Formula: $y = a + b \cdot x$;
$y = W_{dyn}$ (J/min or kpm/min); x = age (years);
W_{dyn} (J/min) = $2.60316 - 6.61534 \cdot 10^{-2} \cdot x$;
SD $y \cdot x = \pm 0.7698$; n = 73; r = –0.35.
W_{dyn} (kpm/min) = $0.26545 - 0.67458 \cdot 10^{-2} \cdot x$;
SD $y \cdot x = \pm 0.0785$.
a = J/min; b = kpm/min.

Table 264. Inspiratory dynamic work of breathing (W_{in}) in relation to age in boys and girls

Age years	W_{in} mean		lower limits		upper limits	
	a	b	a	b	a	b
6	1.100	0.112	0.323	0.033	1.867	0.190
8	1.028	0.104	0.255	0.026	1.795	0.183
10	0.956	0.097	0.188	0.019	1.723	0.175
12	0.884	0.090	0.107	0.011	1.651	0.168
14	0.811	0.082	0.040	0.004	1.579	0.161
16	0.739	0.075	–	–	1.507	0.153
18	0.667	0.068	–	–	1.435	0.146
20	0.595	0.060	–	–	1.363	0.139
22	0.523	0.053	–	–	1.291	0.131
24	0.451	0.046	–	–	1.218	0.124
26	0.379	0.038	–	–	1.146	0.117

Formula: $y = a + b \cdot x$;
$y = W_{in}$ (J/min or kpm/min); x = age (years);
W_{in} (J/min) = $1.31663 - 3.60510 \cdot 10^{-2} \cdot x$;
SD $y \cdot x = \pm 0.3844$; n = 73; r = –0.38.
W_{in} (kpm/min) = $0.13426 - 0.36762 \cdot 10^{-2} \cdot x$;
SD $y \cdot x = \pm 0.0392$.
a = J/min; b = kpm/min.

Table 265. Percentage of inspiratory dynamic from total work of breathing (% W_{in}/W_{tot}) in relation to body height or age in boys and girls

Height cm	% $\frac{W_{in}}{W_{tot}}$ mean	Age years	% $\frac{W_{in}}{W_{tot}}$ mean
115	40.70	6	39.09
116	40.47	8	38.11
120	39.95	10	37.12
124	39.44	12	36.14
128	38.92	14	35.16
132	38.41	16	34.18
136	37.90	18	33.20
140	37.38	20	32.22
144	36.87	22	32.24
148	36.36	24	30.26
152	35.84	26	29.28
156	35.33		
160	34.81		
164	34.30		
168	33.79		
172	33.27		
176	32.76		
180	32.25		
182	32.20		

Formula: $y = a + b \cdot x$;

$y = \% \frac{W_{in}}{W_{tot}}$; $\quad$ $y = \% \frac{W_{in}}{W_{tot}}$;

x = body height (cm); $\quad$ x = age (years);

$\% \frac{W_{in}}{W_{tot}} =$ $\quad\quad$ $\% \frac{W_{in}}{W_{tot}} =$

$55.36631 - 0.12841 \cdot x$; $\quad$ $42.03381 - 0.49042 \cdot x$;

SD $y \cdot x = \pm 7.2$; $n = 73$; $r = -0.29$.

Table 266. Mean values ($\pm$ SD) of work of breathing and its components

	n	Age years	W_{tot} J/l	W_{dyn} J/l	W_{el} J/l	W_{tot} J/min	W_{dyn} J/min	% $\frac{W_{in}}{W_{tot}}$	% $\frac{W_{dyn}}{W_{tot}}$
Healthy	73	6–26	0.324 ±0.098	0.235 ±0.088	0.205 ±0.069	2.45 ±0.98	1.77 ±0.785	36.0 ±7.5	71.4 ±12.4
Bronchial asthma symptom-free	16	6–18	0.412 ±0.098	0.363 ±0.196	0.206 ±0.069	3.82 ±2.16	3.63 ±2.35	45.1 ±9.5	87.8 ±22.6
Cystic fibrosis	12	7–21	0.637 ±0.196	0.539 ±0.196	0.343 ±0.196	5.10 ±2.55	4.41 ±2.55	46.5 ±8.6	84.1 ±14.5
Idiopathic pulmonary fibrosis	12	6–21	0.735 ±0.196	0.186 ±0.078	–	6.18 ±2.84	1.47 ±0.882	–	25.9 ±9.8

Table 267. Alveolar ventilation ($\dot{V}_A$BTPS) (y) in liters per minute in relation to body height (x) in boys and girls

Height cm	$\dot{V}_A$, liters/min		
	mean	lower limits	upper limits
126	3.43	2.34	5.03
131	3.68	2.51	5.39
136	3.93	2.68	5.77
141	4.20	2.86	6.15
146	4.47	3.05	6.55
151	4.74	3.24	6.95
156	5.03	3.43	7.37
161	5.32	3.63	7.80
166	5.62	3.83	8.23
171	5.92	4.04	8.68
176	6.24	4.26	9.14
178	6.36	4.40	9.20

Formula: log y = a + b·log x;
log $\dot{V}_A$ (l/min) = −3.2156·1.7860·log body height (cm);
SD log y·x = ±0.08; n = 46; r = +0.65.

Table 269. Respiratory dead space (V_D) (y) in relation to body height (x) in boys and girls

Height cm	V_D, ml		
	mean	lower limits	upper limits
126	97	35	160
131	107	46	170
136	117	55	180
141	127	64	190
146	137	74	200
151	147	84	210
156	157	94	220
161	167	104	230
166	177	114	240
171	187	124	250
176	197	134	260
178	201	138	264

Formula: y = a + b·x;
$\dot{V}_D$ (ml) = −153.4204 + 1.9907·body height (cm);
SD y·x = ±31.43; n = 46; r = +0.65.

Table 268. Ventilation of respiratory dead space ($\dot{V}_D$ BTPS) (y) in liters per minute in relation to body height (x) in boys and girls

Height cm	$\dot{V}_D$, liters/min		
	mean	lower limits	upper limits
126	2.92	1.29	4.56
131	3.07	1.44	4.71
136	3.22	1.58	4.86
141	3.37	1.73	5.00
146	3.51	1.88	5.15
151	3.66	2.03	2.30
156	3.81	2.17	5.45
161	3.96	2.32	5.59
166	4.11	2.47	5.74
171	4.25	2.62	5.89
176	4.40	2.76	6.04
178	4.45	2.81	6.09

Formula: y = a + b·x;
$\dot{V}_D$ (l/min) = −0.7970 + 0.0295·body height (cm);
SD y·x = ±0.82; n = 46; r = +0.44.

Table 270. Oxygen consumption at rest ($ØiO_2$) (y) in relation to body height (x) in boys and girls

Height cm	O$_2$ consumption					
	mean		lower limits		upper limits	
	a	b	a	b	a	b
126	0.145	195	0.096	129	0.194	262
131	0.154	208	0.105	141	0.203	274
136	0.163	220	0.114	154	0.213	286
141	0.172	232	0.123	166	0.222	299
146	0.182	244	0.132	178	0.231	311
151	0.191	257	0.141	191	0.240	323
156	0.200	269	0.151	203	0.249	335
161	0.209	281	0.160	215	0.258	348
166	0.218	294	0.169	228	0.267	360
171	0.227	306	0.178	240	0.277	372
176	0.236	318	0.187	252	0.286	384
178	0.240	323	0.191	257	0.289	389

Formula: $y = a + b \cdot x$;
$ØiO_2$ (mmol/s) = $-0.085061 + 0.00183 \cdot$ body height (cm);
SD $y \cdot x = \pm 0.0246$; n = 44; r = $+0.72$.
$\dot{V}O_2$ (ml/min STPD) = $-114.3298 + 2.4592 \cdot x$;
SD $y \cdot x = \pm 33.11$.
a = $ØiO_2$ (mmol/s); b = $\dot{V}O_2$ (ml/min STPD).

Table 271. Carbon dioxide output at rest ($ØiCO_2$) (y) in relation to body height (x) in boys and girls

Height cm	CO$_2$ output					
	mean		lower limits		upper limits	
	a	b	a	b	a	b
126	0.113	152	0.064	86	0.161	217
131	0.121	163	0.072	97	0.170	229
136	0.129	174	0.081	109	0.178	240
141	0.138	186	0.089	120	0.187	251
146	0.146	197	0.097	131	0.195	263
151	0.155	208	0.106	143	0.204	274
156	0.163	220	0.114	154	0.212	285
161	0.172	231	0.123	165	0.220	297
166	0.180	242	0.131	177	0.229	308
171	0.188	254	0.140	188	0.237	319
176	0.197	265	0.148	200	0.246	331
178	0.201	270	0.152	204	0.249	335

Formula: $y = a + b \cdot x$;
$ØiCO_2$ (mmol/s) = $-0.0996649 + 0.001689 \cdot$ body height (cm);
SD $y \cdot x = \pm 0.0244$; n = 44; r = $+0.69$.
$\dot{V}CO_2$ (ml/min STPD) = $-133.9583 + 2.2687 \cdot x$;
SD $y \cdot x = \pm 32.85$.
a = $ØiCO_2$ (mmol/s); b = $\dot{V}CO_2$ (ml/min STPD).

Table 272. Lung diffusing capacity (CO single breath method) (DL_{CO}) in relation to total lung capacity (TLC) in boys and girls

TLC ml	DL_{CO} mean		lower limits		upper limits	
	a	b	a	b	a	b
1,600	3.402	10.15	2.353	7.05	4.91	14.61
1,700	3.574	10.66	2.472	7.41	5.16	15.35
1,800	3.743	11.17	2.590	7.76	5.41	16.00
1,900	3.911	11.67	2.706	8.11	5.65	16.80
2,000	4.078	12.17	2.821	8.45	5.89	17.52
2,100	4.243	12.66	2.935	8.79	6.13	18.22
2,200	4.406	13.15	3.048	9.13	6.36	18.93
2,300	4.568	13.63	3.160	9.47	6.60	19.62
2,400	4.729	14.11	3.271	9.80	6.83	20.31
2,500	4.888	14.59	3.382	10.13	7.06	21.00
2,600	5.046	15.06	3.491	10.46	7.29	21.68
2,700	5.203	15.53	3.600	10.79	7.52	22.35
2,800	5.359	16.00	3.707	11.11	7.74	23.02
2,900	5.514	16.45	3.815	11.43	7.97	23.69
3,000	5.668	16.91	3.921	11.75	8.19	24.35
3,100	5.821	17.37	4.027	12.07	8.41	25.01
3,200	5.973	17.82	4.132	12.38	8.63	25.66
3,300	6.124	18.27	4.237	12.69	8.85	26.31
3,400	6.274	18.82	4.341	13.01	9.06	26.95
3,500	6.424	19.17	4.444	13.32	9.28	27.60
3,600	6.672	19.61	4.547	13.62	9.50	28.23
3,700	6.720	20.05	4.649	13.93	9.71	28.87
3,800	6.867	20.49	4.751	14.24	9.92	29.50
3,900	7.014	20.93	4.852	14.54	10.13	30.13
4,000	7.160	21.37	4.953	14.84	10.34	30.76
4,100	7.305	21.80	5.053	15.14	10.55	31.38
4,200	7.449	22.23	5.153	15.44	10.76	32.00
4,300	7.593	22.66	5.253	15.74	10.97	32.62
4,400	7.736	23.08	5.352	16.04	11.18	33.23
4,500	7.878	23.51	5.450	16.33	11.38	33.84
4,600	8.020	23.93	5.548	16.63	11.59	34.45
4,700	8.161	24.36	5.646	16.92	11.79	35.06
4,800	8.302	24.78	5.743	17.21	12.00	35.66
4,900	8.442	25.19	5.840	17.50	12.20	36.27
5,000	8.582	25.61	5.937	17.79	12.40	36.87
5,100	8.721	26.03	6.033	18.08	12.60	37.46
5,200	8.860	26.44	6.129	18.37	12.80	38.06
5,300	8.998	26.85	6.225	18.65	13.00	38.65
5,400	9.135	27.26	6.320	18.94	13.20	39.24
5,500	9.272	27.67	6.415	19.22	13.40	39.83
5,600	9.409	28.08	6.509	19.51	13.60	40.42
5,700	9.545	28.49	6.604	19.79	13.79	41.01
5,800	9.681	28.89	6.698	20.07	13.99	41.59
5,900	9.816	29.29	6.791	20.35	14.18	42.17
6,000	9.951	29.70	6.884	20.63	14.18	42.75
6,100	10.086	30.10	6.978	20.91	14.57	43.33
6,200	10.220	30.50	7.070	21.19	14.77	43.90
6,300	10.353	30.90	7.163	21.46	14.96	44.48
6,400	10.487	31.30	7.255	21.74	15.15	45.05
6,500	10.620	31.69	7.347	22.02	15.35	45.62
6,600	10.752	32.09	7.438	22.29	15.54	46.19
6,700	10.884	32.48	7.530	22.56	15.73	46.76
6,800	11.016	32.87	7.621	22.84	15.92	47.32
6,900	11.147	33.27	7.712	23.11	16.11	47.89

Formula: $\log y = a + b \cdot \log x$;

$y = DL_{CO}$ (mmol/min/kPa or ml/min/Torr); x = TLC (ml);

$\log DL_{CO}$ (mmol/min/kPa) $= -2.06996 + 0.8120 \cdot \log$ TLC;

SD $\log y \cdot x = \pm 0.08$; n = 56; r = +0.82.

$\log DL_{CO}$ (ml/min/Torr) $= -1.5950 + 0.8120 \cdot \log x$;

SD $\log y \cdot x = \pm 0.08$.

a = mmol/min/kPa; b = ml/min/Torr.

Table 273. Membrane component of lung diffusing capacity (CO single breath method) (Dm) in relation to total lung capacity (TLC) in boys and girls

TLC ml	Dm mean		lower limits		upper limits		TLC ml	Dm mean		lower limits		upper limits	
	a	b	a	b	a	b		a	b	a	b	a	b
1,600	4.85	14.49	2.92	8.63	8.05	24.34	4,300	11.57	34.55	6.97	20.57	19.20	58.03
1,700	5.11	15.28	3.08	9.10	8.49	25.67	4,400	11.80	35.26	7.11	20.99	19.59	59.21
1,800	5.38	16.07	3.24	9.57	8.93	26.99	4,500	12.04	35.96	7.25	21.41	19.98	60.39
1,900	5.64	16.85	3.40	10.03	9.36	28.31	4,600	12.27	36.66	7.39	21.83	20.37	61.57
2,000	5.90	17.63	3.55	10.50	9.80	29.61	4,700	12.51	37.36	7.53	22.25	20.76	62.75
2,100	6.16	18.40	3.71	10.96	10.23	30.91	4,800	12.74	38.06	7.67	22.66	21.15	63.92
2,200	6.42	19.17	3.86	11.41	10.65	32.20	4,900	12.97	38.76	7.82	23.08	21.53	65.09
2,300	6.67	19.74	4.02	11.87	11.08	33.48	5,000	13.21	39.45	7.96	23.49	21.92	66.25
2,400	6.93	20.70	4.17	12.32	11.50	34.76	5,100	13.44	40.14	8.09	23.90	22.30	67.42
2,500	7.18	21.45	4.32	12.77	11.92	36.03	5,200	13.67	40.83	8.23	24.31	22.69	68.58
2,600	7.43	22.20	4.48	13.22	12.34	37.29	5,300	13.90	41.52	8.37	24.72	23.07	69.73
2,700	7.68	22.95	4.63	13.67	12.75	38.55	5,400	14.13	42.21	8.51	25.13	23.45	70.89
2,800	7.93	23.70	4.78	14.11	13.17	39.80	5,500	14.36	42.90	8.65	25.54	23.83	72.04
2,900	8.18	24.44	4.93	14.55	13.58	41.05	5,600	14.59	43.58	8.79	25.95	24.22	73.19
3,000	8.43	25.18	5.08	14.99	13.99	42.29	5,700	14.82	44.26	8.93	26.36	24.59	74.34
3,100	8.67	25.92	5.23	15.43	14.40	43.53	5,800	15.05	44.95	9.06	26.76	24.97	75.48
3,200	8.92	26.65	5.37	15.87	14.81	44.76	5,900	15.27	45.63	9.20	27.17	25.35	76.43
3,300	9.16	27.38	5.52	16.30	15.21	45.99	6,000	15.50	46.31	9.34	27.57	25.73	77.77
3,400	9.41	28.11	5.67	16.74	15.62	47.21	6,100	15.73	46.98	9.48	27.98	26.11	78.90
3,500	9.65	28.83	5.81	17.17	16.02	48.43	6,200	15.95	47.66	9.61	28.38	26.48	80.04
3,600	9.89	29.56	5.96	17.60	16.42	49.64	6,300	16.18	48.33	9.75	28.78	26.86	81.17
3,700	10.13	30.28	6.10	18.03	16.82	50.85	6,400	16.41	49.01	9.88	29.18	27.23	82.30
3,800	10.38	31.00	6.25	18.46	17.22	52.05	6,500	16.63	49.68	10.02	29.58	27.60	83.43
3,900	10.61	31.71	6.39	18.88	17.62	53.26	6,600	16.86	50.35	10.15	29.98	27.98	84.56
4,000	10.85	32.42	6.54	19.31	18.02	54.46	6,700	17.08	51.02	10.29	30.38	28.35	85.68
4,100	11.09	33.14	6.68	19.73	18.41	55.65	6,800	17.30	51.69	10.42	30.78	28.72	86.81
4,200	11.33	33.85	6.82	20.15	18.81	56.84	6,900	17.53	52.36	10.56	31.18	29.09	87.93

Formula: $\log y = a + b \cdot \log x$;
$y = Dm$ (ml/min/kPa or ml/min/Torr); $x = TLC$ (ml);
$\log Dm$ (mmol/min/kPa) $= -2.12936 + 0.8787 \cdot \log TLC$;
SD $\log y \cdot x = \pm 0.11$; $n = 56$; $r = +0.73$.
$\log Dm$ (ml/min/Torr) $= -1.6544 + 0.8787 \cdot \log x$;
SD $\log y \cdot x = \pm 0.11$.
a = mmol/min/kPa; b = ml/min/Torr.

Table 274. Lung capillary blood volume (CO single breath method) (Vc) in relation to total lung capacity (TLC) in boys and girls

TLC, ml	Vc, ml			TLC, ml	Vc, ml		
	mean	lower limits	upper limits		mean	lower limits	upper limits
1,600	53.72	27.43	105.19	4,300	80.52	39.77	152.49
1,700	54.95	28.06	107.61	4,400	81.16	40.12	153.82
1,800	56.15	28.67	109.94	4,500	81.79	40.46	155.12
1,900	57.30	29.26	112.20	4,600	82.42	40.79	156.41
2,000	58.41	29.83	114.38	4,700	83.03	41.12	157.67
2,100	59.49	30.38	116.50	4,800	83.64	41.45	158.93
2,200	60.54	30.92	118.55	4,900	84.24	41.77	160.16
2,300	61.56	31.44	120.55	5,000	84.83	42.09	161.38
2,400	62.56	31.95	122.49	5,100	85.42	42.40	162.59
2,500	63.52	32.44	124.38	5,200	86.00	42.71	163.58
2,600	64.47	32.92	126.23	5,300	86.58	43.02	164.95
2,700	65.39	33.39	128.03	5,400	87.14	43.32	166.12
2,800	66.29	33.85	129.79	5,500	87.70	43.62	167.27
2,900	67.16	34.30	131.52	5,600	87.80	43.92	168.40
3,000	68.03	34.74	133.20	5,700	87.86	44.21	169.52
3,100	68.87	35.17	134.85	5,800	87.98	44.50	170.61
3,200	69.70	35.59	136.47	5,900	88.00	44.79	171.74
3,300	70.51	36.01	138.06	6,000	88.26	45.07	172.82
3,400	71.30	36.41	139.62	6,100	88.81	45.35	173.90
3,500	72.08	36.81	141.14	6,200	89.35	45.63	174.97
3,600	72.85	37.20	142.65	6,300	89.89	45.91	176.02
3,700	73.60	37.59	144.12	6,400	90.43	46.18	177.06
3,800	74.34	37.97	145.57	6,500	90.95	46.45	178.10
3,900	75.07	38.34	147.00	6,600	91.48	46.72	179.12
4,000	76.50	38.70	148.41	6,700	92.00	46.98	180.14
4,100	77.19	39.07	149.79	6,800	92.51	47.24	181.14
4,200	77.88	39.42	151.15	6,900	93.02	47.50	182.14

Formula: $\log y = a + b \cdot \log x$;
$y = Vc$ (ml); $x = TLC$ (ml);
$\log Vc = 0.5265 + 0.3757 \cdot \log TLC$;
SD $\log y \cdot x = \pm 0.15$; $n = 56$; $r = +0.34$.

Table 275. Lung diffusing capacity – CO single breath method – (DL_{CO}) (y) in relation to body height (x) in boys and girls

Height cm	DL_{CO} mean		lower limits		upper limits	
	a	b	a	b	a	b
107	3.40	10.17	2.25	6.72	5.15	15.39
108	3.47	10.37	2.29	6.90	5.25	15.59
110	3.60	10.78	2.38	7.17	5.46	16.20
112	3.74	11.19	2.47	7.44	5.67	16.82
114	3.88	11.61	2.56	7.72	5.88	17.46
116	4.03	12.04	2.66	8.01	6.10	18.10
118	4.17	12.48	2.76	8.30	6.32	18.76
120	4.32	12.92	2.85	8.60	6.55	19.43
122	4.48	13.38	2.96	8.90	6.78	20.11
124	4.63	13.84	3.06	9.20	7.01	20.81
126	4.79	14.31	3.16	9.52	7.25	21.51
128	4.95	14.79	3.27	9.84	7.49	22.23
130	5.11	15.27	3.37	10.16	7.74	22.96
132	5.28	15.77	3.48	10.49	7.99	23.71
134	5.44	16.27	3.60	10.82	8.24	24.46
136	5.62	16.78	3.71	11.16	8.50	25.23
138	5.79	17.30	3.82	11.51	8.77	26.01
140	5.97	17.83	3.94	11.86	9.03	26.81
142	6.15	18.37	4.06	12.21	9.30	27.61
144	6.33	18.91	4.18	12.58	9.58	28.43
146	6.51	19.46	4.30	12.94	9.86	29.26
148	6.70	20.02	4.43	13.32	10.14	30.10
150	6.89	20.59	4.55	13.70	10.43	30.96
152	7.08	21.17	4.68	14.08	10.73	31.83
154	7.28	21.75	4.81	14.47	11.02	32.71
156	7.48	22.35	4.94	14.86	11.32	33.60
158	7.68	22.95	5.07	15.26	11.63	34.51
160	7.89	23.56	5.21	15.67	11.94	35.43
162	8.09	24.18	5.35	16.08	12.25	36.36
164	8.30	24.81	5.48	16.50	12.57	37.30
166	8.52	25.44	5.62	16.92	12.89	38.26
168	8.73	26.09	5.77	17.35	13.22	39.22
170	8.95	26.74	5.91	17.79	13.55	40.20
172	9.17	27.40	6.06	18.22	13.88	41.20
174	9.40	28.07	6.21	18.67	14.22	42.20
176	9.62	28.75	6.36	19.12	14.57	43.22
178	9.85	29.43	6.51	19.58	14.92	44.26

Formula: log y = a + b·log x;
log DL_{CO} (mmol/min/kPa) =
  − 3.7042 + 2.0876·log body height (cm);
SD log y·x = ±0.09; n = 56; r = +0.76.
log DL_{CO} (ml/min/Torr) = − 3.2292 + 2.0876·log x;
SD log y·x = ±0.09.
a = mmol/min/kPa; b = mmol/min/Torr.

Table 276. Lung diffusing capacity – CO single breath method – (DL_{CO}) (y) in relation to age (x) in boys and girls

Age years	DL_{CO} mean		lower limits		upper limits	
	a	b	a	b	a	b
5	3.24	9.68	2.04	6.23	5.14	16.04
6	3.81	11.39	2.40	7.32	6.04	17.69
7	4.37	13.06	2.76	8.41	6.93	20.30
8	4.92	14.71	3.10	9.47	7.80	22.86
9	5.47	16.33	3.45	10.51	8.67	25.38
10	6.00	17.94	3.79	11.54	9.52	27.88
11	6.54	19.53	4.12	12.57	10.36	30.34
12	7.06	21.01	4.45	13.58	11.20	32.79
13	7.58	22.66	4.78	14.58	12.02	35.21
14	8.10	24.20	5.11	15.57	12.84	37.61
15	8.62	25.73	5.43	16.56	13.66	39.99
16	9.12	27.25	5.76	17.54	14.46	42.35
17	9.62	28.76	6.07	18.51	15.27	44.70

Formula: log y = a + b·log x;
log DL_{CO} (mmol/min/kPa) =
  − 0.11096 + 0.8898·log age (years);
SD log y·x = ±0.10; n = 56; r = +0.72.
log DL_{CO} (ml/min/Torr) = 0.3640 + 0.8898·log x;
SD log y·x = ±0.10.
a = mmol/min/kPa; b = ml/min/Torr.

Table 277. Lung diffusing capacity – CO single breath method – (DL_{CO}) (y) in relation to body surface (x) in boys and girls

Body surface m^2	DL_{CO} mean		lower limits		upper limits	
	a	b	a	b	a	b
0.68	3.42	10.2	2.26	6.75	5.17	15.46
0.70	3.52	10.5	2.33	6.96	5.34	15.94
0.80	4.06	12.13	2.68	8.01	6.14	18.36
0.90	4.60	13.74	3.04	9.07	6.96	20.79
1.00	5.14	15.35	3.39	10.33	7.78	22.81
1.10	5.68	16.99	3.75	11.43	8.60	25.23
1.20	6.23	18.62	4.12	12.53	9.43	27.66
1.30	6.78	20.26	4.48	13.63	10.27	30.10
1.40	7.33	21.91	4.84	14.74	11.10	32.56
1.50	7.89	23.57	5.21	15.86	11.94	35.02
1.60	8.45	25.23	5.58	16.98	12.79	37.49
1.70	9.01	26.89	5.95	18.10	13.63	39.97
1.80	9.57	28.57	6.32	19.23	14.48	42.46
1.90	10.13	30.25	6.69	20.36	15.34	44.96
1.92	10.25	30.59	6.77	20.59	15.51	45.46

Formula: log y = a + b·log x;
log DL_{CO} (mmol/min/kPa) =
  0.71124 + 1.0568·log body surface (m^2);
SD log y·x = ±0.09; n = 56; r = +0.75.
log DL_{CO} (ml/min/Torr) = 1.1862 + 1.0568·log x;
SD log y·x = ±0.09.
a = mmol/min/kPa; b = ml/min/Torr.

Table 278. Membrane component of lung diffusing capacity – CO single breath method – (Dm) (y) in relation to body surface (x) in boys and girls

Body surface m²	Dm					
	mean		lower limits		upper limits	
	a	b	a	b	a	b
0.68	4.85	14.50	2.79	8.33	8.43	25.17
0.70	5.01	14.98	2.88	8.62	8.71	26.03
0.80	5.85	17.47	3.36	10.06	10.17	30.37
0.90	6.70	20.02	3.85	11.52	11.65	34.79
1.00	7.57	22.61	4.35	13.18	13.16	38.79
1.10	8.45	25.24	4.86	14.71	14.69	43.31
1.20	9.34	27.91	5.38	16.26	16.24	47.89
1.30	10.25	30.61	5.90	17.84	17.82	52.52
1.40	11.17	33.34	6.42	19.43	19.41	57.22
1.50	12.09	36.11	6.96	21.04	21.02	61.96
1.60	13.03	38.90	7.49	22.67	22.64	66.76
1.70	13.97	41.73	8.04	24.32	24.29	71.60
1.80	14.93	44.57	8.59	25.98	25.94	76.48
1.90	15.89	47.44	9.14	27.65	27.62	81.41
1.92	16.08	48.03	9.25	27.99	27.96	82.40

Formula: $\log y = a + b \cdot \log x$;
$\log Dm$ (mmol/min/kPa) =
  $0.87934 + 1.1548 \cdot \log$ body surface (m²);
SD $\log y \cdot x = \pm 0.12$; n = 56; r = +0.70.
$\log Dm$ (ml/min/Torr) = $1.3543 + 1.1548 \cdot \log x$;
SD $\log y \cdot x = \pm 0.12$.
a = mmol/min/kPa; b = ml/min/Torr.

Table 279. Lung capillary blood volume – CO single breath method – (Vc) (y) in relation to body surface (x) in boys and girls

Body surface m²	Vc, ml		
	mean	lower limits	upper limits
0.68	59.10	8.04	110.16
0.70	59.70	8.64	110.76
0.80	62.66	11.60	113.72
0.90	65.63	14.15	116.69
1.00	68.59	17.58	119.64
1.10	71.55	20.49	122.61
1.20	74.51	23.46	125.57
1.30	77.47	26.42	128.53
1.40	80.44	29.38	131.49
1.50	83.40	32.34	134.46
1.60	86.36	35.31	137.42
1.70	89.32	38.26	140.38
1.80	92.29	41.23	143.34
1.90	95.25	44.19	146.30
1.92	95.84	44.78	146.90

Formula: $y = a + b \cdot x$;
Vc (ml) = $38.9658 + 29.6220 \cdot$ body surface (m²);
SD $y \cdot x = \pm 25.53$; n = 56; r = +0.32.

Table 280. 'Specific' lung diffusing capacity – CO single breath method – ($D_{L_{CO}}$/TLC) (y) in relation to body height (x) in boys and girls

Height cm	$D_{L_{CO}}$/TLC					
	mean		lower limits		upper limits	
	a	b	a	b	a	b
107	2.08	6.23	1.43	4.27	2.74	8.19
108	2.08	6.21	1.42	4.26	2.73	8.16
110	2.06	6.18	1.41	4.22	2.72	8.13
112	2.05	6.14	1.40	4.19	2.71	8.10
114	2.04	6.10	1.39	4.15	2.70	8.06
116	2.03	6.07	1.37	4.12	2.69	8.03
118	2.02	6.04	1.36	4.09	2.67	7.99
120	2.01	6.01	1.35	4.05	2.66	7.96
122	2.00	5.97	1.34	4.01	2.65	7.93
124	1.98	5.94	1.33	3.98	2.64	7.89
126	1.97	5.91	1.32	3.95	2.63	7.86
128	1.96	5.87	1.31	3.92	2.62	7.83
130	1.95	5.84	1.29	3.88	2.61	7.79
132	1.94	5.80	1.28	3.85	2.60	7.76
134	1.93	5.77	1.27	3.82	2.58	7.72
136	1.92	5.74	1.26	3.78	2.57	7.69
138	1.91	5.70	1.25	3.75	2.56	7.66
140	1.89	5.67	1.24	3.71	2.55	7.62
142	1.88	5.63	1.23	3.68	2.54	7.59
144	1.87	5.60	1.22	3.65	2.53	7.56
146	1.86	5.57	1.20	3.61	2.52	7.52
148	1.85	5.53	1.19	3.58	2.51	7.40
150	1.84	5.50	1.18	3.55	2.49	7.45
152	1.83	5.47	1.17	3.51	2.48	7.42
154	1.82	5.43	1.16	3.48	2.47	7.39
156	1.80	5.40	1.15	3.44	2.46	7.35
158	1.79	5.36	1.14	3.41	2.45	7.31
160	1.78	5.33	1.13	3.38	2.44	7.28
162	1.77	5.30	1.11	3.34	2.43	7.25
164	1.76	5.26	1.10	3.31	2.41	7.22
166	1.75	5.23	1.09	3.27	2.40	7.18
168	1.74	5.20	1.08	3.24	2.39	7.15
170	1.72	5.16	1.07	3.21	2.38	7.12
172	1.71	5.13	1.06	3.17	2.37	7.08
174	1.70	5.09	1.05	3.14	2.36	7.05
176	1.69	5.06	1.03	3.11	2.35	7.01
178	1.68	5.03	1.02	3.07	2.34	6.98

Formula: $y = a + b \cdot x$;
$D_{L_{CO}}$/TLC (mmol/min/kPa/l) =
  $2.69189 - 5.6615 \cdot 10^{-3} \cdot$ height (cm);
SD $y \cdot x = \pm 0.328$; n = 56; r = -0.28.
$D_{L_{CO}}$/TLC (ml/min/Torr/l) = $8.0355 - 0.0169 \cdot x$;
SD $y \cdot x = \pm 0.98$.
a = mmol/min/kPa/l; b = ml/min/Torr/l.

Table 281. Lung-diffusing capacity (D_L), membrane component (Dm), alveolar capillary blood volume (Vc), and 'specific' values, i.e. D_L/TLC, Dm/TLC, Vc/TLC, in relation to body height (x) in boys and girls (single-breath CO method)

Test (y)	Regression equation	n	r	Height, cm		
				107	150	178
$D_{L_{CO}}$ mmol/min/kPa	log y = – 3.70415 + 2.0876·log x log SD y·x = ± 0.09	56	+ 0.76	3.41	6.90	9.86
Dm mmol/min/kPa	log y = – 3.96376 + 2.2896·log x log SD y·x = ± 0.12	56	+ 0.69	4.82	11.02	15.78
Vc, ml	y = 8.7041 + 0.4656·x SD y·x = ± 25.82	56	+ 0.29	58.5	78.5	91.6
$D_{L_{CO}}$/TLC mmol/min/kPa/l	y = 2.69189 – 5.6615·10^{-3}·x SD y·x = ± 0.328	56	– 0.28	2.08	1.84	1.68
Dm/TLC mmol/min/kPa/l	y = 3.58148 – 5.0250·10^{-3}·x SD y·x = ± 0.730	56	– 0.12*	3.03	2.83	2.69
Vc/TLC ml/l	y = 57.5314 – 0.2424·x SD y·x = ± 7.20	56	– 0.49	31.5	21.2	14.4

n = Number of subjects; r = correlation coefficient between test and body height; * = non-significant r.
For height 107, 150 and 178 cm mean values are given. TLC was measured in a body plethysmograph as a sum of FRC_{box} + IC.

Table 282. Lung-diffusing capacity (D_L), membrane component (Dm), alveolar capillary blood volume (Vc), and 'specific' values, i.e. D_L/TLC, Dm/TLC, Vc/TLC, in relation to age (x) in boys and girls (single-breath CO method)

Test (y)	Regression equation	n	r	Age, years		
				5	11	17
$D_{L_{CO}}$ mmol/min/kPa	log y = – 0.11096 + 0.8898·log x log SD y·x = ± 0.10	56	+ 0.72	3.24	6.54	9.63
Dm mmol/min/kPa	log y = – 0.0489 + 1.0005·log x log SD y·x = ± 0.12	56	+ 0.67	4.39	9.84	15.21
Vc, ml	y = 53.8466 + 2.0816·x SD y·x = ± 26.4	56	+ 0.21	64.3	76.7	89.2
$D_{L_{CO}}$/TLC mmol/min/kPa/l	y = 2.29850 – 0.03863·x SD y·x = ± 0.325	56	– 0.31	2.11	1.87	1.64
Dm/TLC mmol/min/kPa/l	y = 3.13279 – 0.02586·x SD y·x = ± 0.734	56	– 0.10*	3.00	2.85	2.69
Vc/TLC ml/l	y = 40.9142 – 1.6706·x SD y·x = ± 6.95	56	– 0.54	32.5	22.5	12.5

n = Number of subjects; r = correlation coefficient between test and age; * = non-significant r.
For ages 5, 11 and 17 years mean values are given. TLC was measured in a body plethysmograph as a sum of FRC_{box} + IC.

Table 283. Lung-diffusing capacity (D_L), membrane component (Dm), alveolar capillary blood volume (Vc), and 'specific' values, i.e. D_L/TLC, Dm/TLC, Vc/TLC, in relation to body surface (x) in boys and girls (single-breath CO method)

Test (y)	Regression equation	n	r	Body surface, m^2		
				0.68	1.3	1.92
$D_{L_{CO}}$ mmol/min/kPa	log y = 0.71124 + 1.0568·log x log SD y·x = ± 0.09	56	+0.75	3.42	6.78	10.25
Dm mmol/min/kPa	log y = 0.87934 + 1.1548·log x log SD y·x = ± 0.12	56	+0.70	4.85	10.25	16.08
Vc, ml	y = 38.9658 + 29.6220·x SD y·x = ± 25.53	56	+0.32	59.1	77.5	95.84
$D_{L_{CO}}$/TLC mmol/min/kPa/l	y = 2.20721 − 0.27262·x SD y·x = ± 0.332	56	−0.24	2.02	1.85	1.68
Dm/TLC mmol/min/kPa/l	y = 3.06981 − 0.18124·x SD y·x = ± 0.734	56	−0.07*	2.94	2.83	2.72
Vc/TLC ml/l	y = 37.9937 − 12.5714·x SD y·x = ± 7.40	56	−0.45	29.4	21.7	13.9

n = Number of subjects; r = correlation coefficient between test and body surface; * = non-significant r.

For body surface 0.68, 1.3 and 1.92 m^2 mean values are given. TLC was measured in a body plethysmograph as a sum of FRC_{box} + IC.

Subject Index

Airflow
  interruption technique, PV curves 16,
    17, 19
  resistance, subdivision 51, 52
Airway
  conductance 54, 62, 63
    specific 56, 62, 63
  obstruction tests 32
  patency 32
  resistance 52–56, 58–61, 199, 200
    peak flow 59
    specific 56
    total 59
Alveolar ventilation 83, 84, 210

Backlake index 66, 204
Body plethysmography 7, 53, 55–58

Campbell diagram 69, 71, 72
Carbon dioxide elimination 83, 84, 211
Compressed gas during forced expiration
  44
Conductance, upstream airways segment
  39, 42, 187–189
Confidence limits 2

Diaphragm dome 16, 28
Downstream airway segment 35–37

Elastic recoil pressure, lungs 16, 148–163
Esophageal elastance 17, 27, 28
Esophageal pressure 16
Exponential function fitted in PV curve
  26

Flow transients at cough 40, 47
Forced expiratory volume curves 49
FRC_{box} 7, 10, 11

FRC_{He} 7, 10, 11
Functional dead space 83, 84, 210
Functional residual capacity
  measurement 6

Gas exchange, lungs 83

Helium dilution method 4

Inspiratory muscle strength, PV curve 29
Isovolume-pressure-flow curve 45

K-value 32

Loop formation, pressure-flow diagram
  56
Lower limits 2
Lung
  capacities 4
  compliance, dynamic 15, 170–172
    dynamic, specific 15, 23, 172
    static 15, 164–169
      specific 22, 167–169
  diffusing capacity, blood component
    88–90, 214, 216–218
    membrane component 88–90, 214,
      216–218
    specific 91–93, 216–218
    CO method 85
      single breath 86, 212, 215, 217,
      218
      steady state 86
  elasticity 13, 25
  function, children, adolescents VII
  hysteresis 17, 18, 26
  recoil pressure 15, 16
  resistance 63, 202
  tissue resistance 65

Lung (cont.)
   ventilation 5, 146, 147
   volume(s) 4
      dynamic 47, 190–198
      static 4, 114–143
   volume restriction, intraparenchymal
      24
      extraparenchymal 25

Maximum expiratory flow
   rates 32, 40, 173–186
   volume curve 33, 34, 39
Multiple-breath nitrogen washout curve
   66

Nitrogen elimination time 66, 203

Oxygen consumption 83, 84, 211

Partial expiratory flow-volume curve 40,
   46, 47
Pressure-volume curve 15, 16
   expiratory, semistatic 15, 16
   expiratory, static 15, 16
   thorax 72, 78, 80
Pressure-volume loop 17, 70
Pulmonary resistance 63, 202

Regression equation 1
   power 2
Residual nitrogen concentration 66, 67
Rigid lung 13, 24

Slow expiration technique, PV curves
   16–18, 29
Specific maximum expiratory flow rates
   39, 179–183
Spirographic investigation 6
Static and dynamic lung compliance,
   difference between 23
Supramaximal expiratory airflow 40

Thoracic gas volume 10, 11, 57–61
Transfer factor, CO method 85
Transpulmonary pressure 16, 17
Trapped gas/air 7

Units, SI and conventional 145
Upper limits 2
Upstream airway segment 35–37

Ventilation, dead space 83, 84, 210
Vertical pleural pressure gradient 17, 28
Volume of isoflow 39, 43

Work of breathing 68
   'active' 73, 74
   corrected 78–81
   on lungs, dynamic/viscous 69, 206, 208
   on lungs, total 69, 205, 207